New Concepts in Diastasi Recti Surgery

Salvatore Cuccomarino • Ezequiel M. Palmisano
Derlin M. Juárez Muas
Editors

New Concepts in Diastasi Recti Surgery

Minimally Invasive Surgical Techniques and Patient Management

Springer

Editors
Salvatore Cuccomarino
American College of Surgeons
Maria Pia Hospital
Turin, Italy

Ezequiel M. Palmisano
Department of Surgery
Italian University Institute of Rosario (IUNIR)
Rosario, Argentina

Derlin M. Juárez Muas
Department of Surgery
Public Maternal and Children Hospital
Salta, Argentina

ISBN 978-3-031-74949-0 ISBN 978-3-031-74947-6 (eBook)
https://doi.org/10.1007/978-3-031-74947-6

This Springer imprint is published by the registered company Springer Nature Switzerland AG
The registered company address is: Gewerbestrasse 11, 6330 Cham, Switzerland

Preface

This book aims to be the first text to provide readers with clear concepts on the definition and pathophysiology of diastasis of the rectus and a current classification according to its surgical management. It also offers precise indications for surgical rehabilitation, allowing patients to arrive in the best possible condition for surgery. This work offers an insight into multidisciplinary management, providing a comprehensive and modern treatment of this pathology and the abdominal wall.

Ever since one of us, Derlin Marcio Juárez Muas, first described the pre-aponeurotic endoscopic approach for the treatment of diastasis recti, this condition, which until then was considered purely cosmetic and which we now know to be the main (in terms of frequency) pathology of the post-partum abdominal core, has powerfully come into our lives and has profoundly influenced our professional and research activities. Between the three of us, we have examined and operated on more than a thousand patients with diastasis recti, and we have observed how it profoundly alters the physiology of the abdominal core, affecting breathing, the function of the pelvic floor and paravertebral muscles, intra-abdominal pressure, and the correct activity of all the mechanisms that depend on it; we have seen how the surgical repair of diastasis can be rightfully included among the functional interventions, i.e. those interventions that restore one (and in the case of diastasis, more than one) lost function to the organism. The pre-aponeurotic approach, systematised in the 1970s by Chevrel but then demonised by the surgical community, prompted us to study the mechanisms of seroma formation, which is the main postoperative complication of this approach; to identify the causes of seroma dependent on the patient and on the operation; and to establish a preoperative pathway that today allows us to reduce this adverse event to very low percentages compared to even just a few years ago.

We were the first to talk about pre- and post-surgical physiotherapy as an essential element of the functional reconstruction process of the abdominal core; thanks to the intuition of another one of us, Ezequiel Palmisano, together with another editor of this book, Gullermo Di Biasio, we went further and developed a tactic that combines endoscopic repair with 'ancillary'—but still minimally invasive—surgical techniques of subcutaneous fat tissue reduction and skin tightening, thus allowing many patients, previously destined to undergo abdominoplasty, to benefit from minimally invasive methods of treating their condition.

We have systematised and described the use of botulinum toxin for the treatment of large abdominal diastases and aggressively introduced intraoperative analgesia techniques—peripheral nerve blocks—and the principles of ERAS to improve the outcome of our patients. We are convinced that diastasis recti represents an excellent pathophysiological model to study the abdominal core in depth, and we are certain that in the near future, many general surgeons will start to consider this condition no longer as an aesthetic problem, but as a condition that can significantly worsen the quality of life of patients.

Our book is dedicated to these colleagues, hoping that its approach to the definition and treatment of diastasis is clear and practical enough to encourage surgeons who read it to embark on the extraordinary and fascinating journey of diastasis recti surgery.

Turin, Italy Salvatore Cuccomarino
Rosario, Argentina Ezequiel M. Palmisano
Salta, Argentina Derlin M. Juárez Muas

July 13, 2024

Contents

Chapter 1
Why an Abdominal Wall Surgeon Should Operate a Diastasis Recti?

Salvatore Cuccomarino

In 2019 I wrote for the *Revista Hispanoamericana de Hernia* journal, after the invitation of Professor Fernando Carbonell Tatay, who at that time was the president of the Hispano-American Hernia Society, an editorial titled *Why an Abdominal Wall Surgeon Should Operate the Diastasis Recti?*

I had started to be interested in diastasis recti 2 years before, in 2017, when for the first time in Europe I performed the REPA technique by Derlin Juarez Muas. In the 2 years between the first review and writing the article, I learned a lot (but certainly not everything) about diastasis.

Therefore, I wrote the editorial with the enthusiasm (and perhaps the naivety) of the neophyte, clearly establishing some points that would later become more or less "the seven commandments" (forgive me the presumption) in the activities of many (but not of all) general surgeons who are abdominal wall specialists and deal with diastasis recti.

In fact, I wrote that:

Abdominoplasty is not indicated in patients with diastasis recti without a pendulous abdomen

Patients who come to us for diastasis problems present important functional symptoms

Therefore, diastasis is not an aesthetic problem but a functional pathology

Many patients do not accept abdominoplasty as an operation to treat the symptoms associated with diastasis (and this further more demonstrates that we are not talking about an aesthetic problem)

Minimally invasive surgery for abdominal wall defects, as well as the necessary experience in prosthetic meshes, is the heritage of general surgeons

S. Cuccomarino (✉)
General Surgeon, Fellow of the American College of Surgeons, Maria Pia Hospital, Turin, Italy
e-mail: dr.cuccomarino@cuccomarinomd.com

S. Cuccomarino et al. (eds.), *New Concepts in Diastasi Recti Surgery*,
https://doi.org/10.1007/978-3-031-74947-6_1

Endoscopic surgery—REPA—had allowed us to discover that patients with diastasis recti in approximately 90% of cases were carriers of one or more hernias of the *linea alba*
The postoperative physiotherapy is important for the recovery of patients

I recognize at that time it was quite unconscious to write a lot of things in that editorial: it would still be unconscious today. Although these were "rude" statements as I had expressed them, some of them sounded like real heresies. Is not the diastasis a cosmetic problem? So, why aesthetic surgeons would operate it? Is the diastasis a functional pathology as hiatal hernia? But when such enormity has been felt? And the relationship between linea alba hernias and diastasis? Postoperative physiotherapy? A whole sesquipedal nonsense. Specially in my country, where just a couple of years ago, at a congress of the Italian Society of Surgery held in Rome, a very important Neapolitan surgeon, recognized throughout the world for his professional skills, in a session on abdominal wall surgery, shouted that he didn't want to hear about diastasis recti because general surgeons don't perform cosmetic surgery. In the end I will have to recant, I thought at that moment, but I was consoled by the certainty of not being the first to do that in my country.

When I wrote the editorial, aware that I was affirming concepts that, perhaps, at that time, I would not have been able to convincingly support in a public debate; I still felt "protected" by the fact that the *Revista Hispanoamericana de Hernia* journal was almost exclusively distributed in Spanish-speaking countries and which was not indexed in Medline; that is why I was counting on the fact that, probably, I would have had had the famous "25 readers" of the Manzoni's novel *The Betrothed.*

The *Revista Hispanoamericana de Hernia* journal is an open-access journal, whose articles can be read and downloaded by anyone, requiring only a simple free online registration. To date, this editorial has been downloaded more than 53,000 times, according to the publisher's web portal: a result that I would never have expected, which indicates, at least, a concern, the search for a point of reference by the general surgeons who deal with abdominal wall surgery.

Abdominal wall surgery in the last years has been increasingly recognized as a superspecialty of general surgery, like colorectal surgery or hepatobiliary surgery and, therefore, increasingly needs standardization, guidelines and certifications. From this point of view, the REPA, carried out for the first time in 2014 in Salta, Argentina, by Derlin Juarez Muas, represents an intervention very close to the "ideal": it is standardized and reproducible; it has its learning curve that must have a tutor, requires significant technical skills, and, above all, is effective. All of this will be discussed throughout this work, which is probably the first publication, written by super experts in the sector, to talk about diastasis recti as a functional pathology and not as a cosmetic problem.

To understand why diastasis is a functional pathology, it is necessary to know in detail the functional anatomy of the abdominal core and the relationships that exist between the muscles of the abdominal wall and the pelvic floor, the spine, and the diaphragm; it is necessary to understand how intra-abdominal pressures vary as the muscular contraction of the different central components varies in a situation of "altered muscle geometry." That is why I could say that the core of this book is the anatomy chapter, entrusted to an excellent anatomist such as Professor Alfredo Moreno Egea, and physiotherapy chapter, written by Dr. Marcel Caufriez, inventor of hypopressive gymnastics, and by his pupil Dr. Fabrizio Botanica, who coordinates the team of physiotherapists of my surgical organization. These notions help us understand why a general surgeon should deal with diastasis recti and why diastasis recti is not an aesthetic condition but a kind of "forgotten pathology," which essentially consists of an insufficiency of the linea alba: in particular, it is a structural alteration of the linea alba that determines an abnormal separation between the rectus abdominis muscles of at least 2.5 cm, with a protrusion of the abdominal contents over a linea alba thinner and wider than normal, covered by subcutaneous cellular tissue and skin. It is a common opinion that the linea alba is very resistant; however this thesis is currently questioned by various considerations [1]:

The normal linea alba has a variable width, being wider and thinner in women and obese people.
It is one of the areas of the abdominal wall where ventral hernias (umbilical and epigastric) appear most frequently.
Incisional hernias are more frequent if the suture of the abdominal wall is placed without including the edges of the rectus muscles and less frequent if the suture includes the latter, invaginating the linea alba [2].
In laparoscopy, trocar hernias are most frequently located in the linea alba.
Incisional hernias in paramedian or transverse incisions are rare.

From these observations arises the hypothesis of "sick linea alba complex" (SLAC), that is, an intrinsically defective linea alba and, therefore, more frequently subject to pathologies such as hernias, incisional hernias, and diastasis. The molecular basis of these alterations most likely lies in an alteration of type I and type III collagen synthesis [3]. In this context, a series of pathophysiological mechanisms develop, which will be commented on in a specific chapter, that explain the appearance of the clinical manifestations of diastasis recti; at the moment it is enough to say that diastasis recti is an authentic pathology of the abdominal wall whose manifestations are extremely interesting both from an anatomical and pathophysiological point of view, demonstrating the very close synergies that exist between the different muscular components of the abdominal core (abdominopelvic, dorsolumbar, and perineal, together with the diafragm); its treatment, far from being aesthetic, is aimed at reconstructing the correct contraction vectors and re-establishing the balance between the agonist and antagonist muscles of the trunk. The symptoms that patients present are real and are treated with diastasis repair [4, 5], which significantly improves the quality of life of the patients [6]. These symptoms are exhaustively named in the literature [7] and can be divided into symptoms related to instability of the abdominal core (breathing alterations, difficulty in trunk movements), pain (low back pain, joint pain, pelvic pain), dysfunction of the pelvic floor (stress urinary incontinence), fecal incontinence, pelvic organ prolapse, gastrointestinal disorders (constipation, slow transit, and abdominal bloating, gastroesophageal reflux), and linea alba hernias, in particular umbilical hernia [8].

Pain, pelvic floor dysfunction, and intestinal problems are the symptoms most frequently reported by patients and seriously interfere with their quality of life. A Swedish study published by the *British Journal of Surgery* [9] demonstrated that the quality of life of women who suffer diastasis recti is significantly worse than that of the average woman in Sweden and that after surgery this parameter improves significantly ($p < 0.001$), returning to levels comparable with the population average. This is why diastasis recti should be considered a functional pathology and its surgical correction a functional surgery. We must not forget that diastasis recti represents an important risk factor for the recurrence of umbilical hernias when it is not repaired at the same time as the hernia [10, 11], especially in women [12–14]. This fact imposes (or at least should impose) any surgeon can be able to treat both pathologies at the same time—in fact, in these cases the repair is defined as "obligatory," in an article in a monograph on diastasis recti in *Hernia* journal [15]. In all cases with diastasis recti and linea alba hernias, abdominal wall repair with mesh is recommended [7, 11, 16]. Even for umbilical hernia repair alone, the use of mesh is indicated, regardless of the diameter of the hernia port: in a large study on 7849 patients published in 2022, it was observed that, even in hernias with a port < 1 cm (for whose treatment sutures alone were considered sufficient until recently), the use of mesh reduces recurrences in a statistically significant manner [17].

All of the above, together with the fact that diastasis is an obvious factor of weakness of the linea alba and the high incidence of linea alba hernias observed during surgery [8], justifies the assertion that diastasis recti represents a risk factor for the appearance of this type of hernias, particularly umbilical hernias [18]. This is one of the main reasons why a surgeon who deals with abdominal wall surgery should also deal with diastasis recti.

1.1 Preaponeurotic Surgery of the Abdominal Wall and Diastasis Recti

Preaponeurotic (or *onlay*) abdominal wall repair techniques have been known since the late 1970s and involve putting the mesh over the musculofascial layer of the abdominal wall and under the subcutaneous layer. The first to describe it was a French surgeon Jean Paul Chevrel [19, 20]. The validity of the technique is verified by decades of clinical use and stigmatized by various works, including a Cochrane Review [21–27]. Onlay techniques do not show postoperative complications (except the formation of seromas) or recurrences in a statistically higher percentage compared to sublay techniques (such as the Rives technique, today considered the *gold standard* of repair of midline abdominal defects) or intraperitoneal technique. Even more complex wall repair techniques, such as SAC (anatomic separation of components) by Prof. Fernando Carbonell Tatay [28], widely used by Ibero-American surgeons for the repair of large defects of the abdominal midline (remember that the Hispano-American school of wall surgery is historically one of the most important in the world), involve the use of preaponeurotic meshes.

In 2014, Dr. Derlin Juarez Muas, general surgeon at the Maternal and Child Hospital in Salta, in northern Argentina, and co-editor of this book, was "forced" to face a "strange" problem. The gynecologists and physiotherapists at his hospital sent him many patients with diastasis recti, and many of them, even with important symptoms related to the diastasis (low back pain, abdominal pain, urinary incontinence, etc.), did not agree to undergo the classic abdominoplasty surgery.

Under this pressure, Derlin, an advanced laparoscopist surgeon, invented the REPA technique (preaponeurotic endoscopic repair, technique that was later renamed SCOLA (Subcutaneous Onlay Laparoscopic Approach) by English speakers, (with an obvious semantic error because REPA is not a laparoscopic surgery, since it does not imply access to the abdominal cavity), thanks to which, through a subcutaneous access with three trocars colocated in the suprapubic area, it was possible to reach the anterolateral wall of the abdomen and perform the plication of the recti muscles necessary for the treatment of diastasis. Dr. Juarez Muas decided to combine the plication with the placement of a large preaponeurotic mesh, to strengthen the repair and the wall as a whole: so was born what today is probably the most standardized and used minimally invasive surgical treatment in the world for the treatment of diastasis recti associated with linea alba hernias [7]. Dr. Juarez Muas published his technique in 2017 [29], and that same year I realized it for the first time in Europe [30]. This technique has been highly appreciated by patients [6, 23, 31]. Over the years, other minimally invasive techniques have been added to REPA (ELAR, MILAR, MILOS, etc.). However REPA continues to be the preferred technique by surgeons (as reported in the guidelines for the treatment of diastasis recti from the European Hernia Society [28], "*Endoscopic subcutaneous dissection followed by linea alba plication with onlay mesh was the most reported technique*"; the guidelines of the *Hispano-American Hernia Society (SoHAH)* are even more categorical "*endoscopic examination is recommended, except when an abdominoplasty is specified. The REPA technique is associated with better results compared to minimally invasive or mixed options*" [32].

Therefore, if indicated correctly, actually REPA can probably be considered the *gold standard* for the minimally invasive repair of diastasis recti.

One of the most debated topics at abdominal wall surgery congresses and online forums is whether or not diastasis repair should involve the use of mesh: after all, it is said diastasis is not a real defect, so why should mesh be used? And shouldn't plication of the linea alba be enough, as plastic surgeons do?

The considerations set out above should be sufficient to answer this question, but we can add that not using mesh in diastasis recti surgery increases recurrences significantly [8, 33]. This should put an end to all discussions, but on the contrary it opens a new one: which mesh to use for diastasis recti surgery?

To answer this question, it is necessary to return to the characteristics, and in particular the complications, of preaponeurotic techniques from Chevrel onwards. In general, any mesh inserted into the human body behaves like a foreign body: one of the most complex things when planning an operation to repair an abdominal wall defect is the choice of prosthetic material, since an "ideal" mesh does not exist [21]. Meshes can be classified based on their composition (polymeric or synthetic-reticular prostheses, lamellar, composites, and biological or natural prostheses) [34]. Most reticular prostheses are made of polypropylene and are characterized by the presence of pores with a diameter between 1 and 4 mm and by excellent integration in the receiving organism [35]. An important classification parameter of these prostheses is their density, that is, the weight in relation to the area (g/m^2): in this sense, prostheses are recognized, high (>80 g/m^2), medium (50–80 g/m^2), low (35–50 g/m^2), and ultra-low (<35 g/m^2) density prostheses [36, 27].

The importance of prostheses in the repair of wall defects has been clear to surgeons since the late nineteenth century: the statement of Theodore Billroth, who observed that the secret of the radical cure of hernia would be discovered when it would be possible to produce synthetically woven of density and hardness of fascia and tendons. This result, or something very similar, was achieved in the 1950s, thanks to polypropylene, a plastic material synthesized by the Italian chemist Giulio Natta (who won the Nobel Prize for Chemistry for them in 1963). Polypropylene meshes were used for the first time for the repair of abdominal wall defects in the 1950s by the American surgeon F.C. Usher [37]: its routine use has radically changed the natural history of wall surgery in terms of reducing recurrences and other complications, such as chronic postoperative pain, to the point that studies on the evidence of the role of polypropylene prostheses have merited publication in journals of the caliber of the *British Journal of Surgery* [38] and *Annals of Surgery* [39]. Between 1958 and 2007, 287 articles were published on the use of polypropylene as a prosthetic material for the repair of abdominal wall defects (by far, it is the largest number of articles published on a specific material for the creation of abdominal prostheses: in the second place, polyester is found, with "only" 67 articles published) [40].

The success (in terms of recurrences and postoperative complications) of each prosthetic repair of the abdominal wall, assuming that it is technically well performed, depends on both the characteristics of the prosthesis and the recipient organism: while the former can be standardized and they are well known before the surgery, the later ones are not. Each mesh, by behaving like a foreign body, induces an inflammatory reaction, which is the basis of post-surgical complications of abdominal wall prosthetic surgery (pain, seroma formation, etc.), so it depends on the mesh itself (as mentioned, the "weight" of the patient's biological characteristics in determining complications is very difficult to evaluate preoperatively). To reduce the inflammatory response, maintaining the benefits of prosthetic repair, over time there was a tendency to use lighter and more macroporous polypropylene prostheses that induce the formation of a "network" scar instead of a "plaque" [41, 42]. Today we know that this has a solid scientific basis: the biological response induced by polypropylene prostheses is characterized by the inclusion of the mesh in a "mold" of scar tissue; this can cause problems of postoperative discomfort and pain [43], and in particular it is due to its density (i.e., the polymer weight and size of the mesh pores) [35, 44] more than to the prosthetic material. The characteristics of the patient influence, in a very incisive way, the result of the biological processes that lead to the formation of scar tissue. For example, the presence of altered collagen synthesis, particularly type I and III, has been highlighted both in patients with hernia pathology and in women with diastasis recti [3, 40, 45], to the point that some Authors suggest that this abdominal wall pathology is actually a connective tissue pathology [46].

Some postoperative complications are also related to the characteristics of the prostheses. Lightweight meshes are known to cause less pain and foreign body sensation postoperatively than heavy meshes, resulting in a better quality of life after surgery [47–51]. Furthermore, the inflammatory response induced by the prosthetic material is one of the main causes of seroma, another complication of parietal surgery of great importance in preaponeurotic surgery, which is minimized with the use of light macroporous meshes [52–54]. The latter, thanks to the lower induced inflammatory reaction, are less susceptible to the "shrinkage" phenomenon or contraction of the mesh [55], one of the possible causes of recurrence in repairs of abdominal wall defects. It must also be considered that light meshes have an elasticity of 20–35%, much more similar to the abdominal wall (38%) than that of heavy meshes (4–15%) [52]: which, especially when the mesh is large, it has a significant impact on the patient's postoperative comfort.

All of the above has meant that in the preaponeurotic repair (REPA) of diastasis recti, heavy meshes have been abandoned, due to the complications induced, and today light or ultralight meshes are widely used. But the most important consequence that represents one of the reasons why the general surgeon must approach diastasis surgery is that the knowledge of prosthetic materials for the repair of the abdominal wall and the experience in their use is his own and exclusive heritage.

This book aims to explain in detail to general surgeons who deal with abdominal wall surgery why to repair diastasis recti, how to do it, and what results to expect. It is the first book of its kind, and I sincerely hope that this work can help both colleagues in their daily clinical activity and patients to find a satisfactory solution to their problems, which until now have been ignored or underestimated even by doctors for whom abdominal wall surgery has become their professional destiny.

References

1. Naraynsingh V, Maharaj R, Dan D, Hariharan S. Strong linea alba: myth or reality? Med Hypotheses. 2012;78(2):291–2.
2. Naraynsingh V, Ariyanayagam D. Rectus repair for midline ventral abdominal wall hernia. Br J Surg. 1993;80(5):614–5.
3. Blotta RM, Costa SD, Trindade EN, Meurer L, Maciel-Trindade MR. Collagen I and III in women with diastasis recti. Clinics. 2018;73:e319.
4. Juárez Muas DM, Palmisano E, Pou Santoja G, Cuccomarino S, González Higuera G, Mayo P, Martínez Maya JD, Domínguez G, Ayala Acosta JC, Chichizola A. Reparación endoscópica preaponeurótica (REPA) como tratamiento de la diástasis de los músculos rectos asociada o no a hernias de la línea media. Estudio multicéntrico. Rev Hispanoam Hernia. 2019;7(2):59–65.
5. Nervil GG, Paulsen JF, Kalstrup J, Deigaard S, Herbst I, Lambaa S, Hölmich L. Simple plication alleviates physical symptoms in patients with post-gestational rectus diastasis. Hernia. 2023;27(4):957–68.

6. Cuccomarino S, Bonomo LD, Aprà F, Toscano A, Jannaci A. Preaponeurotic endoscopic repair (REPA) of diastasis recti: a single surgeon's experience. Surg Endosc. 2022;36(2):1302–9.
7. Hernández-Granados P, Henriksen NA, Berrevoet F, Cuccurullo D, López-Cano M, Nienhuijs S, Ross D, Montgomery A. European Hernia Society guidelines on management of rectus diastasis. Br J Surg. 2021;108(10):1189–91.
8. Juárez Muas D, Palmisano EM, Pou Santonja G, González Higuera LG, Martínez Maya JD, Domínguez G, Ayala Acosta JC, Blanco M, Cuccomarino S, Cabral Castelli ML. Morbilidad a corto y largo plazo de la reparación endoscópica preaponeurótica en la diástasis de los rectos asociada o no a hernia de la línea media: estudio prospectivo, multicéntrico e internacional. Rev Hispanoam Hernia. 2023;11(3):111–7.
9. Olsson A, Kiwanuka O, Wilhelmsson S, Sandblom G, Stackelberg O. Cohort study of the effect of surgical repair of symptomatic diastasis recti abdominis on abdominal trunk function and quality of life. BJS Open. 2019;3(6):750–8.
10. Köhler G, Luketina RR, Emmanuel K. Sutured repair of primary small umbilical and epigastric hernias: concomitant rectus diastasis is a significant risk factor for recurrence. World J Surg. 2015;39(1):121–6.
11. Nishihara Y, Asami M, Shimada T, Kawaguchi Y, Omoto K. Comorbid rectus abdominis diastasis is a risk factor for recurrence of umbilical hernia in Japanese patients. Asian J Endosc Surg. 2021;14(3):368–72.
12. Katawazai A, Wallin G, Sandblom G. Long-term reoperation rate following primary ventral hernia repair: a register-based study. Hernia. 2022;26(6):1551–9.
13. Zhang Y, Zhou H, Chai Y, Cao C, Jin K, Hu Z. Laparoscopic versus open incisional and ventral hernia repair: a systematic review and meta-analysis. World J Surg. 2014;38(9):2233–40.
14. Nouh T, Ali FS, Krause KJ, Zaimi I. Ventral hernia recurrence in women of childbearing age: a systematic review and meta-analysis. Hernia. 2018;22(6):1067–75.
15. Campanelli G. Umbilical hernia, epigastric hernia and diastasis recti: an open discussion. Hernia. 2021;25(3):559–60.
16. Reinpold W, Köckerling F, Bittner R, Conze J, Fortelny R, Koch A, Kukleta J, Kuthe A, Lorenz R, Stechemesser B. Classification of rectus diastasis-a proposal by the German Hernia Society (DHG) and the International Endohernia Society (IEHS). Front Surg. 2019;6:1.
17. Henriksen NA, Jensen KK, Bisgaard T, Helgstrand F, The Danish Hernia Database. Suture or mesh repair of the smallest umbilical hernias: a nationwide database study. World J Surg. 2022;46(8):1898–905.
18. Ranney B. Diastasis recti and umbilical hernia causes, recognition and repair. S D J Med. 1990;43(10):5–8.
19. Chevrel JP. Traitement des grandes éventrations médianes par plastie en paletot et prothèse. Nouv Press Med. 1979;8(9):695–6.
20. Chevrel JP, Dilin C, Morquette H. Traitement des éventrations abdominales médianes par autoplastie musculaire et prothèse pré-musculo-aponévrotique. A propos de 50 observations. Chirurgie. 1986;112(9):616–22.
21. Korenkov M, Paul A, Sauerland S, Neugebauer E, Arndt M, Chevrel JP, Corcione F, Fingerhut A, Flament JB, Kux M, Matzinger A, Myrvold HE, Rath AM, Simmermacher RK. Classification and surgical treatment of incisional hernia. Results of an experts' meeting. Langenbeck's Arch Surg. 2001;386(1):65–73.
22. Wéber G, Baracs J, Horváth OP. "Onlay" mesh provides significantly better results than "sublay" reconstruction. Prospective randomized multicenter study of abdominal wall reconstruction with sutures only, or with surgical mesh–results of a five-years follow-up. Magy Seb. 2010;63(5):302–11.
23. Pereira C, Gururaj S. Onlay versus sublay mesh repair for incisional hernias: a systematic review. Cureus. 2023;15(1):e34156.
24. Shah DK, Patel SJ, Chaudhary SR, Desai NR. Comparative study of onlay versus sublay mesh repair in the management of ventral hernias. Updates Surg. 2023. https://doi.org/10.1007/s13304-023-01532-5.

25. Haskins IN, Voeller GR, Stoikes NF, Webb DL, Chandler RG, Phillips S, Poulose BK, Rosen MJ. Onlay with adhesive use compared with sublay mesh placement in ventral hernia repair: was chevrel right? An Americas Hernia Society Quality Collaborative Analysis. J Am Coll Surg. 2017;224(5):962–70.
26. Bessa SS, El-Gendi AM, Ghazal AH, Al-Fayoumi TA. Comparison between the short-term results of onlay and sublay mesh placement in the management of uncomplicated para-umbilical hernia: a prospective randomized study. Hernia. 2015;19(1):141–6.
27. den Hartog D, Dur AHM, Tuinebreijer WE, Kreis RW. Open surgical procedures for incisional hernias. Cochrane Database Syst Rev. 2008;3:CD006438. https://doi.org/10.1002/14651858.CD006438.pub2.
28. Carbonell Tatay F, Moreno EA. Eventraciones. Otras hernias de pared y cavidad abdominal. Madrid: Asociación Española de Cirujanos; 2012.
29. Juárez Muas DM, Verasay GF, Martín GW. Reparación endoscópica prefascial de la diástasis de los rectos: descripción de una nueva técnica. Rev Hispanoam Hernia. 2017;5(2):47–51.
30. Pou SG. Historia natural de la reparación endoscópica preaponeurótica (REPA). Rev Hispanoam Hernia. 2018;6(4):165–6.
31. Juárez Muas DM. Preaponeurotic endoscopic repair (REPA) of diastasis recti associated or not to midline hernias. Surg Endosc. 2019;33(6):1777–82.
32. Zorraquino GA. Guía clínica de la diástasis de los músculos rectos del abdomen y pequeños defectos de la línea alba. Rev Hispanoam Hernia. 2021;9(2):118–25.
33. Hickey F, Finch JG, Khanna A. A systematic review on the outcomes of correction of diastasis of the recti. Hernia. 2011;15(6):607–14.
34. Bellon JM. Revisión de una clasificación de materiales protésicos destinados a la reparación herniaria: correlación entre estructura y comportamiento en los tejidos receptores. Rev Hispanoam Hernia. 2014;2(2):49–57.
35. Langer C, Schwartz P, Krause P, Mohammadi H, Kulle B, Schaper A, Füzesi L, Becker H. In-vitro study of the cellular response of human fibroblasts cultured on alloplastic hernia meshes. Influence of mesh material and structure. Chirurg. 2005;76(9):876–85.
36. Earle DB, Mark LA. Prosthetic material in inguinal hernia repair: how do I choose? Surg Clin North Am. 2008;88(1):179–201.
37. Usher FC. Further observations on the use of marlex mesh: a new technique for the repair of inguinal hernias. Am Surg. 1959;25:792–5.
38. Butters M, Redecke J, Köninger J. Long-term results of a randomized clinical trial of Shouldice, Lichtenstein and transabdominal preperitoneal hernia repairs. Br J Surg. 2007;94(5):562–5.
39. Liem MS, van Duyn EB, van der Graaf Y, van Vroonhoven TJ, Coala Trial Group. Recurrences after conventional anterior and laparoscopic inguinal hernia repair: a randomized comparison. Ann Surg. 2003;237(1):136–41.
40. Fachinelli A, Maciel Trindade MR. Qualitative and quantitative evaluation of total and types I and III collagens in patients with ventral hernias. Langenbeck's Arch Surg. 2007;392(4):459–64.
41. Schumpelick V, Klinge U, Rosch R, Junge K. Light weight meshes in incisional hernia repair. J Minim Access Surg. 2006;2(3):117–23.
42. Novitsky YW, Harrell AG, Hope WW, Kercher KW, Heniford BT. Meshes in hernia repair. Surg Technol Int. 2007;16:123–7.
43. Cobb WS, Kercher KW, Heniford BT. The argument for lightweight polypropylene mesh in hernia repair. Surg Innov. 2005;12(1):63–9.
44. Bellón JM, Rodríguez M, García-Honduvilla N, Pascual G, Gómez Gil V, Buján J. Peritoneal effects of prosthetic meshes used to repair abdominal wall defects: monitoring adhesions by sequential laparoscopy. J Laparoendosc Adv Surg Tech A. 2007;17(2):160–6.
45. White B, Osier C, Gletsu N, Jeansonne L, Baghai M, Sherman M, Smith CD, Ramshaw B, Lin E. Abnormal primary tissue collagen composition in the skin of recurrent incisional hernia patients. Am Surg. 2007;73(12):1254–8.
46. Zheng H, Si Z, Kasperk R, Bhardwaj RS, Schumpelick V, Klinge U, Klosterhalfen B. Recurrent inguinal hernia: disease of the collagen matrix? World J Surg. 2002;26(4):401–8.

47. Bona S, Rosati R, Opocher E, Fiore B, Montorsi M, SUPERMESH Study Group. Pain and quality of life after inguinal hernia surgery: a multicenter randomized controlled trial comparing lightweight vs heavyweight mesh (Supermesh Study). Updat Surg. 2018;70(1):77–83.
48. Bakker WJ, Aufenacker TJ, Boschman JS, Burgmans JPJ. Lightweight mesh is recommended in open inguinal (Lichtenstein) hernia repair: a systematic review and meta-analysis. Surgery. 2020;167(3):581–9.
49. Uzzaman MM, Ratnasingham K, Ashraf N. Meta-analysis of randomized controlled trials comparing lightweight and heavyweight mesh for Lichtenstein inguinal hernia repair. Hernia. 2012;16(5):505–18.
50. Li J, Ji Z, Cheng T. Lightweight versus heavyweight in inguinal hernia repair: a meta-analysis. Hernia. 2012;16(5):529–39.
51. Zhong C, Wu B, Yang Z, Deng X, Kang J, Guo B, Fan Y. A meta-analysis comparing lightweight meshes with heavyweight meshes in Lichtenstein inguinal hernia repair. Surg Innov. 2013;20(1):24–31.
52. Amid PK. Classification of biomaterials and their related complications in abdominal wall hernia surgery. Hernia. 1997;1:15–21.
53. Schumpelick V, Klosterhalfen B, Müller M, Klinge U. Minimized polypropylene mesh for preperitoneal net plasty (PNP) of incisional hernias. Chirurg. 1999;70(4):422–30.
54. Kalaba S, Gerhard E, Winder JS, Pauli EM, Haluck RS, Yang J. Design strategies and applications of biomaterials and devices for hernia repair. Bioact Mater. 2016;1(1):2–17.
55. Bilsel Y, Abci I. The search for ideal hernia repair; mesh materials and types. Int J Surg. 2012;10(6):317–21.

Part I
Regions

Chapter 2
Surgical Anatomy of the Anterolateral Wall of the Abdomen and Classification of the Diastasis Recti

Alfredo Moreno Egea

The abdominal wall (AW) is a complex muscular aponeurotic structure that ensures the containment of the abdominal viscera, allows changes in volume and pressure inside the viscera, facilitates trunk movements, and participates in breathing, digestion, defecation, cough, and childbirth. The work of the AW cannot be understood in isolation from its attachments to the diaphragm (roof of the AW) and the perineum (floor of the AW), explaining the stability of the spine and adequate control of the sphincters, among other functions.

The anterior and lateral wall of the abdomen is made up of the rectus abdominis, piriformis, and the broad muscles of the abdomen, which are the internal oblique, external oblique, and transversus abdominis.

2.1 Muscular System

The *rectus abdominis* are two medial muscles with a vertical direction, originating in the body of the pubis through a flattened and quadrilateral tendon 2.5–3 cm wide. The internal fibers ascend vertically and the external fibers obliquely outward, forming a flattened fascicle that gradually widens as it ascends. Finally, it is inserted into three tabs: an external one on the lower edge of the cartilage of the fifth rib, a middle one on the lower edge of the cartilage of the sixth rib, and an internal one on the lower edge of the cartilage of the seventh rib, in the ligament costoxiphoid and in the xiphoid appendage. The muscle usually has three to four aponeurotic

A. M. Egea (✉)
Abdominal Wall Unit, Morales Meseguer University Hospital, Murcia, Spain

Revista Hispanoamericana de Hernia, Valencia, Spain

S. Cuccomarino et al. (eds.), *New Concepts in Diastasi Recti Surgery*,
https://doi.org/10.1007/978-3-031-74947-6_2

intersections: one umbilical, two supraumbilical, and one infraumbilical. They are the main flexors of the abdominal wall; they stabilize the pelvis when walking, protect the abdominal viscera; and help with forced expiration.

The *external oblique muscles* of the abdomen form the most superficial layer of the lateral wall of the abdomen. They originate on the external face of the last six to eight ribs in the form of fingerings that intersect the upper six with the analogues of the serratus major and the lower three with those of the latissimus dorsi. The upper fascicles descend almost horizontally, the lower ones vertical, and the middle ones oblique. It is inserted into the iliac crest, anterior edge of the coxal bone, pubis, and linea alba, intertwining with the aponeurosis of the contralateral muscle. It participates in the control of intra-abdominal pressure but with less influence than the transverse muscle. In addition, it collaborates in ipsilateral inclination, contralateral rotation, and flexion of the trunk. The costal insertions provide an important mechanical advantage to reduce the vertical and lateral dimensions of the rib cage, turning it into a strong expiratory muscle of great importance at the time of childbirth.

The *internal oblique muscles* of the abdomen are located in the intermediate plane of the abdominal wall, perpendicular to the external oblique. It inserts into the lateral half of the inguinal ligament, the iliac crest, the thoracolumbar fascia, and the inferior and posterior borders of the 10th–12th rib. Fibers originating from the inguinal ligament are directed inferomedially to the pubic crest through the conjoint tendon attached to the transversus abdominis. The posterior fibers ascend laterally until they reach the ribs, near the costochondral joint. The intermediate fibers have a superomedial orientation, reaching the linea alba through a bilaminar aponeurosis that mixes with the aponeurosis of the external oblique and transversus abdominis, forming a fascial network that crosses the midline. They contribute to the support of the abdominal viscera and the modulation of intra-abdominal pressure, in a similar way to the transverse one. Due to the orientation of their fibers, they also generate flexion, ipsilateral rotation, and ipsilateral lateral flexion movements.

The *transversus abdominis muscle* is the deepest of the broad muscles of the abdominal wall. It originates from the anterior three-quarters of the iliac crest, the lateral third of the inguinal ligament, the thoracolumbar fascia, and the inner surface of the six lower costal cartilages that interdigitate with fibers of the diaphragm. Below the arcuate line, it inserts into the pubic crest and pectineal line forming the conjoint tendon attached to the internal oblique. The lumbopelvic insertions ensure correct fascial tension that contributes to the stability of the spine. We can differentiate three regions of different morphology: (1) the fibers of the most superior region with transverse orientation, of shorter length and thickness; (2) the middle fibers between the rib cage and the iliac crest with insertions on the thoracolumbar fascia, in an inferomedial direction and of greater length; and (3) the lower fibers that go from the iliac crest to the inguinal ligament, with an inferomedial direction and the thickest. The transversus is essential in lumbopelvic stability, controlling intra-abdominal pressure, tension of the thoracolumbar fascia, and joint compression [1, 2] (Fig. 2.1).

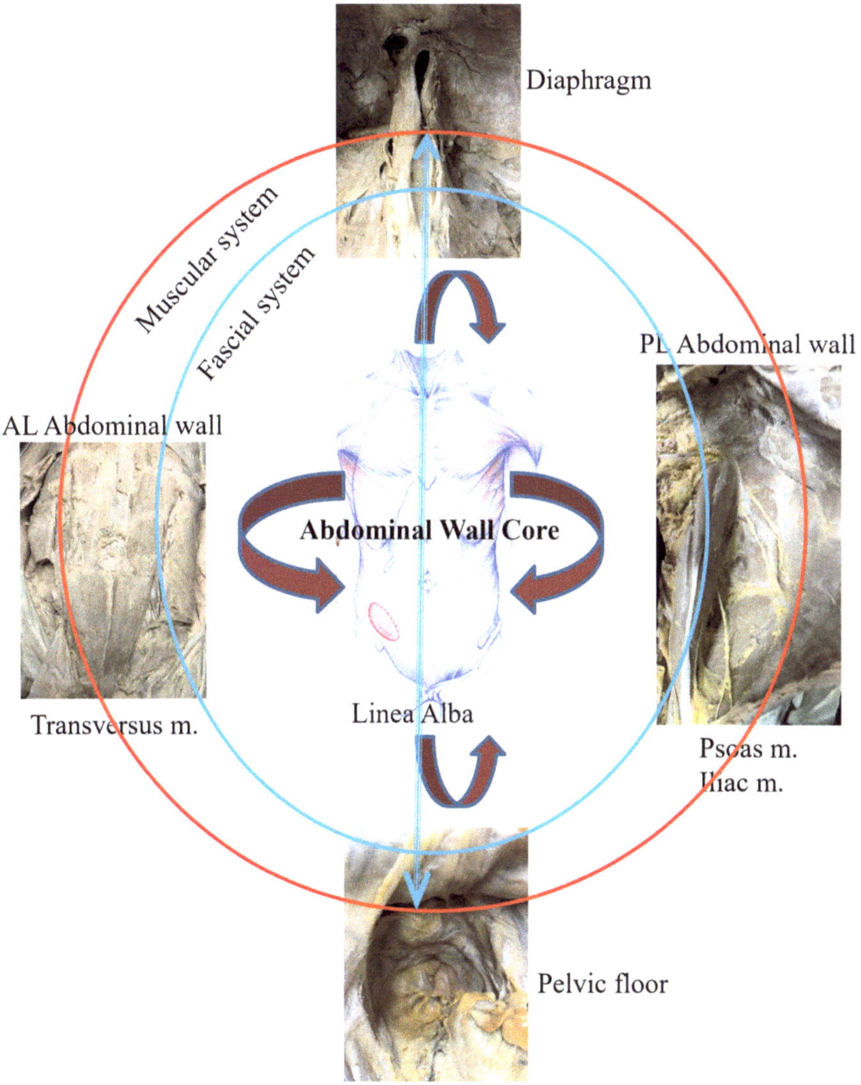

Fig. 2.1 A new concept of abdominal wall core. The components of the muscular and fascial system are shown, including the diaphragm as the roof, the pelvic floor, the abdominal wall (transversus abdominis muscle), and the posterolateral musculature (psoas and iliacus muscle). These components work together to maintain the abdominal wall core (AWC)

Each muscular element of the wall is arranged in a plane with a different orientation so that its forces increase the overall stability of the resulting total structure. The two oblique muscles are almost opposite and complement each other, but the transverse is essential to ensure closure of the abdomen, and its effect is unique; it cannot be compensated by the rest.

2.2 Aponeurotic System

The muscles that form the anterolateral wall of the abdomen have insertion aponeurosis in the form of strong and resistant membranes that continue the muscular body until reaching the midline or the dorsolumbar column, closing a system or unit that ensures the function of the abdominal wall in its entirety set.

2.2.1 Anterior Aponeurosis

The three broad muscles have their own anterior insertion aponeurosis. The muscular portion of the transversus is the one that extends the most until reaching the outer edge of the rectus femoris muscle. The muscular portion of the two obliques is more lateral, the internal one first and the external one more lateral, without overlapping between their muscular borders. In this way, the Spiegel line is formed, which depends above all on the transverse muscle transition. Each anterior aponeurosis is welded to the posterior sheet of the muscle that covers it, making it impossible to separate them, except that of the external oblique, which can be separated in a careful dissection, as it is the most distal and therefore its parietal effect on tension can be discharged global.

The arrangement with respect to the rectus muscle varies depending on the location, forming two portions of different consistency: (1) upper or retromuscular portion (2/3) and (2) lower or premuscular portion (1/3), where all the anterior aponeurosis are arranged superficial to the rectus muscle. The transition level between both portions forms the arch of Douglas, from which it is necessary to section the transverse muscle to address the preperitoneal space, which alters the stability of the abdominal building.

Below this level, a gradual loss of the aponeurosis occurs, and the rectus muscle is covered only by the transversalis fascia.

The aponeurotic structure has a trilaminar arrangement above the umbilicus: two layers of the external oblique and the anterior of the internal and behind it a posterior sheet of the bifurcation of the OI and two layers of the transverse. This trilaminar and crisscross structure is what gives the entire midline its resistance. At a level of 7–8 cm caudals, all the aponeuroses already pass in front, and there is no aponeurotic support.

2.2.2 Posterior Aponeurosis

The posterior transverse aponeurosis is the true tendon that closes the abdominal wall at the vertebral level. This aponeurosis does not have any reinforcement of the oblique muscles or the quadratus lumborum. At the cranial level, it performs costal closure through the lumbocostal ligament of Henle, a structure that is part of the arch of the quadratus lumborum. Although it is considered a trilaminar aponeurosis, the only leaf that has consistency is the middle one that ends at the apex of the transverse processes from the 12th rib to the iliac crest and fuses with the latissimus dorsi aponeurosis, contributing to form the lumbar aponeurosis. It is made up of various types of fibers, the lower ones slightly oblique and the upper ones oblique, never horizontal.

2.2.3 *Linea Alba (LA)*

The linea alba is the tendinous lamina that occupies the midline space between the two rectus abdominis muscles and extends from the xiphoid process to the pubic symphysis. It is a tendinous raphe formed by the insertions of the broad muscles of the abdomen, so that it provides stability to the abdominal wall and the trunk. Like the abdominal aponeurosis, the LA is more resistant below the navel as all the muscles of the abdominal wall come together. For this reason, diastasis recti at the infraumbilical level is less common than at the supraumbilical level. The LA usually has an average height of 35 cm, a thickness of 2–3 mm, and a variable width depending on the level considered. From top to bottom, it progressively widens to the navel, and then one or two fingers below it narrow until almost linearly it reaches the pubic symphysis. Its upper portion (2/3) is membranous and ribbon-like, with a width of 6–7 mm at the top, 10–12 mm in its middle part, and 20–22 mm at the level of the navel. The lower portion (1/3) is about 12–14 cm in length, with a width that reduces to 2–3 mm, ending in a point at the pubis, suddenly widening, like a triangle, the base of which is inserted into its top and back. The superior insertion is carried out by means of vertical fascicles or xiphoid ligament that is inserted at the tip and on the underside of the xiphoid appendage, in a plane posterior to that of the rectus muscle, which does so on the rib cage. Behind this level there is adipose cellulose tissue that rests on the xiphoid insertions of the transverse. The inferior insertion is arranged in two planes in relation to the rectum, in front in a small triangular fibrous fascicle that is inserted into the suspensory ligament of the penis (or clitoris) and behind in a triangular sheet or suprapubic ligament or foot posterior of the LA. This posterior insertion sends an extension to the Colles' ligament and the posterior surface of the horizontal ramus of the pubis to the internal orifice of the subpubic canal. In its lower part, this ligament sometimes presents a small pit in the midline through which one or more branches of the epigastric vessels with their corresponding adipose tissue penetrate [1–3].

Therefore, any operation designed on the abdominal wall must attempt to maintain the integrity of the transversus muscle aponeurosis as it is the only true insertion strap, which ensures solid visceral containment and closure of the cavity. The anatomy suggests that the continuity of the transverse should be understood as a surgical priority.

2.3 Fascial System

The fascia constitutes a primary support element of the organism, a continuous envelope of connective tissue in a craniocaudal and ventrodorsal direction. All of them have the same embryological origin and common functions. We can differentiate them according to their position in superficial fascias (Scarpa), middle, and deep (transverse and thoracolumbar); they join the different tissues together and react as a whole to disturbances.

2.3.1 Superficial Fascia

Superficial fascia is formed by two planes, a layer of subcutaneous adipose tissue or Camper's fascia and a deep layer of loose connective tissue or Scarpa's fascia. Both layers are fused above the navel and are difficult to identify. Below the navel both layers are well defined and have greater surgical interest. *Camper's fascia* is the portion of subcutaneous fat in relation to the lower abdominal wall, limited at its deep edge by a well-marked fascia or condensation, of variable density. It is continuity of the subcutaneous fat of the thoracic region and extends inferiorly and laterally to the thigh, gluteal region, and perineum. At the level of the scrotum, it is more defined and is called Dartos. This plane is formed by bands of cellular tissue in a transverse direction, parallel to the inguinal ligament but without adhering to it or to the iliac crest. Camper's fascia plays a protective and insulating role for the deep organs of the abdomen and serves as a marker to identify superficial epigastric lesions.

Scarpa's fascia is the deep membrane formed by condensation of the previous layer of Camper. It is usually well defined on the aponeurosis of the external oblique muscle, from which it must be differentiated. At a higher level, it continues with the adipose fascia of the pectoral region, forming the anterior limit of the retromammary space. At an inferior level, it is inserted into the fascia lata of the thigh, superiorly and laterally into the pubic crest. It adheres internally to the inguinal arch and the external ring. Its continuation toward the perineum is known as Colles' fascia. This plane must be repaired to reinforce the abdominal wall and reduce tension on the skin, which promotes a resistant scar without abnormalities. Between this plane and Camper's plane, the circumflex iliac vessels, the superficial external pudendal, and the superficial inferior epigastric vessels are located, as well as the lymphatics and nodes of the groin.

2.3.2 *Transversal Fascia (TF)*

It covers the inner surface of the abdomen deep to the transverse and rectus muscles and superficial to the subperitoneal (or preperitoneal) fascia. It is continuity of the endothoracic fascia that covers the internal surface of the rib cage and the diaphragm, to extend down the abdominal wall with an anterior portion (Cooper's) and a posterior portion (iliac and pelvic fascia). The lower part forms a femoral tunnel for the passage of the femoral vessels to the thigh. It is weak and cellulose in its upper portion, where it is confused with the subperitoneal, but increases its density and thickness in its lower portion, with all the characteristics of a true aponeurosis. It is formed by two layers of non-elastic transverse fibers in parallel, although there are also inclined vertical and oblique fibers, between which the inferior epigastric, iliac, or obturator vessels run, on which its vascularization depends. Its fiber arrangement and density explain the higher frequency of DR at the supraumbilical level. In depth it is surrounded by the preperitoneal fascia, separated from each other by the true preperitoneal space (Fig. 2.2).

2.3.3 *Lumboiliac Fascia (LIF)*

It is formed by the fusion of the aponeurosis of the psoas and iliacus muscles. It represents the posterior portion of the internal abdominal endofascia and transversely occupies the entire width of the internal iliac fossa and vertically extends from the superior insertion of the psoas muscle to its trochanteric insertion. At the cranial level, it is thin and formed by a single cellulose layer, but it gradually thickens as it descends to the pelvis, until it acquires the character of an aponeurosis on the iliacus muscle. It is fixed medially to all the lumbar vertebrae, forming arches for the passage of the lumbar vessels and nerves that communicate with the plexuses and ganglia. At the base of the sacrum, the largest arch is formed, which extends from the last lumbar vertebra to the superior stratum and is where the obturator and lumbosacral nerves pass. At the level of the superior inlet of the pelvis, it sends a thin sheet to the external iliac vessels that keeps them at the inner edge of the psoas. Laterally it is continuous with the fascia of the transverse muscle. At a higher level, it ends on the fibrous arch of the psoas muscle, to which the corresponding fascicles of the diaphragm will be inserted. Inferiorly, the transversal fascia is used forming an angle that closes the cavity, internal lip of the iliac crest, ileopectineal eminence, and posterior and external half of the femoral canal and continues to cover the extrapelvic portion of the psoas, joining the femoral aponeurosis of the sartorius and pectineus.

The LIF is made up of two layers of fibers: (1) transversely directed fibers that start from the circumference of the iliac crest and go to the superior inlet of the pelvis and (2) vertically directed fibers that come from the psoas tendon. Both planes of fibers are delimited by two fatty layers that are the link between them and

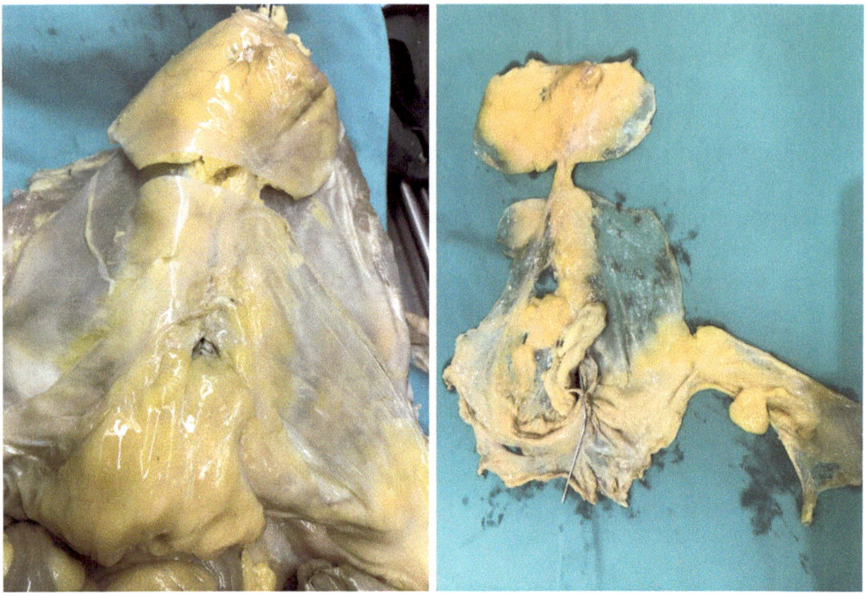

Fig. 2.2 Aponeurosis of the abdominal wall. Preparation of the internal surface of the abdominal wall to see the deep support of the abdominal core: preperitoneal fascia + adipose tissue + transversal fascia (premuscular). This plane (1) facilitates the proper sliding of the entire wall and its mobility independent of the bone framework; (2) protects the abdominal cavity by distributing IAP changes; and (3) distributes the pressure forces or traumas, isolating their content (Laplace and Pascal's law)

offer them elasticity and contractility, properties that they do not have on their own. Based on the predominance of each of these elements, the character of the fascia is modified: more elastic and contractile when the fibers are few or inflexible when they are abundant. This fact explains to the surgeon the difference between its two parts: the thin and transparent lumbar part allows the ilioinguinal nerve to be seen, while the iliac part is thick and doubles to hide the nerves in its thickness (femorocutaneous nerve on the iliac muscle and genitofemoral on the anterior surface of the psoas). The deep blade is inserted around the upper inlet of the pelvis, and the superficial one surrounds the iliac vessels to go down to the pelvis and continue with the pelvic fascia (Fig. 2.3).

2.3.4 *Thoracolumbar Fascia (TLF)*

It is the dense connective tissue membrane that surrounds the deep muscles of the back of the trunk. It extends from the lumbosacral area, where it is very prominent, to the thoracic area where it becomes thinner and ends up joining the nuchal fascia. This connective tissue serves as a muscular retinaculum for the lumbar erector

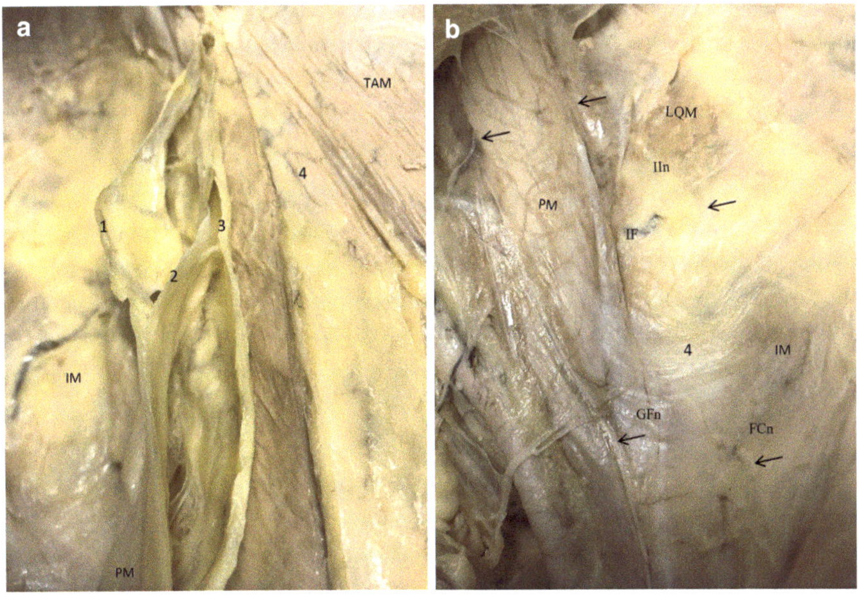

Fig. 2.3 Fascia system. Dissection slide showing the lumboiliac retroperitoneal space. (**a**) Approach planes, (1) peritoneum, (2) preperitoneal fascia, (3) fascia transversalis, (4) lumboiliac fascia. (**b**) The nerve paths under the FLI are shown with arrows for transparency, according to the different thickness

muscles, which it acts as a clamp, and its contraction creates a hydraulic amplification mechanism that stabilizes the lumbar spine. Different immuno-histochemical studies have shown that it is innervated by nociceptive endings and has an essential role in the genesis of low back pain. The TLF is made up of three laminae: anterior, middle, and posterior.

The *anterior lamina* of TLF is the thinnest and thinnest. It covers the anterior surface of the transverse muscle until it reaches the fascia iliaca, covers quadratus lumborum and psoas, and inserts into the anterior surface of the lumbar transverse processes. Its fibers have an oblique direction and continue in a cranial direction, increasing in thickness to form part of the lateral lumbo-costal arch that serves as the insertion of the diaphragm. In this way, it participates in the so-called lumbopelvic intrinsic subsystem, related to intra-abdominal pressure. Its capacity to transmit tension is much lower than that of the other two remaining sheets.

The *middle lamina* covers the posterior surface of the transversus muscle and separates it from the sacrospinalis, behind the quadratus lumborum and psoas, until it inserts into the medial tip of the lumbar transverse processes. Its fibers have an inferior and lateral direction, mostly transverse, but with a small obliquity of 10–25° with respect to the horizontal, so it can generate a small longitudinal tension. The muscle that contributes most to the tension of the TLF due to its extensive insertion is the transverse muscle, although they also participate through their insertions, the IO below the level of L3, and the EO above this level. Although the transverse causes tension mainly on the middle lamina, it also influences the posterior lamina through the lateral raphe where the different laminae join. The insertions of the IO-AT in the middle lamina allow traction of the transverse processes, stabilizing the lumbar spine in the frontal and transverse planes. This middle lamina is designed to transmit a wide range of loads and tensions directly, while the posterior lamina does so less directly from various muscles.

The *posterior lamina* represents the continuation of the aponeurosis of the latissimus dorsi with that of the gluteus maximus, starting from L4 toward the sacrum, until it is inserted into the spinous processes of the lumbar and dorsal vertebrae, into the supraspinous and interspinous ligaments, into the iliac spine, anterosuperior, and in the contralateral iliac bone, behind the erector and multifidus muscles. It is the widest and strongest of the three and the only one that continues into the thoracic region. It is bilaminar (superficial and deep), with the two layers progressively fusing below T12. In the thoracic region, its thickness is reduced, the superficial layer ends on the upper edge of the minor rhomboid, and the deep layer reaches the splenium of the neck. Therefore, it forms a continuous compartment over the entire spinal column. Its fibers have a heterogeneous obliquity, more pronounced in the lower lumbar segments than in the upper ones and greater in the superficial layer than in the deep one. This obliquity means that the transverse tensions produced on it by the abdominal muscles can be converted into longitudinal ones and increase the rigidity of the spine against flexion. It is designed to be an important stabilizer and transmitter of forces between the shoulder girdle, the lumbar spine, the pelvic girdle, and the lower limbs.

The *function of the TLF* is spinal stability, segmental control of the three planes of movement, proprioception, generation of tension, and improvement of the efficiency of paravertebral muscle contraction, force transfer, and protection of the sacroiliac joint. Any alteration of this tissue can lead to a lack of strength, movement, or degeneration, which will have an impact on lumbopelvic stability. It is considered an essential structure to be able to carry out normal daily activity. Tension on the TLF and intra-abdominal pressure require mutual interaction to create effective spinal stability. The abdominal muscles (in addition to the dorsal, gluteus maximus, lumbar erectors, and multifidus) directly increase the tension on the TLF, creating a natural belt that increases the rigidity of the lumbopelvic complex and therefore its stability capacity. The action of the lumbar abdominal muscles undoubtedly contributes to the increase in intra-abdominal pressure and the tension of the TLF. If we compare this structure to that of a tent, the abdominal muscles would be the lateral supports, the column the central mast, and the TLF the fabric of the tent itself. In order to support it, the lateral grips must be under a certain tension and provide stability to the entire structure. Any alteration of this fascia (such as DR) impacts lumbopelvic stability and can cause chronic low back pain. In summary, the TLF should be considered a core or control center that integrates a set of active structures (muscles of the thoracic and lumbar, abdominal, and hip regions) and other passive ones (vertebrae, discs, ligaments, etc.), whose action together allows adequate control of the stability of the trunk, both statically and dynamically, as well as an adequate and optimal transmission of forces between the upper and lower limbs, in a combined or sequential manner. That is, the TLF is the link and relationship with the rest of the structures, and any tension alteration in it automatically affects the entire system, justifying the presence of alterations in body areas far from the area of injury. In fact, the transverse muscle is the one that generates the greatest tension on the TLF, increases intra-abdominal pressure, and stabilizes the lumbar spine [1, 4].

Therefore, the *abdominal core* is an anatomical and functional concept, which encompasses muscular, osteo-ligamentous, and neural control structures related to the dorsolumbar region, pelvis, and hip, whose joint participation allows adequate and optimal control of stability and motion. Any alteration of this fascial system can cause (1) tension and a feeling of stiffness in the lower dorsal region; (2) tightness, spasticity, and increased muscle tone; (3) increased lumbar lordosis; (4) not being able to perform properly and correct form of diaphragmatic breathing; (5) lack of spinal mobility; (6) alteration in gait; and (7) headache.

2.4 Irrigation and Innervation of the Abdominal Wall

2.4.1 Vascularization of the Abdominal Wall

The blood supply to the abdominal wall can be divided into three zones.

2.4.1.1 Zone I

Limits: area that includes the upper and middle central portion of the abdominal wall, above to the xiphoid process and the medial costal margins, lateral to the semilunar line and below to the lower edge of the umbilicus.

Vessels: come from the superior and inferior epigastric arteries, with the inferior artery being dominant. The superior epigastric artery originates from the lateral thoracic artery at the level of the sixth rib. The inferior epigastric artery arises from the inner surface of the external iliac artery above the inguinal ligament, ascends along the inner edge of the deep inguinal ring, pierces the transversal fascia, reaches the outer edge of the rectus sheath, and penetrates it near the semilunar line to divide most frequently into two main branches (Moon and Taylor Type II). In addition to these main branches, it gives pubic, muscular, and umbilical branches. The superior and inferior epigastric arteries run deep to the rectus abdominis muscle, in front of its posterior sheath, but it is not unusual for one or both to have an intramuscular course in some segment of their course. They supply blood to the muscle, skin, and subcutaneous tissue through perforators.

Perforating: they can be subdivided into medial and lateral. They resemble longitudinal rows that run parallel to the abdominal wall. Medial perforators tend to have a broader vascular territory when they cross the midline, while lateral perforators are located on their specific side of the abdomen. Perforators are essential for selecting the type of incision and repair technique. The common midline incision will interrupt the medial perforators that cross the midline, limiting the collaterals in zone I. When the subcutaneous tissue is separated from the anterior rectus sheath, the blood supply to this anterior tissue is affected because much of the blood supply to this region depends on these musculocutaneous perforators.

2.4.1.2 Zone II

Limits: area bounded above by zone I or lower edge of navel, down to lower edge of abdominal wall and laterally reaches midaxillary line.

Vessels: originate from the deep epigastric arcade, the superficial inferior epigastric, the superficial external pudenda, and the superficial circumflex iliac. The area posterior and cephalic to the anterosuperior iliac spine is irrigated by perforators of the deep circumflex iliac artery, branch of zone III.

2.4.1.3 Zone III

Limits: area formed by the lateral abdominal wall and limited superiorly by the costal margin, medially by the semilunar line, and laterally by the midaxillary line.

Vessels: depends on the musculophrenic, lumbar, and lower intercostal arteries; the latter derives from the deep circumflex iliac artery. The musculophrenic artery is the second branch of the internal thoracic artery at its bifurcation. It passes in an inferolateral direction behind the seventh, eighth, and ninth ribs, providing large branches to the intercostal arteries and eventually joining the lumbar artery, supplying the lateral abdominal wall. The lumbar and inferior intercostal arteries lie in the plane between the transverse and internal oblique.

Venous drainage of the abdominal wall follows the same pattern as the arterial drainage with the exception of the paraumbilical vessels, which from the umbilicus reach the round ligament of the liver and drain into the portal vein system.

Lymphatic drainage: cranial lymphatic drainage follows the anterior region via the intrathoracic route, the caudal region follows the inguinal route, and the lateral region follows the lumbar route [1, 5] (Fig. 2.4).

2.4.2 Innervation of the Abdominal Wall

The innervation of the anterior abdominal wall depends on the ventral branches of the intercostal nerves from T7 to L1: anterior and lateral cutaneous branches of the intercostal nerves T7–T11, the subcostal nerve T12, and the iliohypogastric and ilioinguinal branches of L1 accompany the respective vessels in the neurovascular or transverse plane between the internal oblique and transversus abdominis muscles.

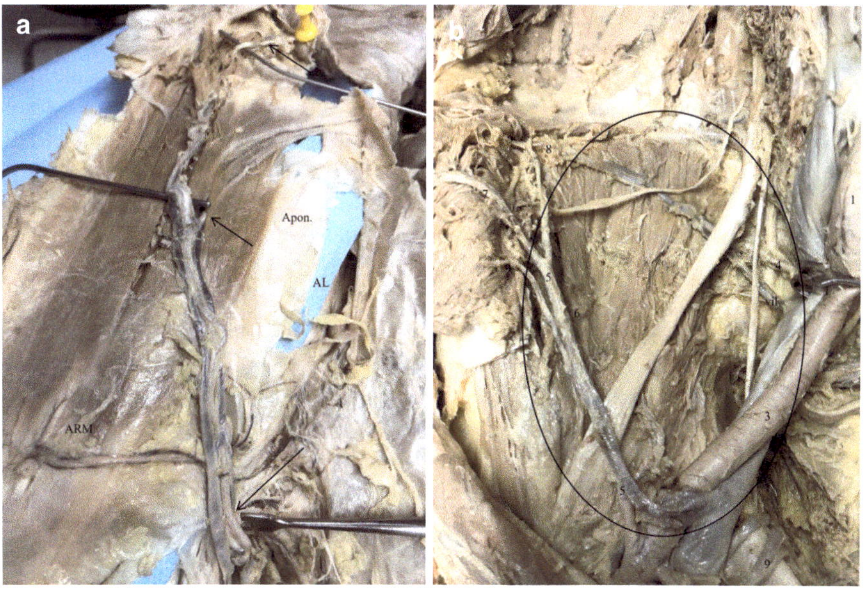

Fig. 2.4 (a) Study of the inferior epigastric artery in relation to a retromuscular approach. Dissection of the vessel in its ascending path over the rectus femoris. Its direction and branches are well appreciated, and cranially its relationship with the subcostal nerve is indicated (yellow pin) as it descends after perforating the posterior sheath. (b) Study of the retroiliac vascular circle in relation to a preperitoneal approach (external iliac and the circumflex, internal iliac and iliolumbar). (1) Primitive iliac artery. (2) Internal iliac artery. (3) External iliac artery. (4) Iliolumbar artery. (5) External iliac circumflex artery. (6) Internal branches for the iliac. (7) Branches for the muscles of the abdomen. (8) Anastomosis with the iliolumbar. (9) Communicating branch from epigastric to obturatrix. (10) Spermatic artery

The segmental nerves from T6 to T9 emerge from the costal margin to enter the plane, between the midline, and the anterior axillary line. T6 enters just lateral to the white line, while T7-8-9 enters from the costal margin, increasing their more lateral location, respectively. The branch of T9 arises medial (85%) or lateral to the anterior axillary line. Within the plane, the nerves have an intense distribution and numerous anastomoses, so that each one can contribute to at least two levels of segmentation. T11 and T12 communicate through small branches with the one immediately above and below. They all contribute in this way to innervate the oblique muscles and the rectus abdominis.

Upon reaching the lateral edge of the rectum, the nerves make an angle of 90° and cross the muscle from the posterior wall to the anterior aponeurosis accompanied by an artery and a vein, surrounded by fat and connective tissue, forming a neurovascular bundle that crosses the rectum. At each level, a total of six exit holes were distributed in both rectus muscles. Once the anterior sheath is reached, they make another right angle to continue along the wall, innervating the skin and subcutaneous cellular tissue, so that they are distributed through various origins of segmentation. Below the umbilicus, there are usually four to six nerves re-formed after these anastomoses between the original ones, which move under the posterior surface of the rectum forming a second nerve plexus that is located in relation to the lateral branch of the inferior epigastric artery or plexus of the rectal sheath that spans from T6 to L1, similar to the transverse plexus. The nerves on the posterior surface in the vicinity of the vessels give muscular branches following the pattern of the arteries and cutaneous branches that travel with the cutaneous arterial branches. The ilioinguinal nerve enters the plane at the level of the anterior superior iliac spine, giving an inferomedial branch that innervates the rectus muscle. The iliohypogastric nerve crosses the internal oblique muscle to lie between both obliques and reach the rectum (Fig. 2.5).

In the midline, branches from T7–9 supply the upper abdominal wall from the xiphoid process to the superior border of the umbilicus, T10 supplies the area around the umbilicus, and T11–L1 supplies the lower abdominal wall. Laterally, branches T7–12 provide sensory innervation. The ilioinguinal and iliohypogastric nerves also provide sensation to the inner thigh, scrotum, and labia majora. In abdominoplasty surgery, lower abdominal numbness due to injury to the ascending branches of the inguinal nerves is common. Low transverse incisions can injure the lateral femoral cutaneous nerve (dissection near the inguinal fold should be avoided). The motor innervation of the abdominal wall muscles follows a similar pattern. The

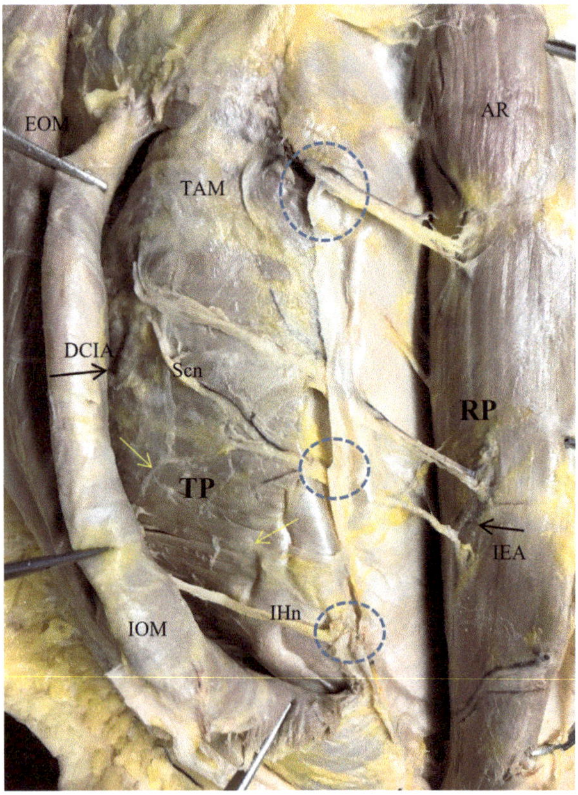

Fig. 2.5 Dissection of the anterolateral abdominal wall to show the two nerve plexuses: (1) neural plexus of the transversus plane (TP) in relation to the external circumflex iliac artery (arrow; DCIA) and (2) neural plexus of the rectal sheath (RP) in relation to the inferior epigastric artery (arrow, IEA). The possible site of injury is marked with a circle

rectus abdominis muscle is innervated by the six lower intercostal nerves. The external oblique, internal oblique, and transversus abdominis muscles are innervated by the inferior intercostal, subcostal, and iliohypogastric and ilioinguinal muscles [1].

2.5 Classification of the Diastasis Recti (DR)

2.5.1 Normal Width of the Distance Between the Rectus Muscles

DR is a global fascial defect, not only of the LA, which involves both the fascial and muscular and aponeurotic systems. Any repair technique must keep this principle in mind. There is no consensus on the inter-rectal distance considered normal. Rath in 1996 proposed a classification of normal linea alba based on radiological measurements where differences in sex (4 mm wider in men) and age (older people over 45 years) were demonstrated:

Rath		
Level	Age <45	Age >45
Above the navel	10 mm	15 mm
At the level of the navel	27 mm	27 mm
Below the navel	9 mm	14 mm

In 2009, Beer et al. conducted an anatomical study in 150 nulliparous women between 20 and 45 years old with a body mass index (BMI) <30 kg/m^2, excluding women with a recent weight loss of more than 10 kg, previous surgeries, or abdominal wall hernias. Ultrasound measurements were taken at three reference points: at the level of the xiphoid process, 3 cm above the navel, and 2 cm below. No significant differences were demonstrated between the width of the linea alba and weight or age. The linea alba reached its maximum width at 3 cm above the navel and then at 2 cm below and at its origin at the level of the xiphoid appendix (31 mm), this difference being statistically significant ($p \leq 0.0001$). The 10th and 90th percentiles were used to establish the definition of normality: at the level of the xiphoid appendix from 2 to 15 mm; 3 cm above the navel from 6 to 22 mm; and 2 cm below from 2 to 16 mm.

Beer	
Level	Width
At the level of the xiphoid	≤15 mm
At 3 cm above the navel	≤22 mm
At 2 cm below the navel	≤16 mm

In primiparous women during pregnancy and postpartum, Mota et al. have published a longitudinal study on 84 primiparous women, measuring the inter-rectal distance sonographically at 4 times during pregnancy: weeks 35–41 of gestation and weeks 6–8, 12–14, and 24–26 postpartum. As a reference they used the center of the navel: 2 cm below and 2–5 cm above. The normal width of the linea alba was established using the 20th and 80th percentiles. The linea alba was widest at 2 cm above the umbilicus during pregnancy (86 mm) and at 6 months postpartum (28 mm). During pregnancy, the width of the linea alba at 2 cm above the navel was significantly greater than at 5 cm above ($p < 0.001$) and at 6 months postpartum also compared to measurements at 2 cm below ($p < 0.001$) and 5 cm above ($p < 0.001$). The authors conclude that a width of the linea alba during pregnancy of 44–79 mm at 5 cm from the navel, of 54–86 mm at 2 cm above the navel, and of 49–79 mm at 2 cm below can be considered normal. At 6 months postpartum, the width of the linea alba considered normal is 12–24 mm at 5 cm from the navel, 17–28 mm at 2 cm from the navel, and 9–21 mm below.

2.5.2 *Pathological Diastasis Recti*

2.5.2.1 Nahas Classification

Based on the myofascial deformity, the author considers four groups of diastasis to which he assigns the most appropriate surgical treatment for its correction. The most common group is Type A.

Nahas		
Diastasis	Etiology	Repair
Type A	Secondary to pregnancy	Plication of the anterior rectus sheath (PVR)
Type B	DR and myoaponeurotic laxity	PVR + plication of the external oblique aponeurosis
Type C	DR and congenital lateralized insertion of the rectus	Medialization of the rectus muscles, release of the posterior sheaths
Type D	DR and waist loss (obesity)	PVR and medialization of the aponeurosis of the external obliques

2.5.2.2 Ranney Classification

It is based on the degree of separation between the rectus abdominis muscles and differentiates diastasis into three degrees: mild (<3 cm), moderate (3–5 cm), and severe (>5 cm).

Ranney	
Mild	<3 cm

Ranney	
Moderate	3–5 cm
Severe	>5 cm

2.5.2.3 Brauman Classification

Brauman et al. demonstrate that there is a transverse stretch limit of the linea alba, regardless of the circumference of the abdomen, and that it ranges between 1 and 2 inches (2.54–5.08 cm). However, DRs of up to 12 cm have been reported, although it is not indicated whether it is associated with a medial hernia.

2.5.2.4 Classification of the German Hernia Society (DHG) and International Endohernia Society (IEHS)

Based on the European Hernia Society (EHS) classification of ventral hernia, the length of the diastasis is defined as M1–M5 and its width applying the Ranney classification as W1-2-3. In addition, the presence of previous surgeries, the number of pregnancies, the condition of the skin of the abdomen (laxity and skin folds), the diagnostic procedure (clinical, radiological), and the presence of pain in the preoperative period are taken into account [6–13].

Surgical Anatomy Tips

- The anatomy of the AW is complex and elegant. Understanding the fascia planes, vascular, nerve, and lymphatic supply is critical to obtain the best aesthetic results with minimal morbidity.
- The best surgical option is one that restores the anatomy and function of the AW, understanding functional repair as one that reconstructs the linea alba.
- The benefit of functional surgery in DR can only be explained based on the aponeurotic and fascial muscle complex of the AW as a single entity or core (abdominal wall core).
- Tension on the LA and the fascial and muscular integrity of the transversus abdominis are necessary for the maintenance of normal function of the abdominal core.
- The preperitoneal fascial plane is the only global compartment, without limits under the AW.
- Superficial dissection must preserve the perforating vessels so as not to damage the blood circulation of the skin and subcutaneous tissue. The best dissection plane is the avascular plane between both oblique muscles.
- The extreme spaces, retroxiphoid and retropubic, should be prolonged to ensure overlapping of the retromuscular approach, and conversely, the lateral edge of the rectus sheath should be avoided to avoid damaging the neurovascular pedicles.

- Knowledge of neural and vascular anatomical variants is essential to reduce surgical complications.
- During dissection of the AW and preperitoneal space, the surgeon must remember the anastomoses between the epigastric vessels, the retropubic branches of both obturator arteries, the suprapubic branches of the inferior epigastric arteries, and the retropubic and suprapubic branches of the obturator.

References

1. Moreno-Egea A. Anatomía quirúrgica para especialistas en pared abdominal. In: Atlas fotográfico de disección. Valencia: SOHAH; 2021.
2. Ger R. The clinical anatomy of the anterolateral abdominal wall musculature. Clin Anat. 2009;22(3):392–7.
3. Hellinger A, Roth I, Biber FC, Frenken M, Witzleb S, Lammers BJ. Surgical anatomy of the abdominal wall. Chirurg. 2016;87(9):724–30.
4. Poulose BK. Abdominal core health: what is it? Surg Clin North Am. 2023;103(5):827–34.
5. Kostov S, Dineva S, Kornovski Y, Slavchev S, Ivanova Y, Yordanov A. Vascular anatomy and variations of the anterior abdominal wall - significance in abdominal surgery. Prague Med Rep. 2023;124(2):108–42. https://doi.org/10.14712/23362936.2023.9.
6. Zorraquino A. Guía clínica de la diástasis de los músculos rectos del abdomen y pequeños defectos de la línea alba. Rev Hispanoam Hernia. 2021;9(2):118–25.
7. Rath AM, Attali P, Dumas JL, Goldlust D, Zhang J, Chevrel JP. The abdominal linea alba: an anatomo-radiologic and biomechanical study. Surg Radiol Anat. 1996;18:281–8.
8. Beer GM, Schuster A, Seifert B, Manestar M, Mihic-Probst D, Weberg SA. The normal width of the linea alba in nulliparous women. Clin Anat. 2009;22:706–11.
9. Mota P, Pascoal AG, Carita AI, Bø K. Normal width of the inter-recti distance in pregnant and postpartum primiparous women. Musculoskelet Sci Pract. 2018;35:34–7.
10. Nahas FX. An aesthetic classification of the abdomen based on the myoaponeurotic layer. Plast Reconstr Surg. 2001;108(6):1788–95.
11. Ranney B. Diastasis recti and umbilical hernia causes, recognition and repair. S D J Med. 1990;43(10):5–8.
12. Brauman D. Diastasis recti: clinical anatomy. Plast Reconstr Surg. 2008;122(5):1564–9.
13. Reinpold W, Köckerling F, Bittner R, Conze J, Fortelny R, Koch A, et al. Classification of rectus diastasis—a proposal by the German Hernia Society (DHG) and the International Endohernia Society (IEHS). Front Surg. 2019;6:1.

Chapter 3
Epidemiology and Causes of Diastasis Recti

Salvatore Cuccomarino

A useful outline of the epidemiology and causes of diastasis recti may be as follows:

- Factors that influence interrectal distance (IRD)
  - Gender (in men the supraumbilical IRD is higher than in nulliparous women)
  - Pregnancies (in women who have had pregnancies, the IRD is higher than in nulliparous women)
  - Anatomical location (supraumbilical IRD > subumbilical IRD)
  - Trunk position (at rest or flexed)
- Risk factors
  - Age
  - Multiparity
  - Having raised children
  - Cesarean section
  - Weight gain (obesity)
  - Previous abdominal operations (with incision in the linea alba)

The prevalence of diastasis recti varies in the literature; in general, this coincides with Sperstad's data [1], but there are very interesting studies in which, in multiparous women, the prevalence of diastasis reaches 52%, with a notable 35% in nulliparous women [2], and can reach 59% in multiparous women [3].

The risk of diastasis depending on age is controversial: in a study on abdominal CT scans of 644 adult women [4], the overall prevalence of diastasis recti was 24.6% between 45 and 59 years and 22.7% in patients over 60 years old; however

S. Cuccomarino (✉)
General Surgeon, Fellow of the American College of Surgeons, Maria Pia Hospital, Turin, Italy
e-mail: dr.cuccomarino@cuccomarinomd.com

S. Cuccomarino et al. (eds.), *New Concepts in Diastasi Recti Surgery*,
https://doi.org/10.1007/978-3-031-74947-6_3

Rath et al. [5] found a significantly greater widening of the linea alba above and below the umbilicus in subjects older than 45 years.

Pregnancy, and in particular the number of pregnancies, is probably the greatest risk factor for the appearance of diastasis recti, due to the prolonged increase in pressure caused by the pregnant uterus and the hormonal changes that occur during this period; cesarean section (and again the number of cesarean sections) is an additional risk factor [6].

The prevalence of diastasis recti increases with the increase toward pathological values of BMI [4], probably due to the increase in intra-abdominal pressure due to visceral fat deposits and also probably because the concentration of collagen in the supraumbilical linea alba of the obese patients is lower than that of the non-obese population [7].

Even in patients with metabolic diseases related to the metabolic syndrome, such as diabetes, the prevalence of diastasis recti appears increased [4].

There is little data on the prevalence of diastasis recti in men, among other things in works that do not directly refer to diastasis recti but in patients with abdominal aortic aneurysm (AAA); in particular, in a 2008 study, diastasis recti was detected in 67.7% of a group of patients with AAA [8], to the point that a second study, from 2010, went so far as to recommend AAA screening in all male patients with diastasis recti [9]. The basis of this association could lie in the alteration of collagen synthesis found in both groups of patients.

There is no relationship between intense physical activity and the appearance of diastasis recti [10, 11], although it is a common experience of those who treat this pathology to have visited professional athletes (e.g., bodybuilders) with diastasis recti with no apparent causes other than their own physical activity.

On the other hand, lifting loads (among which we can also include the point mentioned above such as "having raised children") is undoubtedly a recognized risk factor for the development of diastasis recti [12, 13].

References

1. Sperstad JB, Tennfjord MK, Hilde G, Ellström-Engh M, Bø K. Diastasis recti abdominis during pregnancy and 12 months after childbirth: prevalence, risk factors and report of lumbopelvic pain. Br J Sports Med. 2016;50(17):1092–6.
2. Spitznagle TM, Leong FC, Van Dillen LR. Prevalence of diastasis recti abdominis in a urogynecological patient population. Int Urogynecol J Pelvic Floor Dysfunct. 2007;18(3):321–8.
3. Turan V, Colluoglu C, Turkyilmaz E, Korucuoglu U. Prevalence of diastasis recti abdominis in the population of young multiparous adults in Turkey. Ginekol Pol. 2011;82(11):817–21.
4. Wu L, Gu Y, Gu Y, Wang Y, Lu X, Zhu C, Lu Z, Xu H. Diastasis recti abdominis in adult women based on abdominal computed tomography imaging: prevalence, risk factors and its impact on life. J Clin Nurs. 2021;30(3-4):518–27.
5. Rath AM, Attali P, Dumas JL, Goldlust D, Zhang J, Chevrel JP. The abdominal linea alba: an anatomo-radiologic and biomechanical study. Surg Radiol Anat. 1996;18(4):281–8.

6. Cavalli M, Aiolfi A, Bruni PG, Manfredini L, Lombardo F, Bonfanti MT, Bona D, Campanelli G. Prevalence and risk factors for diastasis recti abdominis: a review and proposal of a new anatomical variation. Hernia. 2021;25(4):883–90.
7. Grossi JV, Nicola FF, Zepeda IA, Becker M, Trindade EN, Diemen VV, Cavazzola LT, Trindade MR. Linea alba collagen assessment in morbidly obese patients. Arq Bras Cir Dig. 2016;29(Suppl 1):8–11.
8. McPhail I. Abdominal aortic aneurysm and diastasis recti. Angiology. 2008;59(6):736–9. https://doi.org/10.1177/0003319708319940.
9. De'Ath HD, Lovegrove RE, Javid M, Peter N, Magee TR, Galland RB. An assessment of between-recti distance and divarication in patients with and without abdominal aortic aneurysm. Ann R Coll Surg Engl. 2010;92(7):591–4.
10. Davenport MH, Ruchat SM, Sobierajski F, Poitras VJ, Gray CE, Yoo C, Skow RJ, Jaramillo Garcia A, Barrowman N, Meah VL, Nagpal TS, Riske L, James M, Nuspl M, Weeks A, Marchand AA, Slater LG, Adamo KB, Davies GA, Barakat R, Mottola MF. Impact of prenatal exercise on maternal harms, labour and delivery outcomes: a systematic review and meta-analysis. Br J Sports Med. 2019;53(2):99–107.
11. Kimber ML, Meyer S, McHugh TL, Thornton J, Khurana R, Sivak A, Davenport MH. Health outcomes after pregnancy in elite athletes: a systematic review and meta-analysis. Med Sci Sports Exerc. 2021;53(8):1739–47.
12. Candido G, Lo T, Janssen PA. Risk factors for diastasis of the recti abdominis. J Assoc Chartered Physiother Women's Health. 2005;97:49.
13. Joueidi Y, Vieillefosse S, Cardaillac C, Mortier A, Oppenheimer A, Deffieux X, Thubert T. Impact of the diastasis of the rectus abdominis muscles on the pelvic-perineal symptoms: review of the literature. Prog Urol. 2019;29(11):544–59.

Chapter 4
Pathophysiology and Clinical Aspects of Diastasis Recti

Salvatore Cuccomarino

If we ask a doctor who is not an expert in abdominal wall surgery to give us a definition of the latter, it is not unusual for him to answer that it is the "lid" of a kind of "box" that contains a noble material, the abdominal viscera. After all, the abdomen—according to common thinking—is just a "container"; what is important is the content.

A surgeon expert in wall surgery, however, could respond that the abdomen is "a magic box" in which structure and function are perfectly interdependent, contributing to processes fundamental to life such as breathing, maintenance of orthostatic position, pregnancy, and, of course, visceral protection.

However, the limits of this "box" are usually vague even for an expert surgeon. Where does the abdomen end and the pelvis begin? We rarely venture into the area under the peritoneal reflection of the pouch of Douglas, as well as into the retroperitoneum. Surgeons, and especially those experienced in abdominal wall surgery, know the anatomy of the latter very well but do not go much further.

For this reason, the concept of abdominal core is not yet extended among surgeons in general and has only recently become part of the professional life of surgeons who are experts in abdominal wall surgery.

The abdominal core was initially defined as a soft tissue "shell" bounded above by the diaphragm, anterolaterally by the abdominal wall and hips, and below by the pelvic floor [1]. The importance of defining this "new anatomical entity" soon seemed crucial, so much so that according to *JAMA Surgery* "most members of the board of governors at the Americas Hernia Society aim to redefine the field of hernia care as abdominal core health, the discipline as abdominal core surgery, and the identity of associated clinicians as abdominal core surgeons" [1].

S. Cuccomarino (✉)
General Surgeon, Fellow of the American College of Surgeons, Maria Pia Hospital, Turin, Italy
e-mail: dr.cuccomarino@cuccomarinomd.com

S. Cuccomarino et al. (eds.), *New Concepts in Diastasi Recti Surgery*,
https://doi.org/10.1007/978-3-031-74947-6_4

Diastasis of the rectus muscles (such as hernias, athlete's pubalgia, injuries to the abdominal core muscles, benign and malignant tumors of the abdominal wall, eventrations, etc.) is part of the pathologies of the abdominal core [2].

However, if we return to the definition of that soft tissue "shell," we will see that it is open posteriorly: a posterior wall is open. This limit has recently been overcome by the proposal to recognize the soft tissues in relation to the lumbosacral portion of the spine as an integral part of the abdominal core [2].

Muscles of crucial importance are part of the abdominal core so defined: first of all the diaphragm, then that complex musculo-tendinous structure represented by the pelvic floor, obviously the muscles of the abdominal wall (rectus, external and internal obliques, transverse) and also the psoas minor and major and iliac (or iliopsoas) muscles, the quadratus lumborum, and the lumbar portion of the sacrospinalis and multifidus muscles.

It is not possible to understand the pathophysiology and clinical features of diastasis recti if we do not have a clear understanding of the anatomy and function of these muscles; however, to have a clear understanding of how and why diastasis recti is a functional pathology (probably the main one in terms of frequency) of the abdominal core, it is advisable to proceed with the principles of the Galilean inductive method: why patients with diastasis rectum suffer from low back pain, stress urinary incontinence, transit disorders, etc.?

4.1 The Diastasis Recti Clinical Manifestations

We can define diastasis recti as an insufficiency of the linea alba caused by its thinning and widening that provokes a separation of the rectus abdominal muscles of at least 2.5 cm.

Much has been written and said about the clinical definition of diastasis recti, but the two fundamental works remain are Sperstad in 2016 [3] and Mota in 2012 [1].

The latter gives a sonographic definition of the normal linea alba: measured sonographically for an extension of 2 cm below the navel, the linea alba should have, at rest, a width no greater than 2 cm above the navel and no more than 85 mm per below the navel.

Sperstad, on the other hand, gives a clinical, non-instrumental definition of diastasis recti, saying that, in a section that goes from 4.5 cm above to 4.5 cm below the navel, the separation between the rectus muscles (or interrectal distance, IRD) is normal if less than two fingers of the examiner enter between the rectums, there is a mild diastasis if two to three fingers enter, a moderate diastasis if the IRD is between three and four fingers, and, finally, a severe diastasis if it is greater than four fingers.

The definitions of diastasis proposed by Sperstad and Mota are evidently in conflict with each other: Sperstad's two fingers (unless the surgeon has a very small hand) are certainly larger than Mota's 2 cm. There are other definitions of diastasis recti [4, 5], but nowadays it is generally accepted to speak of diastasis when the IRD is at least 2 cm; this parameter is accepted both by the guidelines of the *European*

Hernia Society [6] (which explicitly define diastasis recti as "a widening of the linea alba exceeding 2 cm") and by those of the *Hispano-American Hernia Society* [6] and of the *German Hernia Society-International Endohernia Society* [7].

The insufficiency of the linea alba causes a protrusion in the midline of the abdominal contents, covered by the teguments (skin, subcutaneous tissue) and by the linea alba itself. This protrusion is especially evident under stress, but there are patients in whom the diastasis is perfectly visible even at rest (Fig. 4.1).

Diastasis recti is closely related to pregnancy and childbirth. It usually appears in the second trimester of pregnancy and, in most cases, is diagnosed in the third trimester [8]; IRD continues to increase until partum [9], and its spontaneous resolution occurs between the first day and 8 weeks after partum [10].

That said, when defining the symptoms of diastasis recti, there are three key points of great importance to take into account:

1. Approximately one-third of women, 1 year after giving birth, will have diastasis recti that does not will improve over time [11].
2. In more than 95% of cases, these patients present symptoms directly related to diastasis [12].
3. In almost all cases, the diastasis is associated with a hernia of the linea alba, mainly umbilical [13], of which it is not unreasonable to say that the diastasis itself is the cause [4].

The main symptoms related to diastasis, the associated pathologies, and their relative frequencies [12] can be summarized as follows:

- Lower back pain (72.6%)
- Stress urinary incontinence (37.9% incidence, in fact; it is reported up to more than 50% of cases [14])

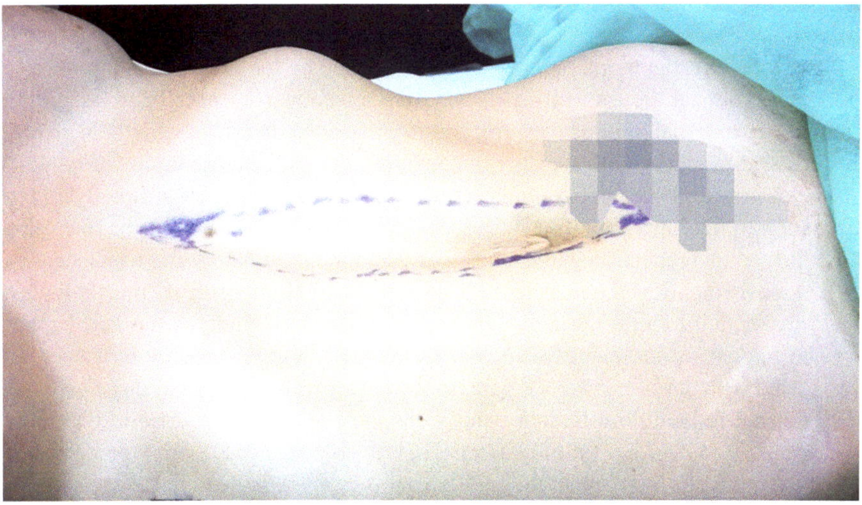

Fig. 4.1 Patient with evident ab-crack

- Digestive disorders (constipation, GE reflux, slow transit) (54.8%)
- Umbilical hernia (96.8%)
- Epigastric hernia (8.9%)
- Lumbopelvic instability [15]

Abdominal bloating is almost constant. In general, diastasis recti is a symptomatic condition in more than 95% of cases [12]; 1 month after surgery, 80% of patients report significant improvement or complete regression of low back pain; 89.8% a disappearance of stress urinary incontinence [16].

Lumbar pain is the most frequent and disabling disorder reported by patients during a visit for diastasis recti. The "normal" history of these patients (who are generally young women, often very athletic, and absolutely "healthy" before their pregnancies) is that, after giving birth, they began to suffer lower back pain, which worsened over time until becoming, in some cases, insupportable. Many of them come to the visit after having already been evaluated by an orthopedist or a physiatrist (which are not infrequently the specialists who send them for surgical evaluation).

The pathophysiological mechanisms that lead to the appearance of low back pain can be summarized as follows: correct posture normally results from the balance between flexor forces, which tend to bend the spine forward and are mainly due to the rectus abdominis muscles, and the extensor forces, which instead tend to accentuate lumbar lordosis and are due to the paraventral muscles, in particular the erector spinae muscles. In patients in whom the action of the erector spinae muscles prevails over that of the rectus muscles, the angles of lumbar and lumbosacral lordosis increase: this causes an increase in pressure, a "crushing," on the lumbosacral intervertebral discs and, therefore, the appearance of low back pain. In diastasis recti, through a very complex mechanism mediated by an anatomical structure known as the thoracolumbar fascia, the activity of the erector spinae muscles prevails over that of the rectus abdominis muscles. Diastasis repair surgery allows rebalancing the flexor and extensor forces of the spine, thus treating low back pain [17].

Anatomically, the thoracolumbar fascia is formed by longitudinal and transverse fibers that connect the aponeurosis of the transverse muscles, internal obliques and (much less) external obliques, the rib, and the iliac crest, laterally, with the vertebral column and medially with the sacrum, covering the paraspinal muscles (Fig. 4.2). As is known, both the oblique and transverse muscles participate directly in the formation of the linea alba (Fig. 4.3): the widening and weakening of the linea alba are reflected in a reduction in the tension of the thoracolumbar fascia, which causes, as previously mentioned, the increase in the lumbar and lumbosacral lordosis angles.

Plication of the rectus muscles significantly reduces the angles of thoracic kyphosis and lumbar lordosis and the lumbosacral angle, in patients with diastasis recti associated with chronic low back pain. In the postoperative period of these patients, a significant reduction in lumbar pain is observed [17]. In a postoperative survey conducted by our group on 63 patients [12], to the question "giving preoperative low back pain a 5, how much do you think it is now?," the patients' response was (on average) 1.24.

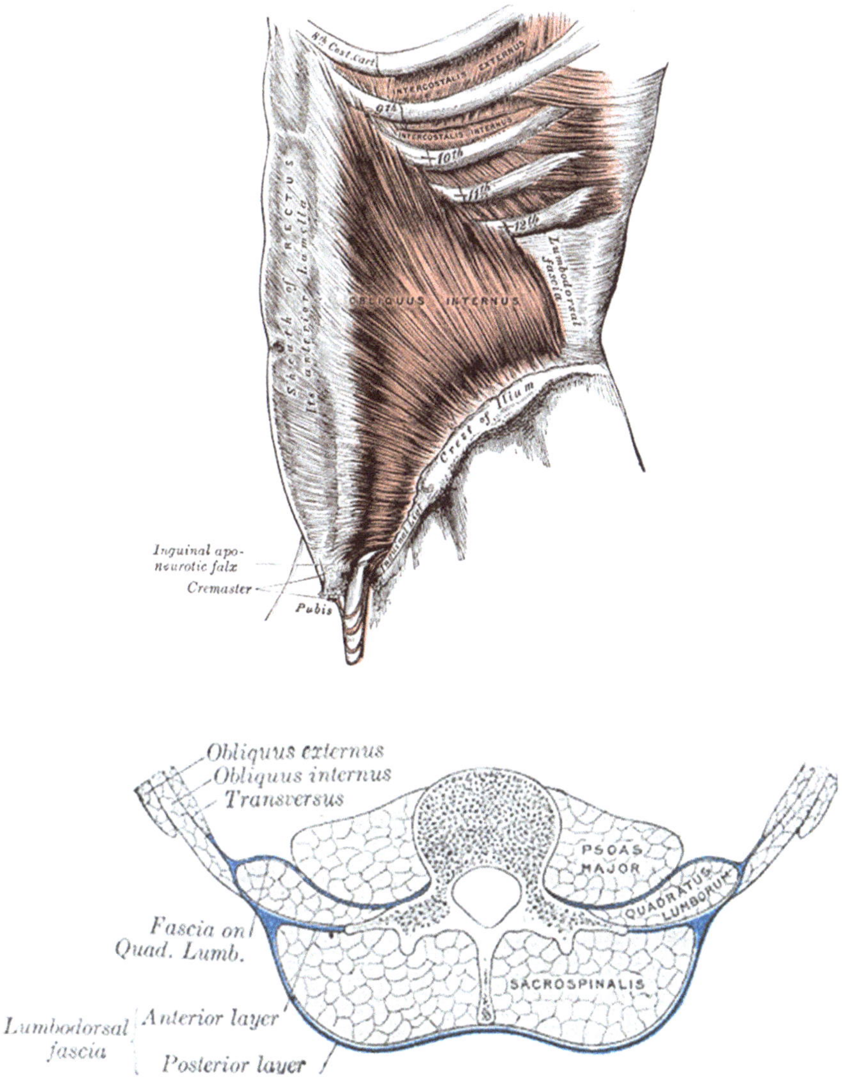

Fig. 4.2 The thoracolumbar (or lumbodorsal) fascia. From: *Henry Gray (1918) Anatomy of the Human Body*, plates 388 and 395. Public domain

This is mainly due to the action of the transverse abdominis muscle, the only one among the muscles of the abdominal wall with double aponeurosis (anterior and posterior) and double insertion in the anterior (sheath of the rectus and linea alba) and posterior (dorsal-lumbar fascia) midline.

These results are generally comparable to those published by Olsson et al. [18] and encourage continued studies in this direction.

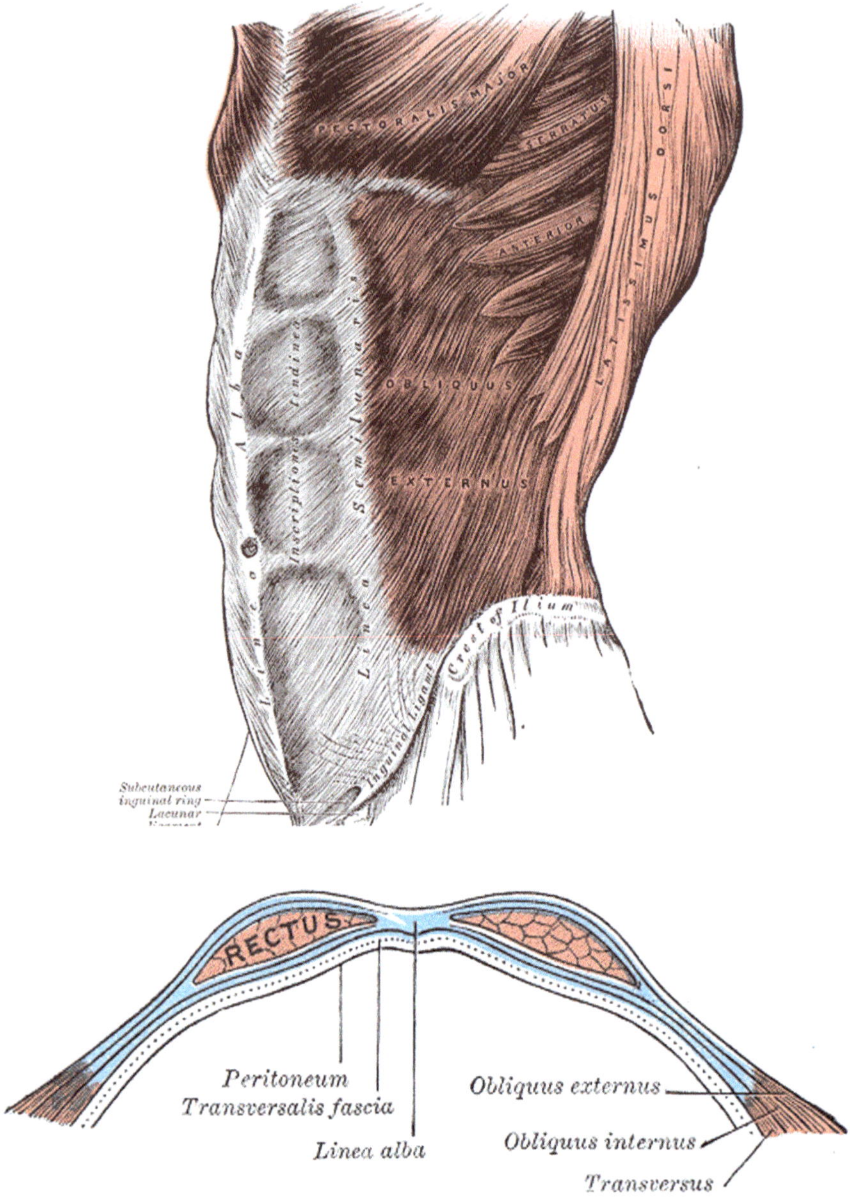

Fig. 4.3 Structure of the linea alba; the participation of the oblique muscles in its constitution is clearly evident. From: *Henry Gray (1918) Anatomy of the Human Body*, plates 392 and 399. Public domain

Regarding stress urinary incontinence, we know that it improves significantly after diastasis correction surgery [16, 18–23], which again encourages us to delve deeper into the pathophysiological mechanisms responsible for both of incontinence and its post-surgical improvement.

These mechanisms have not yet been completely clarified. The works published worldwide indicate that the repair of diastasis recti plays a key role in the reconstruction of the functional stability of all parts of the abdominal core, including the pelvic floor. Already in 1984 Gordon et al. had observed that, non-specifically, physical activity can prevent the appearance of urinary incontinence, thus highlighting the role of muscles other than those of the pelvic floor in the control of urinary continence [24]. The increased strength and stability of the abdominal muscles after surgical repair appear to improve pelvic floor function, to a significantly greater degree than with physical therapy alone. This emphasizes again, if necessary, that the abdominal core is an integrated system of muscle groups that work together.

The literature tells us that there is, in women, a statistically significant correlation between chronic low back pain and stress urinary incontinence [25] that a reduction in the functionality of the muscles of the abdominal wall (particularly the rectus, obliques internal and transverse [26]) results a reduction in the activity of the pelvic floor muscles [27] related in a statistically significant way with the appearance of stress urinary incontinence [28], which the functional deficit of the pelvic floor itself alone is not enough to motivate stress urinary incontinence and that the control and coordination of the function of the abdominal muscles are essential for correct control of this [24] and that contribute to the appearance of urinary incontinence of effort, an alteration of collagen is found, as in diastasis recti [25]. Sapsford et al.[26] have observed how the contraction of the abdominal wall muscles (particularly the external oblique and transverse muscles) is associated with an increase in urethral pressure, contributing to the mechanism of urinary continence. Furthermore, it has been observed that stress urinary incontinence is associated, in women, with abnormal electrical activity of the rectus abdominal muscles [27]. Variations in intra-abdominal pressure probably play a central role in the appearance of stress urinary incontinence in patients with diastasis recti: Martinez Bustelo et al. [28] have proposed that there is, in patients with diastasis recti, a rotation of the intra-abdominal pressure vectors, which, being normally oriented toward the coccyx, would move, in these patients, toward the anterior portion of the pelvic floor: this would favor a weakening of the pelvic floor and the subsequent appearance of stress urinary incontinence and organ pelvic prolapses.

In short, it seems legitimate to postulate that, by controlling intra-abdominal pressure, the muscles of the abdominal core, and in particular the transverse ones and, less, external oblique and rectus, are capable of modulating functions such as maintaining correct posture, urinary continence, gastrointestinal transit (we will not dwell, as seems quite obvious, on how a dysfunction of the abdominal muscles influences abdominal tension), and also on the "emerging" symptoms of diastasis recti, such as gastroesophageal reflux. Without a doubt, this will represent, in the coming years, a fertile field of study for surgeons specialized in abdominal core health and surgery.

References

1. Reinpold W, Köckerling F, Bittner R, Conze J, Fortelny R, Koch A, Kukleta J, Kuthe A, Lorenz R, Stechemesser B. Classification of rectus diastasis-a proposal by the German Hernia Society (DHG) and the International Endohernia Society (IEHS). Front Surg. 2019;6:1.
2. Hernández-Granados P, Henriksen NA, Berrevoet F, Cuccurullo D, López-Cano M, Nienhuijs S, Ross D, Montgomery A. European Hernia Society guidelines on management of rectus diastasis. Br J Surg. 2021;108(10):1189–91.
3. Zorraquino GA. Guía clínica de la diástasis de los músculos rectos del abdomen y pequeños defectos de la línea alba. Rev Hispanoam Hernia. 2021;9(2):118–25.
4. Boissonnault JS, Blaschak MJ. Incidence of diastasis recti abdominis during the childbearing year. Phys Ther. 1988;68(7):1082–6.
5. Gilleard WL, Brown JM. Structure and function of the abdominal muscles in primigravid subjects during pregnancy and the immediate postbirth period. Phys Ther. 1996;76(7):750–62.
6. Coldron Y, Stokes MJ, Newham DJ, Cook K. Postpartum characteristics of rectus abdominis on ultrasound imaging. Man Ther. 2008;13(2):112–21.
7. Cuccomarino S, Bonomo LD, Aprà F, Toscano A, Jannaci A. Preaponeurotic endoscopic repair (REPA) of diastasis recti: a single surgeon's experience. Surg Endosc. 2022;36(2):1302–9.
8. Juárez Muas DM. Preaponeurotic endoscopic repair (REPA) of diastasis recti associated or not to midline hernias. Surg Endosc. 2019;33(6):1777–82.
9. Spitznagle TM, Leong FC, Van Dillen LR. Prevalence of diastasis recti abdominis in a urogynecological patient population. Int Urogynecol J Pelvic Floor Dysfunct. 2007;18(3):321–8.
10. Benjamin DR, van de Water AT, Peiris CL. Effects of exercise on diastasis of the rectus abdominis muscle in the antenatal and postnatal periods: a systematic review. Physiotherapy. 2014;100(1):1–8.
11. Juárez Muas DM, Palmisano E, Pou Santoja G, Cuccomarino S, González Higuera G, Mayo P, Martínez Maya JD, Domínguez G, Ayala Acosta JC, Chichizola A. Reparación endoscópica preaponeurótica (REPA) como tratamiento de la diástasis de los músculos rectos asociada o no a hernias de la línea media. Estudio multicéntrico. Rev Hispanoam Hernia. 2019;7(2):59–65.
12. Temel M, Türkmen A, Berberoğlu Ö. Improvements in vertebral-column angles and psychological metrics after abdominoplasty with rectus plication. Aesthet Surg J. 2016;36(5):577–87.
13. Olsson A, Kiwanuka O, Wilhelmsson S, Sandblom G, Stackelberg O. Cohort study of the effect of surgical repair of symptomatic diastasis recti abdominis on abdominal trunk function and quality of life. BJS Open. 2019;3(6):750–8.
14. Taylor DA, Merten SL, Sandercoe GD, Gahankari D, Ingram SB, Moncrieff NJ, Ho K, Sellars GD, Magnusson MR. Abdominoplasty improves low back pain and urinary incontinence. Plast Reconstr Surg. 2018;141(3):637–45.
15. Carruthers KH, Kocak E, Hulsen JH, McMahan JD. Improvement in stress urinary incontinence after abdominoplasty. Aesthet Surg J. 2014;34(7):1091–8.
16. Carrara A, Catarci M, Fabris L, Zuolo M, Pellecchia L, Moscatelli P, Dorna A, Motter M, Pertile R, Tirone G. Prospective observational study of abdominal wall reconstruction with THT technique in primary midline defects with diastasis recti: clinical and functional outcomes in 110 consecutive patients. Surg Endosc. 2021;35(9):5104–14.
17. Manetti G, Lolli MG, Belloni E, Nigri G. A new minimally invasive technique for the repair of diastasis recti: a pilot study. Surg Endosc. 2021;35(7):4028–34.
18. Olsson A, Kiwanuka O, Sandblom G, Stackelberg O. Evaluation of functional outcomes following rectus diastasis repair-an up-to-date literature review. Hernia. 2021;25(4):905–14.
19. Gordon H, Logue M. Perineal muscle function after childbirth. Lancet. 1985;2(8447):123–5.
20. Bush HM, Pagorek S, Kuperstein J, Guo J, Ballert KN, Crofford LJ. The Association of Chronic Back pain and stress urinary incontinence: a cross-sectional study. J Womens Health Phys Ther. 2013;37(1):11–8.

21. Madill SJ, McLean L. Relationship between abdominal and pelvic floor muscle activation and intravaginal pressure during pelvic floor muscle contractions in healthy continent women. Neurourol Urodyn. 2006;25(7):722–30.
22. Neumann P, Gill V. Pelvic floor and abdominal muscle interaction: EMG activity and intra-abdominal pressure. Int Urogynecol J Pelvic Floor Dysfunct. 2002;13(2):125–32.
23. Sapsford RR, Hodges PW. Contraction of the pelvic floor muscles during abdominal maneuvers. Arch Phys Med Rehabil. 2001;82(8):1081–8.
24. Smith MD, Coppieters MW, Hodges PW. Postural response of the pelvic floor and abdominal muscles in women with and without incontinence. Neurourol Urodyn. 2007;26(3):377–85.
25. Petros PE, Ulmsten UI. An integral theory and its method for the diagnosis and management of female urinary incontinence. Scand J Urol Nephrol Suppl. 1993;153:1–93.
26. Sapsford RR, Hodges PW. The effect of abdominal and pelvic floor muscle activation on urine flow in women. Int Urogynecol J. 2012;23(9):1225–30.
27. Ptaszkowski K, Paprocka-Borowicz M, Słupska L, Bartnicki J, Dymarek R, Rosińczuk J, Heimrath J, Dembowski J, Zdrojowy R. Assessment of bioelectrical activity of synergistic muscles during pelvic floor muscles activation in postmenopausal women with and without stress urinary incontinence: a preliminary observational study. Clin Interv Aging. 2015;10:1521–8.
28. Martinez Bustelo S, Ferri Morales A, Patiño Nuñez S, Viñas Diz S, Martinez RA. Entrevista clínica y valoración funcional del suelo pélvico. Fisioterapia. 2004;26(5):266–80.

Chapter 5
Diagnosis and Surgical Indications

Ezequiel M. Palmisano

5.1 Introduction

In recent years, diastasis of the rectus muscles has aroused the interest of surgeons, especially those dedicated to abdominal wall pathology [1, 2].

Diastasis of the rectus muscles has been the exclusive heritage of plastic surgery for a long time as part of the abdominoplasty technique.

The greater knowledge of the pathophysiology of diastasis of the rectus muscles, the understanding of the associated symptoms, the need to completely restore and reinforce the midline in the presence of a hernia [3], the advancement of mini-invasive techniques, the training of surgeons in laparoscopic surgery, the desire of patients to avoid large scars arrived with the development of different surgical alternatives that meet these objectives [4–6].

The therapeutic indications for diastasis of the rectus muscles were not immune to these changes, and for this we must consider multiple aspects, on the one hand the exclusively cosmetic indication, the presence of symptoms, and finally a combination of both, in short a correct indication based on an adequate evaluation (diagnosis).

5.2 Diagnosis

The diagnosis of diastasis of the rectus muscles is based on a thorough clinical history:

E. M. Palmisano (✉)
Italian University Institute of Rosario (IUNIR), Rosario, Argentina

S. Cuccomarino et al. (eds.), *New Concepts in Diastasi Recti Surgery*,
https://doi.org/10.1007/978-3-031-74947-6_5

Interrogation [7]	Symptoms
	Lower back pain (50–83.3%)
	Constipation (33.3–36%)
	Mild urinary incontinence (32.3–50%)
	Cosmetic (100%)

The physical examination requires a correct assessment in the standing and supine position, the latter, at rest and effort, with or without cervical flexion (Fig. 5.1):

Physical exam [8]	Findings
	Distended abdomen
	Abdominal sagging
	Diastasis of rectus muscles
	Midline hernias
	Lumbar hyperlordosis

These findings will be confirmed ultrasonographically, for which we have developed a protocol that we call dynamic and dedicated ultrasound intended for the functional assessment of diastasis of the rectus muscles. It is developed in two stages:

1. Stage I: assessment of the midline and rectus muscles, aimed at evaluating the function/containment of the rectus muscles. At this stage we classify diastasis of the rectus muscles and midline hernias (Fig. 5.2).
2. Stage II: assessment of broad muscles, where we evaluate the function of the deep system/activation of the transverse abdominis muscle. This stage allows for monitoring during pre- and postoperative rehabilitation (Fig. 5.3).

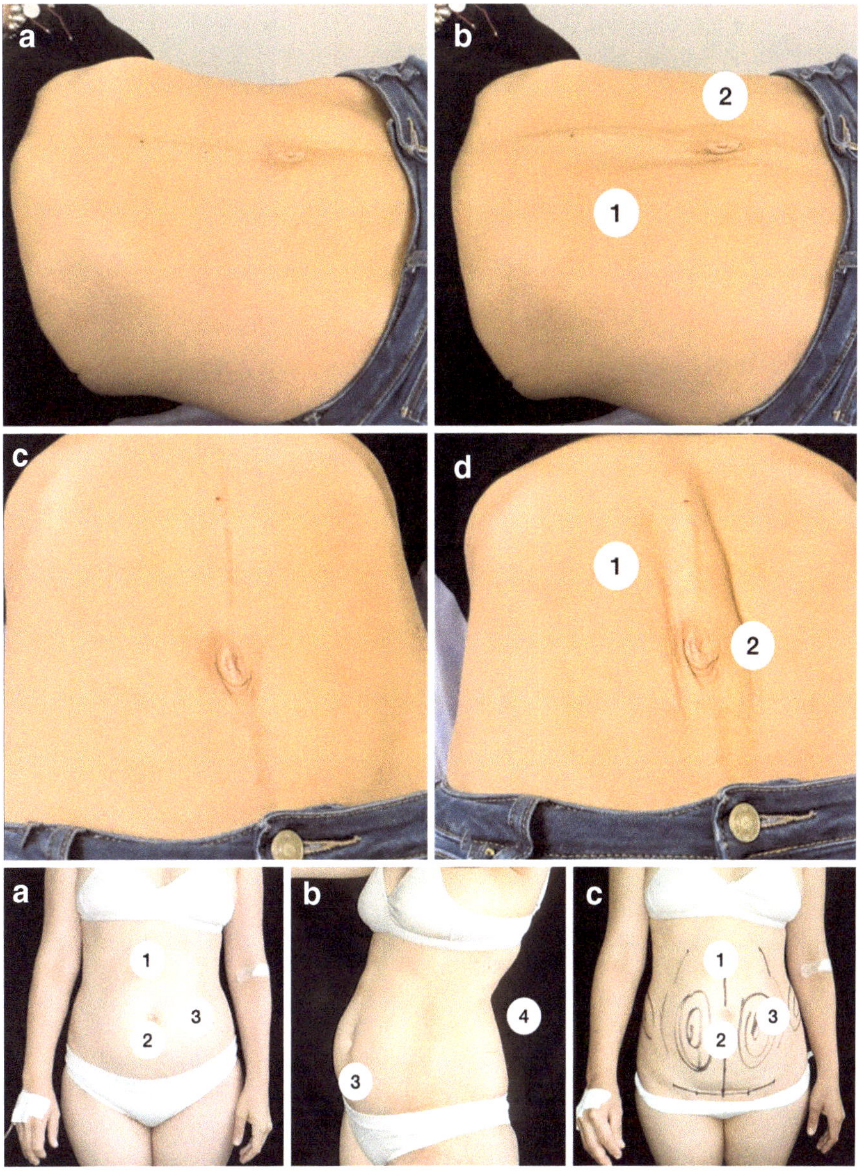

Fig. 5.1 (**a**) Dorsal recumbent right profile at rest. (**b**) Dorsal recubitus right profile with cervical flexion: (1) abdominal diastasis (M1-M5), (2) umbilical hernia (M3). (**c**) Dorsal recubitus front at rest. (**d**) Dorsal recubitus front with flexion cervical (1) abdominal diastasis (M1-M5), (2) umbilical hernia (M3). (**a**) Patient standing in front (1) abdominal diastasis (M1-M5), (2) umbilical hernia (M3), (3) abdominal flaccidity/localized lipodystrophy. (**b**) Patient standing leftprofile (3) abdominalflaccidity/localized lipodystrophy, (4) lumbar hyperlordosis. (**c**) Patient standing in front (1) abdominal diastasis (M1-M5), (2) umbilical hernia (M3), (3) abdominalflaccidity localized lipodystrophy

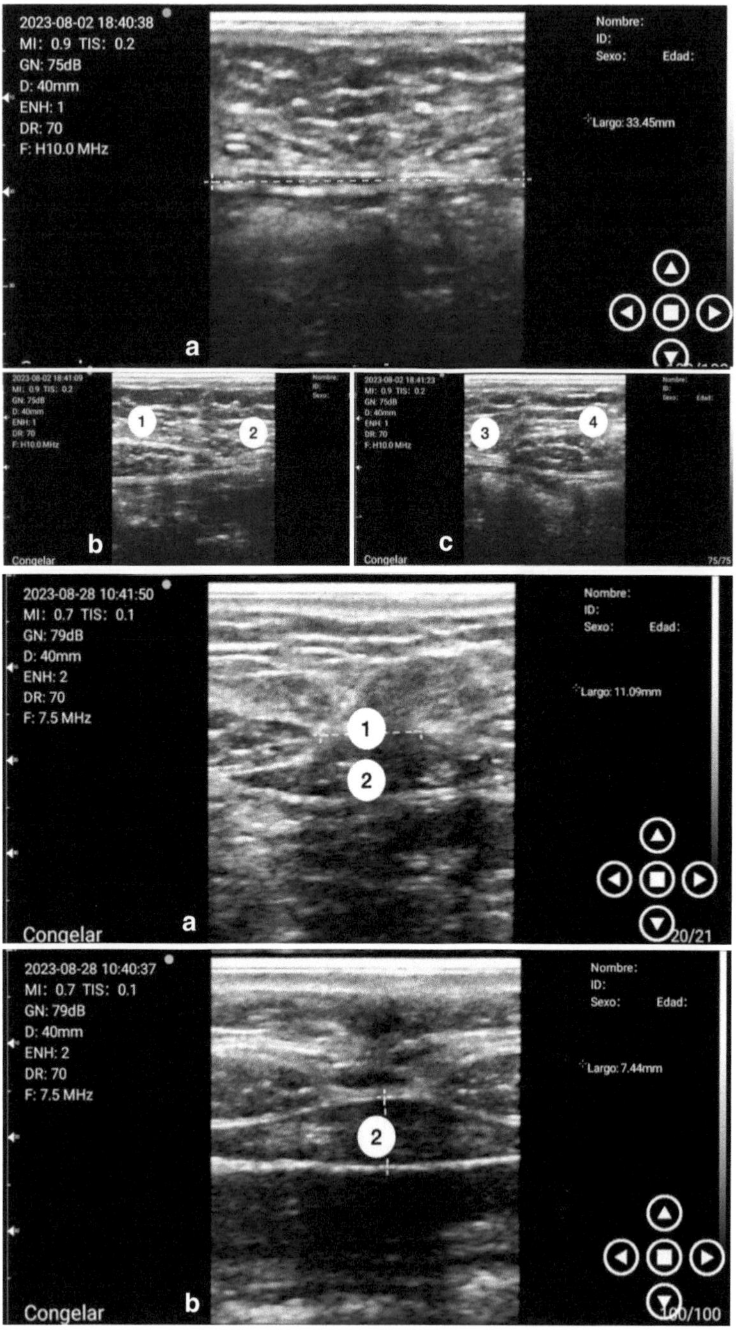

Fig. 5.2 (**a**) Dynamic and dedicated ultrasound. Stage I: Assessment of the midline and rectus muscles, (A) diastasis of the rectus muscles, (B) (1) medial edge of the right rectus muscle, (2) diastasis of the rectus muscles, (C) (3) diastasis of the rectus muscles, (4) medial edge of the left rectus muscle. (**b**) Dynamic and dedicated ultrasound. Stage I: Assessment of the midline and rectus muscles, (A) (1) umbilical hernia M3W1, (2) preperitoneal fat, (B) (2) preperitoneal fat

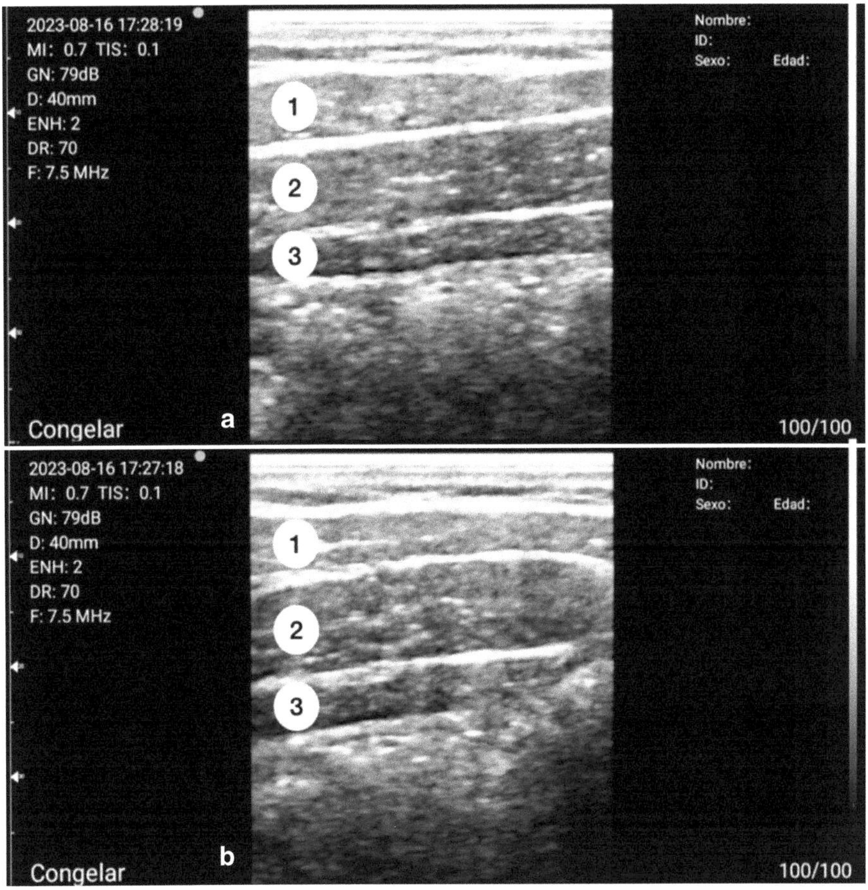

Fig. 5.3 Dynamic and dedicated ultrasound. Stage II: Assessment of broad muscles (**a**) without activation, (1) external oblique muscle, (2) internal oblique muscle, (3) transverse muscle. (**b**) With activation (1) external oblique muscle, (2) internal oblique muscle, (3) transverse muscle. Note the difference in muscle thickness, specifically of the transverse muscle

5.3 Classifications

In the next session, we will describe the different classifications that will be useful in your daily practice every time you explore an abdominal diastasis.

The German Hernia Society and the International Endohernia Society [9] have proposed a classification that divides them as follows

Diastasis recti classification	
Midline	M1 subxiphoidal
	M2 epigastric
	M3 umbilical
	M4 infraumbilical
	M5 suprapubic

Diastasis recti classification	
Width	W1 < 3 cm
	W2 3 < o = 5 cm
	W3 > 5 cm
Width (cm)	
Length (cm)	

Juarez Muas proposes defining a width with limits higher than the previous classification [10].

Width	Small (W1) < 3 cm
	Medium (W2) 3 < o = 5 cm
	Big (W3) 5 < o = 8 cm
	Giant (W3) > 8 cm

The vast majority are concentrated up to 5 cm (small/intermediate). This classification allows for the inclusion of larger diastasis recti muscles that, adequately prepared with botulinum toxin, could benefit from minimally invasive treatment [10].

The European Hernia Society [11] proposed classifying midline and lateral hernias as follows:

Hernia classification	
Midline	M1 subxiphoidal
	M2 epigastric
	M3 umbilical
	M4 infraumbilical
	M5 suprapubic
Lateral	L1 subcostal
	L2 flank
	L3 iliac
	L4 lumbar
Width	W1 < 4 cm
	W2 4 < o = 10 cm
	W3 > 10 cm
Width (cm)	
Length (cm)	
Recurrent (yes/no)	

Abdominal lipodystrophy was classified by Matarazzo into four categories [8]:

Category	Skin (laxity)	Fat	Muscle (flaccidity)
I	Minimal	Variable	Minimal
II	Mild	Variable	Mild (anterior)

Category	Skin (laxity)	Fat	Muscle (flaccidity)
III	Moderate	Variable	Moderate (anterior and superior)
IV	Severe	Variable	Severe (inferior and/or superior)

This classification has its correlation with the indication for treatment:

Category	Treatment
I	Lipectomy with suction
II	Minilipoabdominoplasty
III	Modified abdominoplasty
IV	Classic abdominoplasty with lipectomy and suction

5.4 Indications

After a correct diagnosis, the indications for the treatment of diastasis recti muscles are based on three perspectives: (1) clinical presentation, (2) cosmetic desire, and (3) both.

From the perspective of the general surgeon or with dedication to the pathology of the abdominal wall, the fundamental and priority objective consists of an anatomical and functional repair of the midline [12].

In general we could say that the indications for surgical correction of diastasis recti muscles are the following:

1. Patients with symptomatic midline hernias associated with diastasis of the rectus muscles > or = 2.5 cm. The evidence suggests repair in a single stage, since a higher incidence of recurrence has been demonstrated if the hernia defect is treated separately [3].
2. Patients with symptomatic rectus muscle diastasis > or = 2.5 cm associated with midline hernias (W1 < 4 cm).

Their treatments, as we said previously, have been evolving from the open to the mini-invasive approach; therefore this is also a factor to take into account in decision-making (Fig. 5.4):

1. Diastasis of the rectus muscles associated with abdominal flaccidity, with cosmetic desire regardless of scar and eventual neo-navel, open surgery
2. Diastasis of the rectus muscles associated with abdominal flaccidity, with cosmetic desire and without desire for a scar and eventual neo-navel, minimal approach surgery associated with liposuction and skin tightening systems
3. Diastasis of rectus muscles associated with abdominal flaccidity and without cosmetic desire (including scar and eventual neo-navel), minimal approach surgery
4. Diastasis of rectus muscles not associated with abdominal flaccidity, minimal approach surgery

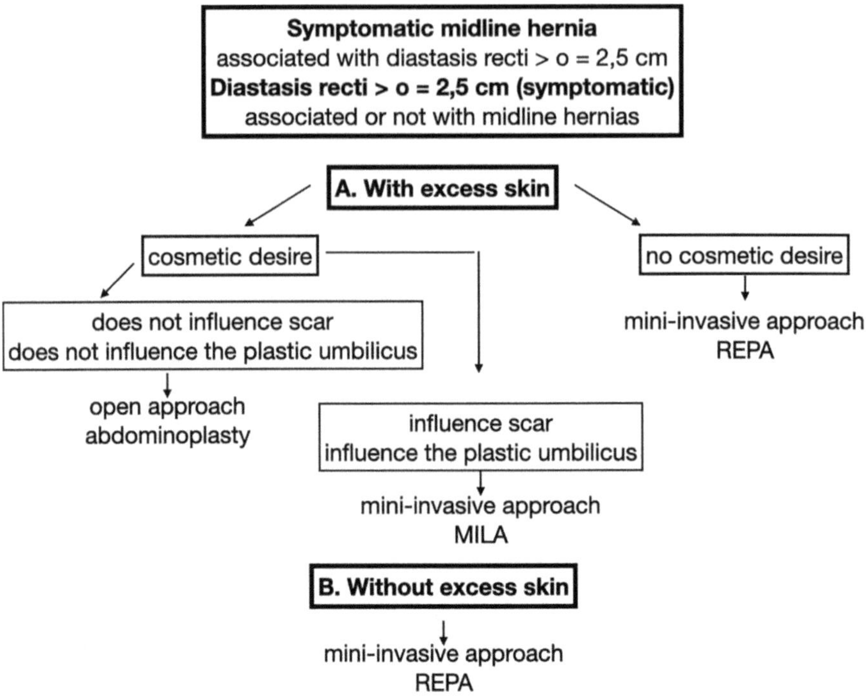

Fig. 5.4 Abdominal diastasis management algorithm. The examples used in this algorithm depend on the experience of each surgeon and may vary depending on the case

The ideal size recommended for repair by minimally invasive approaches is for diastasis of rectus muscles W1W2 with hernia defects up to W1; however, the feasibility of performing it in larger sizes of diastasis in patients previously prepared with botulinum toxin has been published in the literature.

Other factors taken into account when indicating surgical treatment are the following:

- Family planning [14]: the incidence of recurrence increases with pregnancy after hernia repair, so it is suggested to perform it after the last planned pregnancy.
- Distribution of body fat [15, 16]: obesity and high body mass index are considered risk factors for an abdominal wall hernia. However, body fat distribution appears to be a better indicator.
- Finally we must understand that this chapter has been intended for diagnosis and indications by the surgeon; however we strongly recommend joint evaluation with:
  - Kinesiology/physiotherapy
  - Nutritionist
  - Dedicated imaging specialist
  - Plastic surgery

References

1. Palmisano EM. Proposal for a single name in the endoscopic treatment of abdominal diastasis: a scientific need. Rev Hispanoam Hernia. 2023;11(1):1–3.
2. Malcher F, Lima DL, Lima RNCL, Cavazzola LT, Claus C, Dong CT, et al. Endoscopic onlay repair for ventral hernia and rectus abdominis diastasis repair: why so many different names for the same procedure? A qualitative systematic review. Surg Endosc. 2021;35(10):5414–21.
3. Cuccomarino S. Why an abdominal wall surgeon should opérate a diastasis recti? Rev Hispanoam Hernia. 2019;7(2):43–6.
4. Juárez Muas DM, Verasay GF, Garcia WM. Endoscopic prefascial repair of the recti diastasis description of new technique. Rev Hispanoam Hernia. 2017;5(2):47–51.
5. Claus CMP, Malcher F, Cavazzola LT, Furtado M, Morrell A, Azevedo M, et al. Subcutaneous onlay laparoscopic approach (SCOLA) for ventral hernia and rectus abdominis diastasis repair: technical description and initial results. Arq Bras Cir Dig. 2018;31(4):e1399.
6. Juárez Muas DM. Preaponeurotic endoscopic repair (REPA) of diastasis recti associated or not to midline hernias. Surg Endosc. 2019;33(6):1777–82.
7. Juárez Muas DM, Palmisano E, Pou Santoja G, Cuccomarino S, González Higuera G, Mayo P, Martínez Maya JD, Domínguez G, Ayala Acosta JC, Chichizola A. Reparación endoscópica preaponeurótica (REPA) como tratamiento de la diástasis de los músculos rectos asociada o no a hernias de la línea media. Estudio multicéntrico. Rev Hispanoam Hernia. 2019;7(2):59–65.
8. Palmisano EM, Di Biasio G. Minimally invasive management alternative for the treatment of patients with abdominal diastasis and dermo-fat flap using the VER tactic: Vaser® + endoscopy + Renuvion®. Rev Hispanoam Hernia. 2022;10(4):167–71.
9. Reinpold W, Köckerling F, Bittner R, Conze J, Fortelny R, Koch A, Kukleta J, Kuthe A, Lorenz R, Stechemesser B. Classification of rectus diastasis—a proposal by the German Hernia Society (DHG) and the International Endohernia Society (IEHS). Front Surg. 2019;6:1. https://doi.org/10.3389/fsurg.2019.00001.
10. Juárez Muas DM, Palmisano EM, Santonja GP, Paz OR. Adjuvant botulinum toxin for endoscopic management (preaponeurotic endoscopic repair) of severe diastasis recti. Int J Abdom Wall Hernia Surg. 2021;4:45–50.
11. Muysoms FE, Miserez M, Berrevoet F, et al. Classification of primary and incisional abdominal wall hernias. Hernia. 2009;13:407–14. https://doi.org/10.1007/s10029-009-0518-x.
12. Claus C, Palmisano EM. MILA (Minimally invasive lipoabdominoplasty) for diastasis recti. Are general surgeons and plastic surgeons fighting or playing together? Rev Argent Cir. 2023;115(4):393–5. https://revista.aac.org.ar/index.php/RevArgentCirug/article/view/637.
13. Gernot K, Ruzica-Rosalia L, Klaus E. Sutured repair of primary small umbilical and epigastric hernias: concomitant rectus diastasis is a significant risk factor for recurrence. World J Surg. 2015;39:121–6. https://doi.org/10.1007/s00268-014-2765-y.
14. Oma E, Henriksen NA, Jensen KK. Ventral hernia and pregnancy: a systematic review. Am J Surg. 2019;217(1):163–8. https://doi.org/10.1016/j.amjsurg.2018.04.016.
15. Xv Y, Tao Q, Cao N. The causal association between body fat distribution and risk of abdominal wall hernia: a two-sample Mendelian randomization study. Hernia. https://doi.org/10.1007/s10029-023-02954-1.
16. Baastrup NN, Jensen KK, Christensen JK, Jorgensen LN. Visceral obesity is a predictor of surgical site occurrence and hernia recurrence after open abdominal wall reconstruction. Hernia. 2022;26(1):149–55. https://doi.org/10.1007/s10029-021-02522-5. Epub 2021 Oct 29.

Chapter 6
Gender-Specific Differences in Etiology, Symptomatology, Indication, and Choice of Technique for Treating Rectus Diastasis Associated with Midline Hernias

Jan F. Kukleta

6.1 Introduction

For decades, the diagnosis of rectus diastasis (RD) was not worthy of professional discussion. There was no indication warranting surgical correction other than an aesthetic one. The most common cause of RD is physiological adaptation of the female abdominal wall during pregnancy. In more than 40% of these women, the widening linea alba fails to return to its pre-pregnancy condition leading to lasting changes in posture and further sequelae. Given the social changes, emerging population behavioral patterns, surgical advances in minimally invasive techniques, and the fact that men can be compromised by RD as well, the previously neglected issue of RD following pregnancy has graduated to a controversial abdominal wall repair topic.

The majority of scientific reports pertaining to RD cover the post-gestational form. Literature focusing on male RD is scarce and non-specific, as RD patients of both genders are grouped together as a homogenous group. Some of the following statements or comments are based on the author's personal experience exceeding three decades of minimal invasive hernia repair and abdominal wall reconstruction. Published data in the reference list are distinguished from the author's personal opinion (PO) and are marked accordingly.

The following important statements are worthy of reader attention:

Male RD and female RD share etiological differences. The indications for surgery differ. Surgical treatment for both sexes differs frequently. Therefore, the results of corrective techniques need to be evaluated separately [1, 2].

Patients with small midline primary or incisional hernias associated with RD have a higher recurrence rate if only the hernia is repaired [3].

J. F. Kukleta (✉)
Klinik Im Park, Hirslanden Group, Zurich, Switzerland

S. Cuccomarino et al. (eds.), *New Concepts in Diastasi Recti Surgery*,
https://doi.org/10.1007/978-3-031-74947-6_6

The degree to which patients with large RDs suffer from decreased abdominal core functionality differs among women and men. Lumbopelvic instability, chronic back pain, limited urinary continence, distorted perception of body image, and impaired quality of life may be the consequences of acquired muscular imbalance [4–7].

Linea alba reconstruction (LAR) with concomitant repair of midline hernias decreases the recurrence rate and improves abdominal core functionality [4, 8].

Various approaches to LAR have been published with different philosophies and variable results [9].

Functional improvements following linea alba reconstruction may have a long-lasting impact on quality of life [5, 8, 10–12].

It is time to analyze the existing data, to collect prospective data, and to follow the existing preliminary recommendations [13–15].

6.2 Rectus Diastasis: Update 2024. Finally, a Recognized Surgical Problem

In the last three decades, dramatic changes in understanding and treatment of abdominal wall defects have occurred, from repairing the defects to taking care of the entire abdominal core. It ranges from general surgery to visceral surgery to herniology and from parietology to abdominal core health care. The success of any of these treatment options should be judged not merely by the low recurrence rate but also by the improvement of (overall) quality of life.

The abdominal core is a functionally and anatomically complex entity. The muscles of the abdominal core and its connective tissue enable stability, tension, torso movements, respiration, and support for the gastrointestinal tract. The straight and oblique muscles, diaphragm, pelvic floor, erector spinae, multifidus, latissimus dorsi, gluteus, psoas, and other hip muscles all belong to the core. The transfer in muscle force hinges on the "quality" of connective tissue. The strength of the abdominal core may be limited by hereditary factors or may be weakened as a result of pregnancy, abdominal obesity, advanced age, or high BMI. Muscle weakness of the abdominal core contributes to abdominal wall laxity, deformation, and functional deficits. Thinning and widening of both the anterolateral muscles and the linea semilunaris can lead to body image impairment as well as a variety of facets pertaining to decreased quality of life (QoL). The complexity of the term QoL has been demonstrated in various existing scoring systems attempting to quantify the extent of disability and justify (indicate) the need for therapy.

Rectus diastasis affects both men and women but in different ways. The anatomical changes may appear quite similar; however, functional deficits vary considerably between the sexes. The impact of RD on QoL differs between the sexes [1, 16].

6.3 Etiology, Abdominal Core, Linea Alba, Collagen

6.3.1 Gender Differences

The hereditary etiology of RD can arise from differences in collagen composition and linea alba architecture. There are structural differences in the linea alba between men and women [1, 17, 18]. Inborn separation of the recti muscles was described by Nahas [19], and an autosomal dominant inheritance pattern was reported by Digilio et al. [17].

The acquired etiology of RD is most commonly a consequence of pregnancy, long-term increase in intra-abdominal pressure in individuals with visceral obesity, chronic obstructive pulmonary disease, or weight lifting or improper exercise. Gender differences can also play a role in symptoms of body image and core stability [1].

The importance of collagen properties was highlighted by Henriksen et al. [20]. Connective tissue consists of an extracellular matrix (ECM) and cells. Collagen is synthesized by fibroblasts and represents the main component of the ECM. The collagen turnover profile is altered in patients with inguinal and incisional hernias [20]. Among the 28 distinct collagen types, types I and III are the most important [20, 21]. The collagen ratio between the two types correlates with the strength of the connective tissue. Low levels of both types were demonstrated in women with rectus diastasis [22]. The three different zones of the linea alba exhibited different fiber orientations. In the female infra-umbilical region, there are more transverse fibers than oblique fibers, and these fibers are less thick, resulting in an increased width of the infra-umbilical linea alba [21].

There is abundant evidence of sex-specific differences in the amount, composition, turnover, and metabolism of collagen parallel to the sex-biased mRNA and miRNA expression in abdominal and gluteal adipose tissues. Karastergiou et al. explained the classical difference between "apples and pears" concerning fat distribution in both sexes [23].

Collagen disorders were demonstrated in abdominal aortic aneurysms (AAAs), and there were distinct differences in the course of the disease between males and females. A fourfold increase in rectus diastasis was observed in males with AAA compared to patients with occlusive disease [24]. The different amounts and compositions of collagen in men and women are highly important for understanding the degenerative process [25].

A recent paper by Ugurlu et al. reported a significantly greater incidence of RD in patients with inguinal hernia (46.9% vs. 21.6%, $p < 0.001$). This finding supports the hypothesis that RD and inguinal and umbilical hernias have a common denominator – a systemic defect in collagen metabolism [26]. These results are difficult to interpret due to the unequal number of men and females in the inguinal hernia group.

There are additional unresolved suspicions of sex distinctions ranging from molecular reactions to human behavior patterns. Howard et al. reported sex disparities in the treatment and outcomes of ventral and incisional hernia repair. Women are more likely to experience adverse events after surgery [27]. Schlosser et al. stated in his "Outcomes specific to patient sex after open ventral hernia repair" that female patients experience worse outcomes after open ventral hernia repair [28].

In a systematic review and meta-analysis, Oliveira et al. described the impact of sex on ventral hernia repair outcomes. Female sex is associated with a higher risk of postoperative chronic pain following ventral hernia repair. Postoperative chronic pain was significantly greater in females (OR 1.9; 95% CI 1.64–2.2; $p < 0.001$) [29].

Grossi et al. [30] reported that, in a cadaver study, the amount of collagen fibers in the linea alba was lower in morbidly obese individuals than in nonobese individuals. The amount of collagen fibers becomes significantly smaller in older individuals. A decrease in collagen content with age may cause general distension of the muscle and weakening of the abdominal wall [31]. This may explain the difference in the "apple shape" of the abdomen in male because men with RD and small midline hernias consulted doctors two decades later than women with RD.

The anatomy and function of the abdominal core may differ between sexes. There is a sex difference in the thickness of the lateral abdominal wall in asymptomatic adults [32].

Interesting data on differences in abdominal muscle activation in hypopressive exercises between women and men were published by Da Cuña-Carrera et al. [33]. These exercises were developed for women with pelvic floor or abdominal dysfunctions. This approach seems to be useful for men with urinary incontinence after prostatectomy.

The abdominal wall is anisotropic. Anisotropy ratios of 8–9 have been reported for the human linea alba. The biomaterials used for repair only reached a ratio of 1–3. Mismatches between the properties of implants (suture, meshes, fixation devices) and the host tissue are the most likely causes of failure [34]. As the linea alba, rectus sheath, and other tissues of the abdominal wall exhibit different characteristics, the location of implantation and mesh orientation are important.

The anisotropy of the human linea alba was analyzed in the study of Grässel et al. Compliance in the transverse direction was significantly lower in women than in men. Sex-dependent differences were demonstrated, reflecting the distribution of fiber orientation in the linea alba [35]. Astruc et al. confirmed the variability in the mechanical properties of linea alba according to sex and location [36].

The puzzle pieces of growing knowledge about RD and the abdominal core presented in this paragraph support gender-specific differences. This should translate into decision-making about the indication, type of therapy, and most appropriate technique for repair. A better understanding of sex-related outcomes should result in tailoring of the operative approach and improved guidance regarding postoperative outcomes [29]. Howard et al. described sex as a biological variable in hernia research and demonstrated different results when men and women were analyzed separately [2].

6.4 Prevalence of RD

The presence of diastasis recti abdominis during pregnancy and 12 months after childbirth was examined in 300 Scandinavian primiparas. Sperstad et al. reported RD prevalence rates of 33.1%, 60.0%, 45.4%, and 32.6% at gestation week 21, 6 weeks, 6 months, and 12 months after delivery, respectively [37].

The overall prevalence of RD in males is not well documented. Ninety-four out of 1691 (5.5%) RD patients in the review by Mommers et al. were males [18]. Jessen et al. found 224 men (9.8%) with RD among 2291 patients in a review of 47 studies [38].

6.5 Classifications

Despite several existing classifications, the definition of rectus diastasis is still under debate. The inter-recti distance (IRD), a cutoff for the diagnosis of RD, varies between 20 and 34 mm depending on the source of information [14, 15, 19, 39–41], location, patient size, BMI, and ethnicity [42]. This represents the first of many other obstacles in the evaluation of pathophysiology, symptomatology, indication for therapy, results, and final patient satisfaction.

The Ranney classification (1990) is based on measurements of 1700 postpartum women [43]. The Rath classification (1996) was built on a cadaver study of both sexes, with a focus on the level of weakness relative to the umbilicus and age [39]. The Nahas aesthetic classification (2001) recognizes four types of body appearance based on deformation of the abdominal wall [19], and the Beer classification (2009) is based on the normal width of nulliparous women [41].

Kaufmann et al. defined individuals with a normal IRD up to 34 mm analyzing men and women aged >20–90 years as one group. The 34 mm width corresponds to the age of 75 years [40]. Qu et al. reported that the mean IRD of nulliparous Chinese women 3 cm above the umbilicus was 6.20 ± 5.58 m, with a mean BMI of 21.97 ± 3.86 kg/m^2 [42].

Obviously, these studies demonstrate the variability between sexes and ethnicities. More differentiated data need to be collected and evaluated to enable any future conclusions [13, 14].

A proposal for a classification of RD by the German Hernia Society and International Endohernia Society (2019) used several elements of the Ranney classification and the EHS incisional hernia classification, adding sex, concomitant hernias of the midline, previous abdominal surgery, number of pregnancies and multiple births, spontaneous birth or caesarian section, skin condition, diagnostic procedures, preoperative pain rate, and pain localization as the data that should be recorded [14].

The latest tentative guidelines for the management of rectus diastasis were established by the European Hernia Society in 2021. The low or very low quality of evidence and nearly missing recommendations demonstrate how little we know about a frequently impaired health condition [15].

6.6 Effects of Pregnancy

Pregnancy impacts the whole abdominal core, not only the linea alba. Hormonal changes with increased levels of progesterone and relaxin decrease the tensile strength of the rectus fascia and increase the laxity of the linea alba to facilitate progressive stretching of the abdominal wall [44]. Stretched and displaced muscles lead to weakness, and accentuated lumbar lordosis compensates for the shift in the center of gravity, resulting in low back pain [7, 45, 46]. A distended pelvic floor may cause postpartum deficits in urinary continence and prolapse in later years [7, 47]. Striae, excessive skin folds, abdominal bulging, torso movement limitations, and still looking like pregnant may develop into psychological and social burdens with low body image and impairment of interpersonal relationships [16, 45, 48].

The severity of postpartum symptoms and deterioration in QoL are logical indications for active repair based on the restoration of abdominal core functionality.

6.7 Treatment

6.7.1 Non-surgical Therapy for RD

Jessen et al. summarize the treatment options for RD. The published non-surgical therapies aim to reinforce abdominal wall muscles through prenatal and postnatal exercises, physiotherapist-guided training, specific exercises for the pelvic floor, postural and back care education, and mechanical support with corsets or bandages. In their own words, "the success rate is questionable and not possible to state, as no identified studies report on the long-term effects of physiotherapy" [38].

According to Benjamin et al., in a systematic review of the effect of physiotherapy, recommending physiotherapy in general or in a specific exercise routine is not possible due to the low level of evidence in existing studies [49].

An RCT by Gluppe et al. [50] revealed no effect of postpartum training on RD. An RCT by Emanuelsson et al. [8] compared an intensive physiotherapy group with a surgical treatment group. All participants in the training group opted for surgery due to unsatisfactory results. Another systematic review by Gluppe et al. [51] revealed very low-quality scientific evidence for recommending specific exercise programs to treat postpartum RD.

However, the study of Thabet [52] suggested that a deep core stability program and abdominal binder led to a significant decrease of inter-recti distance and improved QoL.

6.7.2 Surgical Therapy for RD

Both open and endoscope-assisted or endoscopic techniques have yielded good results. The published recurrence rates are close to 0%, and the morbidity rate is low.

The most popular open technique is classical abdominoplasty. Plication can be performed with or without mesh reinforcement [12, 53]. Meshes are more often used for midline hernias associated with RD. There are different plication techniques including single-layer or double-layer methods, interrupted or running suturing, and absorbable or non-absorbable suture material.

In RCTs comparing different suture and suture techniques, none were found to be better than the other [8, 54].

The material used for laparoscope-assisted, laparoscopic, or endoscopic-extraperitoneal RD repairs is similar. There was a low recurrence rate and low morbidity. There is no consensus on the appropriate approach, mesh position (supra-aponeurotic onlay, retromuscular or preperitoneal sublay, underlay), mesh or suture absorbability, or seroma prevention. The preferred choice of technique depends on patient characteristics (sex, RD width, symptoms, age, BMI, skin excess, soft tissue condition), surgeon skills and experience, and realistic expectations.

The driving force of indication for surgical treatment is the achievable improvement in QoL.

6.7.3 Surgical Treatment Outcomes

Symptomatic postpartum diastasis recti are better suited for minimally invasive correction than male RD [11, 55].

Improving posture while reducing the mean lumbosacral angle ($p < 0.001$) was demonstrated 6 months after repair by Temel [56].

Dumanian [57] significantly improved chronic back pain and urinary incontinence in postpartum women following abdominoplasty. Taylor et al. [58] reported that abdominoplasty improved low back pain and urinary incontinence.

Olsson, Carrara, Taylor, Cuccomarino, and Manetti [5, 7, 11, 58, 59] evaluated urinary incontinence. Significant improvements in incontinence severity after 6–8 months were reported. The results remain consistent even after 3 years [5].

Significant improvement in lower back pain (LBP) after surgery was documented by Bellido Luque, Carrara, Manetti, and Taylor [5, 7, 58–60]. However, a systematic review by Gbolabo Sokunbi [61] could not confirm the association between LBP pain and RD. The most positive correlation between LBP and RD was found in studies with a high number of patients (664, 400, 866 vs. 33, 40, 72).

Poorer outcomes were reported in men. A high recurrence rate in severe male diastasis was communicated by Bellido Luque [62]. Similarly, Signorini et al. [63]

reported that seromas were significantly more common in males (55.2%) than in females (24%) ($p = 0.002$).

6.7.4 The Next Steps to Be Implemented

There is an urgent need to standardize the data necessary to measure the quality of outcomes [6, 13]. The sex differences mandate a separate analysis of the techniques used and results achieved respecting the true patient need as a basis for decision-making for indication for any kind of intervention.

Patient-reported outcome measures (PROMs) seem to be good instruments for validating outcomes. The functional and psychological benefits of abdominoplasty and body-contouring procedures for bariatric patients after massive weight loss are well recognized. The BODY-Q by Klassen et al. is recommended as the most appropriate tool for bariatric/body-contouring surgery (PROM) [63]. However, such PROMs in postpartum women seeking abdominoplasty are still missing [63, 64].

References

1. Nienhuijs SW, et al. The male rectus diastasis: a different concept? Hernia. 2021;25:951–6.
2. Howard R, Telem D. Gender matters: mandating sex as a biologic variable in hernia research. Ann Surg. 2019;270(1):10–1.
3. Kohler G, Luketina RS, Emmanuel K. Sutured repair of primary small umbilical and epigastric hernias: concomitant rectus diastasis is a significant risk factor for recurrence. World J Surg. 2015;39:121–6.
4. Olsson A, et al. Cohort study of the effect of surgical repair of symptomatic diastasis recti abdominis on abdominal trunk function and quality of life. BJS Open. 2019;3:750–8.
5. Olsson A, Kiwanuka O, Wilhelmsson S, Sandblom G, Stackelberg O. Surgical repair of diastasis recti abdominis provides long-term improvement of abdominal core function and quality of life: a 3-year follow-up. BJS Open. 2021;5(5):zrab085.
6. Olsson A, Kiwanuka O, Sandblom G, Stackelberg O. Evaluation of functional outcomes following rectus diastasis repair-an up-to-date literature review. Hernia. 2021;25(4):905–14.
7. Carrara A, et al. Prospective observational study of abdominal wall reconstruction with THT technique in primary midline defects with diastasis recti: clinical and functional outcomes in 110 consecutive patients. Surg Endosc. 2021;35:5104–14.
8. Emanuelsson P, et al. Operative correction of abdominal rectus diastasis (ARD) reduces pain and improves abdominal wall muscle strength: a randomized, prospective trial comparing retromuscular mesh repair to double-row, self-retaining sutures. Surgery. 2016;160:1367–75.
9. ElHawary H, Abdelhamid K, Meng F, Janis JE. A comprehensive, evidence-based literature review of the surgical treatment of rectus diastasis. Plast Reconstr Surg. 2020;146(5):1151–64.
10. Swedenhammar E, Strigård K, Emanuelsson P, Gunnarsson U, Stark B. Long-term follow-up after surgical repair of abdominal rectus diastasis: a prospective randomized study. Scand J Surg. 2020;110(3):283–9.
11. Cuccomarino S, Bonomo LD, Aprà F, et al. Preaponeurotic endoscopic repair (REPA) of diastasis recti: a single surgeon's experience. Surg Endosc. 2022;36:1302–9.

12. Nervil GG, et al. Simple plication alleviates physical symptoms in patients with post-gestational rectus diastasis. Hernia. 2023;27:957–68.
13. Köckerling F, Lorenz R, Stechemesser B, Conze J, Kuthe A, Reinpold W, Niebuhr H, Lammers B, Zarras K, Fortelny R, Mayer F, Hoffmann H, Kukleta JF, Weyhe D. Comparison of outcomes in rectus abdominis diastasis repair - which data do we need in a hernia registry? Hernia. 2021;25:891–903.
14. Reinpold W, Köckerling BR, Conze J, Fortelny R, Koch A, Kukleta JF, Kuthe A, Lorenz R, Stechemesser B. Classification of rectus diastasis—a proposal by the German Hernia Society (DHG) and the International Endohernia Society (IEHS). Front Surg. 2019;6:1.
15. Hernández-Granados P, et al. European Hernia Society guidelines on management of rectus diastasis. Br J Surg. 2021;108(10):1189–91.
16. Smith OA, et al. Health related quality of life in abdominal wall hernia: let's ask patients what matters to them? Hernia. 2022;26:795–808.
17. Digilio MC, Capolino R, Dallapiccola B. Autosomal dominant transmission of nonsyndromic diastasis recti and weakness of the linea alba. Am J Med Genet A. 2008;146(2):254–6.
18. Mommers EHH, Ponten JEH, Al Omar AK, de Vries Reilingh TS, Bouvy ND, Nienhuijs SW. The general surgeon's perspective of rectus diastasis. A systematic review of treatment options. Surg Endosc. 2017;31(12):4934–49.
19. Nahas FX. An aesthetic classification of the abdomen based on the myoaponeurotic layer. Plast Reconstr Surg. 2001;108(6):1787–95.
20. Henriksen NA, et al. The collagen turnover profile is altered in patients with inguinal and incisional hernia. Surgery. 2015;157:312–21.
21. Axer H, et al. Collagen fibers in linea alba and rectus sheaths. General scheme and morphological aspects. J Surg Res. 2001;96(1):127–34.
22. Blotta RM, et al. Collagen I and III in women with diastasis recti. Clinics. 2018;7(73):e319.
23. Karastergiou A, et al. Sex differences in human adipose tissues – the biology of pear shape. Biol Sex Differ. 2012;3:13.
24. McPhail I. Abdominal aortic aneurysm and diastasis recti. Angiology. 2009;59(6):736–9.
25. Villard C. The composition of collagen in the aneurysm wall of men and women. J Vasc Surg. 2017;66:579–85.
26. Ugurlu C. Prevalence of rectus diastasis is higher in patients with inguinal hernia. Hernia. 2023;27:943–56.
27. Howard R, et al. Sex disparities in the treatment and outcomes of ventral and incisional hernia repair. Surg Endosc. 2023;37:3061–8.
28. Schlosser KA, et al. Outcomes specific to patient sex after open ventral hernia repair. Surgery. 2020;167(3):614–9.
29. Eduarda SC. Oliveira impact of sex on ventral hernia repair outcomes: a systematic review and meta-analysis. Am J Surg. 2023;226:385–92.
30. Grossi JV, et al. Linea alba collagen assessment in morbidly obese patients. Arq Bras Cir Dig. 2016;29(1):8–11.
31. Calvi ENC. Collagen fibers in the rectus abdominis muscle of cadavers of different age. Hernia. 2014;18:527–33.
32. Rho M, et al. Gender differences on ultrasound imaging of lateral abdominal muscle thickness in asymptomatic adults: a pilot study. PM R. 2013;5(5):374–80.
33. Da Cuña-Carrera I, et al. Are there any differences in abdominal activation between women and men during hypopressive exercises? Int J Environ Res Public Health. 2021;18:6984.
34. Deeken CR, et al. Mechanical properties of the abdominal wall and biomaterials utilized for hernia repair. J Mech Behav Biomed Mater. 2017;74:411–27.
35. Grässel D, et al. Anisotropy of human linea alba: a biomechanical study. J Surg Res. 2005;124(1):118–25.
36. Astruc L, et al. Characterization of the anisotropic mechanical behavior of human abdominal wall connective tissues. J Mech Behav Biomed Mater. 2018;82:45–50.

37. Sperstad JB, et al. Diastasis recti abdominis during pregnancy and 12 months after childbirth: prevalence, risk factors and report of lumbopelvic pain. Br J Sports Med. 2016;50:1092–6.
38. Jessen ML, Öberg S, Rosenberg J. Surgical techniques for repair of abdominal rectus diastasis: a scoping review. J Plast Surg Hand Surg. 2021;55(4):195–201.
39. Rath AM, Attali P, Dumas JL, Goldlust D, Zhang J, Chevrel JP. The abdominal linea alba: an anatomo-radiologic and biomechanical study. Surg Radiol Anat. 1996;18(4):281–8.
40. Kaufmann RL, et al. Normal width of the linea alba, prevalence, and risk factors for diastasis recti abdominis in adults, a cross sectional study. Hernia. 2022;26(2):609–18.
41. Beer GM, et al. The normal width of the linea alba in nulliparous women. Clin Anat. 2009;22:706–11.
42. Qu E, et al. The ultrasound diagnostic criteria for diastasis recti and its correlation with pelvic floor dysfunction in early postpartum women. Quant Imaging Med Surg. 2021;11:706–13.
43. Ranney B. Diastasis recti and umbilical hernia causes, recognition and repair. S D J Med. 1990;43:5–8.
44. Samuel CS, et al. The effect of relaxin on collagen metabolism in the nonpregnant rat pubic symphysis: the influence of estrogen and progesterone in regulating relaxin activity. Endocrinology. 1996;137(9):3884–90.
45. Mughal M, Ross D. Management of the post pregnancy abdomen: the plastic surgical perspective. Hernia. 2021;25:929–38.
46. Doubkova L, et al. Diastasis of rectus abdominis muscles in low back pain patients. J Back Musculoskelet Rehabil. 2018;6:107–12.
47. Joueidi Y, et al. Impact of the diastasis of the rectus abdominis muscles on the pelvic-perineal symptoms: review of the literature. Prog Urol. 2019;29:544–59.
48. Hills NF, et al. Comparison of trunk muscle function between women with and without diastasis recti abdominis at 1 year postpartum. Phys Ther. 2018;1:891–901.
49. Benjamin DR, et al. Effects of exercise on diastasis of the rectus abdominis muscle in the antenatal and postnatal periods: a systematic review. Physiotherapy. 2014;100:1–8.
50. Gluppe SL, et al. Effect of a postpartum training program on the prevalence of diastasis recti abdominis in postpartum primiparous women: a randomized controlled trial. Phys Ther. 2018;98:260–8.
51. Gluppe SL, et al. What is the evidence for abdominal and pelvic floor muscle training to treat diastasis recti abdominis postpartum? A systematic review with meta-analysis. Braz J Phys Ther. 2021;25:664675.
52. Thabet AA. Efficacy of deep core stability exercise program in postpartum women with diastasis recti abdominis: randomized controlled trial. J Musculoskelet Neuronal Interact. 2019;19(1):62–8.
53. Cheesborough JE, Dumanian GA. Simultaneous prosthetic mesh abdominal wall reconstruction with abdominoplasty for ventral hernia and severe rectus diastasis repairs. Plast Reconstr Surg. 2015;135:268–76.
54. Emanuelsson P, et al. Early complications, pain, and quality of life after reconstructive surgery for abdominal rectus muscle diastasis: a 3-month follow-up. J Plast Reconstr Aesthet Surg. 2014;67:1082–8.
55. Juarez Muas DM. Preaponeurotic endoscopic repair (REPA) of diastasis recti associated or not to midline hernias. Surg Endosc. 2018;33:1777–82.
56. Temel M, Türkmen A, Berberoğlu Ö. Improvements in vertebral-column angles and psychological metrics after abdominoplasty with rectus plication. Aesthet Surg J. 2016;36:577–87.
57. Dumanian GA. Mesh abdominoplasty for rectus diastasis in women and men. Hernia. 2021;25:863–70.
58. Taylor DA, et al. Abdominoplasty improves lower back pain and urinary incontinence. Plast Reconstr Surg. 2018;141(3):637–45.
59. Manetti G, Lolli MG, Belloni E, Nigri G. A new minimally invasive technique for the repair of diastasis recti: a pilot study. Surg Endosc. 2021;35(7):4028–34.

60. Bellido LJ. Totally endoscopic surgery on diastasis recti associated with midline hernias. The advantages of a minimally invasive approach. Prospective cohort study. Hernia. 2015;19:493–501.
61. Gbolabo Sokunbi. Is diastasis recti abdominis associated with low back pain? World Neurosurg. 2023;2023(174):119–25.
62. Bellido Luque J, et al. Severe rectus diastasis with midline hernia associated in males: high recurrence in mid-term follow-up of minimally invasive surgical technique. Hernia. 2023;27:335–45.
63. Klassen AF, et al. The BODY-Q: a patient-reported outcome instrument for weight loss and body contouring treatments. Plast Reconstr Surg Glob Open. 2016;13(4):e679.
64. Edmondson SJ, Ross DA. The postpartum abdomen: psychology, surgery and quality of life. Hernia. 2021;25:939–50.

Chapter 7
Preparing the Patient for Surgery

Derlin M. Juárez Muas

Abdominal wall repair in patients with diastasis of the abdominal muscles (DRA) associated or not with midline hernias and in those patients who wish to improve the image of the body contour can be integrated with dermolipectomy or liposuction. In all situations it is an elective surgical intervention, which allows patients to enter a prehabilitation program and to implement multimodal and multidisciplinary measures from the diagnosis of a surgical pathology to the moment of surgery. Through this program we can carry out a personalized study of each case and analyze various factors that influence the outcome such as age, corrected comorbidities, albumin level, toxic habits, family planning, state of muscle mass, and preparation of the abdominal wall and pelvic floor to obtain maximum benefit for patients and arrive at surgery in the best conditions [1]. The aggression caused by a surgical act triggers an inflammatory response due to the activation of the immune system through the release of neuroendocrine hormones and the stimulation of the hypothalamic-sympathetic system, with the release of catecholamines and cortisol. This determines the onset of an initial phase of peripheral insulin resistance and increased protein catabolism [2–4].

The biological response of the organism will depend on the physiological reserve of the patients, which will depend on the multiple factors mentioned above [3]. Furthermore, the extent of the inflammatory response is proportional to the degree of surgical aggressiveness; therefore the size of the wound, tissue dissection, flaps, organ manipulation, energy consumption, etc. influence. The greater the aggression, the greater the metabolic response triggered [2, 4].

D. M. Juárez Muas (✉)
Argentine Hernia Association of Surgery, Salta, Argentina

Argentine Hernia Association, Salta, Argentina

Hispano-American hernia Society, Salta, Argentina

Public Maternal-Child Hospital, Salta, Argentina

National University of Tucumán, Tucumán, Argentine

S. Cuccomarino et al. (eds.), *New Concepts in Diastasi Recti Surgery*,
https://doi.org/10.1007/978-3-031-74947-6_7

Correct preoperative planning and preparation of patients is one of the key points to optimize the outcome of surgery, allow adequate recovery in the shortest possible time, correct and adapt pre-existing medications, and reduce the risk of postoperative complications in the surgical field short and long term, with shorter hospitalization times [1–8].

Preoperative patient management should begin between 30 and 60 days before surgery [4, 9]. It is not advisable to plan the surgery hastily, without taking all the necessary precautions.

It is essential that the patient clarifies all doubts before the procedure, especially if he has no experience with previous surgeries. This increases trust in the surgeon and the operating team, reduces preoperative stress, and is important for an adequate doctor-patient relationship.

There are several important factors that patients must take into account before surgery: it is necessary to plan the time necessary for hospitalization and rest in the postoperative period, so as not to return to usual activities before the time necessary for proper healing and recovery. You will not be able to do physical exertion or lift heavy objects in the first few days after surgery (including your child, if you have recently become a mother). Furthermore, it must be kept in mind that DRA repair with minimally invasive or conventional means is a surgical procedure that requires patient assistance from a family member or trained personnel, to facilitate recovery at least for the first week and not constitute an unpleasant experience.

The recommended position for rest during the first days of the operation is the elevated position of the headboard and the hips flexed to ensure relaxation of the abdominal wall and adequate rest. Therefore, it is important to adapt your bed or use articulated chairs or beds to facilitate the postoperative period.

7.1 Physical Activity Assessment

The habit of performing physical exercises regularly on the part of patients is of great importance, which will allow them to arrive at surgery in good health, with an improvement in cardiopulmonary capacity, reduction in blood pressure, increase in muscle mass and reduced stress and anxiety levels. In addition, it helps to reduce peripheral insulin resistance and promotes a lower inflammatory response to trauma [2, 10], leading patients to better cope with the postoperative period and will facilitate their return to usual activities in the shortest possible time and will help to maintain the body figure.

A program of simple exercises, such as walking 30 min a day and breathing exercises, demonstrated high adherence, with a significant improvement in the 6-min walk test (6WT) [2, 11], which favors strengthening of the respiratory muscles in a short period of time, and is recommended in patients with concomitant lung pathology or a very poor initial physical condition [2, 12, 13].

Cardiorespiratory stress testing (ergospirometry) provides an in-depth evaluation of the patient's cardiopulmonary function and gas exchange [13, 14].

Abdominopelvic physiotherapy is used with curative intent in patients with small (W1), primary DRA, without associated hernia, and with medium (W2) or larger DRA who refuse surgical treatment. It can be framed as conservative management or as a fundamental pillar in the preoperative management of DRA and allows the correct preparation of the abdominal wall (anterior and posterior) and the pelvic floor. It is performed by trained physical therapists and kinesiologists to achieve abdominal core strengthening with the use of isometric abdominal exercises, which have been shown to improve the length of the DRA; hypopressive exercises [15] that specifically strengthen the transverse and pelvic floor muscles; and exercises for Kegel incontinence [15], as the association of DRA with stress urinary incontinence is common. This situation often motivates a consultation with the urologist before the abdominal wall surgeon. A kinesic treatment modality is neuromuscular electrostimulation, which consists in applying electric current to one or more muscles to excite them and obtain their contraction, allowing the re-education of the abdominal wall, pelvic floor, and skin, obtaining muscle strengthening and rehabilitation of the abdominal wall, many times, with an excellent anatomical, functional, and aesthetic result. Another gesture performed by kinesiologists is manual lymphatic drainage, a functional dermatological treatment, which improves superficial lymphatic and vascular microcirculation and provides a lower sensation of swelling and skin sensitivity with greater well-being for patients by providing better healing and a reduction in the incidence of seromas in the postoperative period [9, 16].

7.2 Nutritional Assessment

The nutritional component is an important factor. A good nutritional plan with a healthy and balanced diet is essential for a successful surgery. Consultation with specialists is essential to execute an appropriate nutritional plan for each patient, since malnutrition increases the incidence of intraoperative and postoperative complications and infection of the surgical wound [2, 17–19]. A nutritional assessment of body composition is used through different tests to identify patients with nutritional risk and as a parameter with predictive value for morbidity and mortality [2, 20–22]. At the other extreme, it is overweight and obese. It is well established that BMI greater than 30 is directly related to adverse postoperative outcomes. Patients' weight loss for elective surgeries can positively influence the postoperative period. Several studies have shown that a low-calorie, low-fat diet for 1 week was associated with a decrease in hepatic steatosis and a concomitant decrease in intra- and postoperative hemorrhage. It is common to see overweight women in consultation as a consequence of pregnancy, often with a dermofat flap who seek surgery for a quick solution to recover their pre-pregnancy body shape. In these cases, it is essential to encourage weight loss, change eating habits, adjust the diet in terms of calories and protein balance, and supplement with a complex of vitamins A, E, and C and minerals. However, the use of nutritional supplements in normonourished patients does not seem to present a significant difference [2, 23, 24], so its standardization within prehabilitation programs still requires more evidence. It is advisable to avoid the consumption of coffee and alcohol in the days before surgery, which would promote high blood pressure and bleeding during the intervention and postoperatively.

7.3 Skin Preparation

Another important factor is the preparation of the skin with adequate hydration using moisturizing creams with a high content of vitamin A and E. In addition, we indicate a complex of vitamins A, E, and C orally 30 days prior to the intervention and continue for 30 days postoperative, which would produce better microvascular and lymphatic circulation of the abdominal wall, which would favor lymphatic drainage and reduce postoperative edema and seroma, causing a benefit for better healing.

Vitamin A intervenes in the formation and regeneration of cells and repairs cells that are damaged. All skin cells depend on vitamin A for their multiplication and shedding. This renewal process visibly improves the condition and appearance of the skin.

One of the main benefits of vitamin E for the skin is its antioxidant power. This can be translated into many properties, the first of which is that it delays premature aging, allowing the deterioration of skin cells and the appearance of wrinkles to be delayed. Vitamin C acts as an antioxidant in the body, that is, it fights free radicals. In addition, the body needs this vitamin to produce collagen, which is the protein responsible for the healing, elasticity, and strength of the skin [9, 16].

An important aspect to take into account is the characteristic of the skin. It should be evaluated if there is a local skin condition (dermatitis, mycosis, etc.), to avoid possible infection in the postoperative period. It is recommended to use bacteriostatic solution to bathe 48 h before surgery.

7.4 Assessment of Toxic Habits

It is important to document tobacco use and to inform patients that its use is totally discouraged. This includes nicotine patches, including nicotine-based gum or vapor cigarettes. It is advisable to quit smoking 1 or 2 months before and after surgery, with the aim of reducing intra- and postoperative respiratory complications and the alteration of microcirculation that favors pulmonary thromboembolism, cardiovascular pathology, surgical site infection, and wound dehiscence due to poor perfusion [2, 16, 25–27].

7.5 Clinical Antecedents

A detailed clinical history remains the best document to record existing morbidities such as diabetes mellitus and metabolic syndrome that are the most important factors due to their high frequency. It is estimated that the prevalence of diabetes mellitus is 20% in surgical patients. It has been shown that hyperglycemia, either due to uncontrolled DM or response to surgical stress, is a risk factor for the development of postoperative infections; cardiovascular, respiratory, and microcirculation complications; etc. altering the immune response and producing a pro-inflammatory state in the perioperative period [28]. Glycosylated hemoglobin (HbA1c) is an indicator of metabolic control in the last 3 months [29, 30]; it could be used as a predictive value for SSI since different studies showed an increase in HbA1c was associated with an increase in SSI between 15 and 18% [29, 31]. On the day of surgery, if the HbA1c is less than 7.5% (optimal control) or between 7.5 and 9% (suboptimal control), it is possible to continue with surgery. If its value is greater than 9%, it is recommended to reschedule the surgery until glycemic control improves. Other factors to take into account are obesity, hypothyroidism, hypoproteinemia, high blood pressure, collagenopathies, antiphospholipid syndrome, history of embolisms, surgical site infection, and hematological disorders such as coagulation disorders and anemia, which is evident in 30% of patients undergoing elective surgery (in up to 75% of cases, the anemia is unknown to the patients and their doctors). The current recommendations of the ERAS protocols suggest treating anemia with oral iron during the 14 days prior to surgery [2, 32–34] and limiting the use of intravenous administration and blood transfusions or erythropoiesis-stimulating agents to special situations [2, 35, 36]. These conditions are important to document and carry out the appropriate treatment, in order to arrive in the best conditions for the procedure.

7.6 Psychological Assessment

It is important to take into account the psychological aspect of the patients, which must be evaluated at the time of preoperative management. It will be essential to evaluate whether the patient is suitable for surgery and aware of the expected result as well as the possible complications that may occur. If the case requires it, a psychological consultation should be carried out with the aim of correcting anguish, anxiety, and/or depression, manifestations frequently observed in patients with DRA, associated with alterations in their body image and cosmetics. The correction of the parietal defect improves the aesthetic image of the abdomen and body contour, as well as the function of the abdominal wall, increasing the patients' self-esteem and improving their personal and social quality of life [1, 9, 16, 37, 38].

7.7 Cardiovascular Assessment

Correct pre-surgical cardiovascular examination is of fundamental importance to detect high blood pressure, arrhythmias, ischemic cardiomyopathies, etc. often unknown to patients. Also important is the assessment of surgical risk according to ASA (American Society of Anesthesiologist) to determine if the patient is able to withstand the intervention. It is associated with a pulmonary examination as needed and a correct pre-surgical anesthetic evaluation.

7.8 Usual Medication

It is important to know the routine use of different medications by patients, such as aspirin, anticoagulants, corticosteroids, contraceptives, hypoglycemic agents, antihypertensives, etc. not only for correct management but to avoid drug interactions.

If the patient has a high risk or previous history of DVT (deep vein thrombosis) or PTE (pulmonary thromboembolism) or is obese, antiembolic compression stockings and early ambulation in the postoperative period should be placed. In certain cases, they must be evaluated by hematology due to the need for low-molecular-weight heparin and suspension of anticoagulants or antiplatelet agents at the time corresponding to each medication.

Before planning a tactic and/or surgical technique that we are going to use, it is important to take into account the following points:

- Know the desire for future pregnancies in the short term on the part of patients. If pregnancy is a possibility, surgery is ruled out until the maternity stage has ended. Surgery to correct DRA does not prevent you from having children, but a subsequent pregnancy can alter the aesthetic result of your body image. Therefore, if an intervention is performed to restore the abdominal midline and there is a probability of future pregnancy in the short or medium term, it does not make sense to perform a procedure to improve body contour.
- A fundamental question when planning the intervention is to know how much time has passed since the partum (vaginal or cesarean section), since the minimum recommended time to perform a DRA repair after delivery is 6 months [9, 16, 37]. The closer we get to the postpartum year, the better, since the changes produced by pregnancy have recovered to the maximum. If there is no desire for future pregnancies, a consultation with a family planning service can be carried out, in order to planify a tubal sterilization surgery, since it is feasible to perform both procedures simultaneously.
- The selection of the patient for conventional or mini-invasive surgery will depend on the size of the DRA, whether it is primary or recurrent, whether it is associated with a midline hernia or not, whether the parietal repair requires a prosthesis, and the presence of a dermofatty flap, history of previous surgeries, or if you

are considering liposuction or the use of skin retraction energy in the same procedure.

- An important point to take into account is the patient's expectation regarding the aesthetic result and body contour, as well as the functionality of the abdominal wall in the postoperative period, especially in athletic patients.
- It is important the assessment of the muscle masses of the rectus abdominis and broad abdominal muscles. Above all, in patients with a history of multiple surgeries (denervation, muscle atrophy, etc.), evaluating the presence of scars from previous surgeries allows us to opt for a specific surgical technique, whether conventional, laparoscopic, or endoscopic and robotic in the search of a better anatomical—functional—cosmetic result. In cases with multiple previous surgeries, there may be parietal loss, scar retraction, or deformity of the dermofatty tissue, in which the use of muscle-cutaneous expanders may be necessary.
- It is important to assess the need for dermolipectomy, complex abdominoplasty, or the use of liposuction and use of energy to produce skin retraction in small dermofatty flaps associated with DRA, as occurs in the MILA (minimally invasive lipoabdominoplasty) tactic recommended by Palmisano and Di Biasio [39, 40]. Like the previous situation, it motivates you to work as a team with plastic surgeons.
- Explain to patients the use of a prosthesis; we must always be clear about the benefits of using a mesh and its possible complications.
- Warn patients that every minimally invasive procedure has the possibility of conversion to conventional surgery, due to a possible intraoperative adverse event or technical impossibility of completing the procedure minimally invasive [9, 16, 37].
- Abdominal girdle. An element to take into account is the use of an abdominal binder in the postoperative period. Choosing the correct girdle, material, size, position, and correct compression is an important factor; therefore, it is essential to try it on before surgery to determine comfort, adapt it to each case, and evaluate it in different positions, since it is an element that will be used between 30 and 60 days. Correct use reduces postoperative seroma, avoids skin imperfections or wrinkles, minimizes shearing between the subcutaneous cellular tissue and the aponeurosis-prosthesis, favors its adherence, and provides greater postoperative safety and comfort [9, 16, 37].

In summary, the prehabilitation of a patient must begin at the moment of the decision to operate until the surgery is performed. The programs are multimodal and multidisciplinary, involving behavior modification, physical exercise, nutritional and psychological support, correct clinical alterations, and toxic habits. The goal is to educate them about their pathology and empower them to participate in their recovery. Set logical expectations. Try to achieve optimal physical condition to reduce morbidities and allow a good surgical experience.

References

1. Burch J, Balfour A. Preoperative patient education. Preoperative preparation. In: Ljungqvist O, et al., editors. Enhanced recovery after surgery, part II. Cham: Springer; 2020. p. 37–49. https://doi.org/10.1007/978-3-030-33443-7_5.
2. López Rodriguez-Arias F, et al. Revisión narrativa de la prehabilitación en cirugía: situación actual y perspectivas futuras. Cir Esp. 2020;98(4):178–86. https://doi.org/10.1016/j.ciresp.2019.11.005.
3. Muñoz M, Acheson AG, Auerbach M, Besser M, Habler O, Kehlet H, et al. International consensus statement on the peri-operative management of anaemia and iron deficiency. Anaesthesia. 2017;72:233–47. https://doi.org/10.1111/anae.13773.
4. Balague C, Arroyo A. La prehabilitación, un paso maás en la optimización del paciente quirúrgico. Cir Esp. 2020;98(4):175–7. https://doi.org/10.1016/j.ciresp.2019.06.009.
5. Currie A, Burch J, Jenkins JT, Faiz O, Kennedy RH, Ljungqvist O, et al. The impact of enhanced recovery protocol compliance on elective colorectal cancer resection: results from an international registry. Ann Surg. 2015;261:1153–9. https://doi.org/10.1097/SLA.0000000000001029.
6. Gustafsson UO, Hausel J, Thorell A, Ljungqvist O, Soop M, Nygren J. Adherence to the enhanced recovery after surgery protocol and outcomes after colorectal cancer surgery. Arch Surg. 2011;146:571–7. https://doi.org/10.1001/archsurg.2010.309.
7. Pedziwiatr M, Mavrikis J, Witowski J, Adamos A, Major P, Nowakowski M, et al. Current status of enhanced recovery after surgery (ERAS) protocol in gastrointestinal surgery. Med Oncol. 2018;35:95. https://doi.org/10.1007/s12032-018-1153-0.
8. Ramírez Rodríguez JM, Ocon Breton J, Arroyo SA. Nutrition surgery and programmes of multimodal rehabilitation. Nutr Hosp. 2015;32:2–3. https://doi.org/10.3305/nh.2015.32.1.9203.
9. Juárez Muas D, Palmisano EM, Pou Santonja G, González Higuera LG, Martínez Maya JD, Domínguez G, Ayala Acosta JC, Blanco M, Cuccomarino S, Cabral Castelli ML. Morbilidad a corto y largo plazo de la reparación endoscópica preaponeurótica en la diástasis de los rectos asociada o no a hernia de la línea media: estudio pros- pectivo, multicéntrico e internacional. Rev Hispanoam Hernia. 2023;11(3):111–7.
10. Yariberygi H, Atkin SL, Simental-Mendıa LE, Sahebkar A. Molecular mechanisms by which aerobic exercise induces insulin sensitivity. J Cell Physiol. 2019;234(8):12385–92. https://doi.org/10.1002/jcp.28066.
11. Carley EJ, Steidley DE, Agel BA, Byme T, Mekeel KL, Rakela J, et al. Six-minute walk distance predicts mortality in liver transplant candidates. Liver Transpl. 2010;16:1373–8. https://doi.org/10.1002/lt.22167.
12. Dronker JJ, Lamberts H, Reutelingsperger IM, Naber RH, Dronkers-Landman CM, Veldman A, et al. Preoperative therapeutic programme for elderly patients scheduled for elective abdominal oncological surgery: a randomized controlled pilot study. Clin Rehabil. 2010;24:614–22. https://doi.org/10.1177/0269215509358941.
13. Moran J, Wilson F, Guinan E, McCorminck P, Hussey J, Moriarty J. The preoperative use of field tests of exercise tolerance to predict postoperative outcome in intraabdominal surgery: a systematic review. J Clin Anesth. 2016;35:446–55. https://doi.org/10.1016/j.jclinane.2016.09.019.
14. Snowden CP, Prentis J, Jacques B, Anderson H, Manas D, Jones D, et al. Cardiorespiratory fitness predicts mortality and hospital length of stay after major elective surgery in older people. Ann Surg. 2013;257:999–1004. https://doi.org/10.1097/SLA.0b013e31828dbac2.
15. Sánchez Sánchez B. Efectividad de la gimnasia abdominal hipopresiva frente al entrenamiento perineal clásico en el fortalecimiento del suelo pélvico de la mujer: revisión sistemática. Universidad de Alcalá. Facultad de Fisioterapia. Departamento de Fisioterapia. 2012.
16. Juárez Muas DM, Palmisano E, Pou Santoja G, Cuccomarino S, González Higuera G, Mayo P, Martínez Maya JD, Domínguez G, Ayala Acosta JC, Chichizola A. Reparación endoscópica

preaponeurótica (REPA) como tratamiento de la diástasis de los músculos rectos asociada o no a hernias de la línea media. Estudio multicéntrico. Rev Hispanoam Hernia. 2019;7(2):59–65.
17. Bruns ERJ, Argillander TE, van der Heuvel B, Buskens CJ, van Duijvendij P, Winkels RM, et al. Oral nutrition as a form of pre-operative enhancement in patients undergoing surgery for colorectal cancer: a systematic review. Surg Infect. 2018;19:1–10. https://doi.org/10.1089/sur.2017.143.
18. Burden S, Hill J, Shaffer JL, Todd CJ. Nutritional status of preoperative colorectal cancer patients. Hum Nutr Diet. 2010;23:402–7. https://doi.org/10.1111/j.1365-277X.2010.01070.x.
19. Fukuma Y, Yamamoto K, Hirao M, Nishikawa K, Maeda S, Haraguchi N, et al. Prevalence of malnutrition among gastric cancer patients undergoing gastrectomy and optimal preoperative nutritional support for preventing surgical site infections. Ann Surg Oncol. 2015;22(3):778–85. https://doi.org/10.1245/s10434-015-4820-9.
20. Pecorelli N, Capretti G, Sandini M, Damascelli A, Cristel G, de Cobelli F, et al. Impact of sarcopenic obesity on failure to rescue from major complications following pancreaticoduodenectomy for cancer: results from a multicenter study. Ann Surg Oncol. 2018;25:308–17. https://doi.org/10.1245/s10434-017-6216-5.
21. Cespedes Feliciano EM, Avrutin E, Caan BJ, Borojan A, Mourtzakis M. Screening for low muscularity in colorectal cancer patients: a valid, clinic-friendly approach that predicts mortality. J Cacchexia Sarcopenia Muscle. 2018;9:898–908. https://doi.org/10.1002/jcsm.12317.
22. Brown JC, Bj C, Meyerhardt JA, Weltzen E, Xiao J, Cespedes Feliciano EM, et al. The deterioration of muscle mass and radiodensity is prognostic of poor survival in stage I-III colorectal cancer: a population-based cohort study (CSCANS). J Cachexia Sarcopenia Muscle. 2018;9:664–72.
23. Giger-Pabst U, Lange J, Maurer C, Bucher C, Schreiber V, Schlumpf R, et al. Short-term preoperative supplementation of an immunoenriched diet does not improve clinical outcome in well-nourished patients undergoing abdominal cancer surgery. Nutrition. 2014;29:724–9. https://doi.org/10.1016/j.nut.2012.10.007.
24. Fujitani K, Tsujinaka T, Fujita J, Miyashiro I, Imamura H, Kimura Y, et al. Prospective randomized trial of preoperative enteral immunonutrition followed by elective total gastrectomy for gastric cancer. Br J Surg. 2012;99:621–9. https://doi.org/10.1002/bjs.8706.
25. Yoshida N, Baba Y, Hiyoshi Y, Shigaki H, Kursashige J, Sakamoto Y, et al. Duration of smoking cessation and postoperative morbidity after esophagectomy for esophageal cancer: how long should patients stop smoking before surgery? World J Surg. 2016;40:142–7. https://doi.org/10.1007/s00268-015-3236-9.
26. Sharma A, Deeb AP, Lannuzzi JC, Rickles AS, Monson JR, Fleming FJ. Tobacco smoking and postoperative outcomes after colorectal surgery. Ann Surg. 2013;258:296–300. https://doi.org/10.1097/SLA.0b013e3182708cc5.
27. Stead LF, Koilpillai P, Fanshawe TR, Lancaster T. Combined pharmacotherapy and behavioural interventions for smoking cessation. Cochrane Database Syst Rev. 2016;3:CD008286. https://doi.org/10.1002/14651858.CD008286.pub3.CD008286.
28. Nazar J, Claudio HF, Christian, González A, Alejandro. Manejo preoperatorio de pacientes con Diabetes Mellitus. Rev Chilena Cirug. 2013;65(4):354–9. https://doi.org/10.4067/S0718-40262013000400013.
29. Carranza-Lira S, Serrano-Estrada FD, López-Muñoz E, Hernández-Jiménez LM, Chavarría-Olarte ME. Concentración de hemoglobina glucosilada en pacientes no diabéticas con y sin infección de sitio quirúrgico posterior a la histerectomía. Cir Cir. 2020;88(3):344–8. https://doi.org/10.24875/ciru.19001411.
30. Goldstein DE, Little RR, Wiedmeyer HM, England JD, McKenzie EM. Glycated hemoglobin: methodologies and clinical applications. Clin Chem. 1986;32(10):64–70.
31. Humphers JM, Shibuya N, Fluhman BL, Jupiter D. The impact of glycosylated hemoglobin and diabetes mellitus on wound-healing complications and infection after foot and ankle surgery. J Am Podiatr Med Assoc. 2014;104:320–9.

32. Shander A, Knight K, Thurer R, Adamson J, Spence R. Prevalence and outcomes of anemia in surgery: a systematic review of the literature. Am J Med. 2004;116(7A):58S–69S. https://doi.org/10.1016/j.amjmed.2003.12.013.
33. Grupo de trabajo. Vía Clínica de Recuperación Intensificada en Cirugía Abdominal (RICA). Ministerio de Sanidad, Servicios Sociales e Igualdad. Zaragoza. 2015. http://portal.guiasalud.es/contenidos/iframes/documentos/opbe/2015-07/ViaClinica-RICA.pdf.
34. Scott MJ, Baldini G, Fearon KC, Feldheiser A, Feldman LS, Gan TJ, et al. Enhanced recovery after surgery (ERAS) for gastrointestinal surgery, part 1: pathophysiological considerations. Acta Anaesthesiol Scand. 2015;59:1212–31. https://doi.org/10.1111/aas.12601.
35. García Erce JA, Laso Martínez MJ. "Patient blood management" en la vía clínica de recuperación intensificada en cirugía abdominal. Cir Esp. 2017;95:552–4. https://doi.org/10.1016/j.ciresp.2017.02.001.
36. Froessler B, Rueger AM, Connolly MP. Assessing the costs and benefits of perioperative iron deficiency anemia management with ferric carboxymaltose in Germany. Risk Manage Healthc Policy. 2018;24:77–82. https://doi.org/10.2147/RMHP.S157379.
37. Juárez Muas D. Preaponeurotic endoscopic repair (REPA) of diastasis recti associated or not to midline hernias. Surg Endosc. 2018. https://doi.org/10.1007/s00464-018-6450-3.
38. Holubar S, Soop M. Perioperative optimization of patient nutritional status. In: Ljungqvist O, et al., editors. Enhanced recovery after surgery, part II. Cham: Springer; 2020. p. 51–8. https://doi.org/10.1007/978-3-030-33443-7_6.
39. Palmisano EM, Di Biasio G. Alternativa de manejo miniinvasivo para el tratamiento de pacientes con diástasis abdominal y colgajo dermograso mediante la táctica VER: Vaser® + endoscopia + Renuvion®. Rev Hispanoam Hernia. 2022;10(4):167–71.
40. Claus C, Palmisano EM. MILA (Minimally invasive lipoabdominoplasty) for diastasis recti. Are general surgeons and plastic surgeons fighting or playing together? Rev Argent Cir. 2023;115(4):393–5.

Part II
Plant Profiles

Chapter 8
Open Diastasis Recti Surgery: Abdominoplasty

Mauro Dalmiro Soriano and Ezequiel M. Palmisano

8.1 Introduction

One of the components to be treated in abdominoplasties is abdominal diastasis, being an almost mandatory step. This is achieved through the reapproximation of the rectus muscles, which seeks to relocate them to the midline, restoring it and improving the silhouette.

Abdominoplasty techniques have been constantly evolving since Demars and Marx reported their first dermolipectomy in 1880 [1].

Since 1967, when Pitanguy [2] described the vertical "plication" of the midline with non-absorbable sutures, different techniques were used for the repair of diastasis of the rectus muscles, with different designs in order to give firmness to the muscular wall of the abdomen, adapting them to individual anatomical variations.

Despite the large absolute reduction in surgical procedures performed during the coronavirus pandemic, abdominoplasties and liposuctions remained among the five most performed surgical procedures in both sexes in 2021 according to the 2022 Cosmetic Surgery National Data Bank report [3, 4].

The most common indication for abdominoplasty in women is the sequelae or changes in the postpartum abdominal region that include excess skin, stretch marks, flaccidity, changes in adipose distribution, muscle stretching and weakness, and of course diastasis of the rectus abdominis muscles [5].

Another increasingly important group is made up of patients who have undergone bariatric or metabolic surgeries with the consequent massive weight loss and the consequences that this generates to the abdominal wall due to the overdistension

M. D. Soriano (✉)
IAMEL, Rosario, Argentina

E. M. Palmisano
Italian University Institute of Rosario (IUNIR), Rosario, Argentina

S. Cuccomarino et al. (eds.), *New Concepts in Diastasi Recti Surgery*,
https://doi.org/10.1007/978-3-031-74947-6_8

to which the abdominal muscles and the legs were subjected alba and semilunar lines, in addition to the possible and frequent associations of secondary pathology due to abdominal surgical incisions.

Many controversies have arisen about the duration of the correction, the best type of suture, and the consequences on intra-abdominal pressure and subsequent pregnancy.

There has been a long debate between the use of absorbable sutures and non-absorbable for diastasis correction. The former have the advantage of not generating palpable indurations through the skin in thin patients and a lower risk of granulomas, extrusion, and infections; however, long-term correction is questionable due to the pressures to which is subjected the linea alba, such as muscle contractions, scar retraction, tissue elasticity, and increases in intra-abdominal pressure caused by the organs themselves, physical activities, or conditions such as obesity.

The first to carry out a comparative study between sutures for the correction of abdominal diastasis was Birdsell, who in 1981 demonstrated that there were no differences in the separation of the clips using an absorbable suture versus an non-absorbable one. Despite being a comparative study, it has the disadvantage of having a small sample, short-term follow-up and an operator-dependent method such as radiography [6–8].

8.2 Patient Selection (Personal Approach)

With the aim of decreasing probable complications and bad results, I prefer to do at least two preoperative consults in which I document medical and surgical history, physical examination, and other considerations to take into account concerns such as psychiatric disorders (BDD), unreal expectations with regard to the liposculpture, and relevant details.

Patients that are considered suitable for this procedure must be healthy and understand the treatment completely. Furthermore they must be conscious about their active role in the postoperative stages, and lastly they must follow the surgeon's postoperative instructions.

People under 18 years of age, active smokers who have more than five cigarettes a day, people with a body mass index (BMI) over 30, people who are diagnosed with diabetes, people who present with blood dyscrasia, blood thinners, anti-aggregates, people with a history of coronary artery disease, history of deep vein thrombosis and stroke, and history of pulmonary thromboembolism are excluded.

The procedure will be explained in detail by the surgeon, and both the operating surgeon and the patient must sign the preoperative consent form.

The surgeon takes pictures of the patient, and also the patient will be marked when standing with indelible ink before entering the operation room either the day before the surgery or on the same day [9].

8.3 Preparation

Decontamination of the skin and nasal passages is indicated with daily baths with chlorhexidine soap and intranasal mupirocin for 7 days prior.

Pre-surgical antithrombotic prophylaxis with low-molecular-weight heparin is administered 12 h prior according to the patient's weight and risk factors, which is continued postoperatively under the same criteria, both in dosage and treatment time [10].

Patient should maintain good hydration for 5 days previously with isotonic drinks, and furthermore on the day that the procedure is done, the person must remain on clear fluids for up to 3 h before and 6 h fasting for solids according to the ERAS (Enhanced Recovery After Surgery) protocol, in which it is allowed to ingest solid food even 6 h before the procedure and also drink tea, coffee, and fruit juice without pulp up until 2 h before the procedure, so as to decrease peripheral insulin resistance that is produced by preoperative fasting, without increasing the risk of bronchial aspiration, and moreover decreasing thirst, hunger, and preoperative anxiety [9, 11].

8.4 Marking

The midline is marked as a reference and 6 cm above the anterior vulvar fold, a horizontal line of between 8 and 12 cm is drawn extending along the line of the lower abdominal fold to ensure that no excess skin is left at the ends that cause the called "dog ears," and if there is a lot of lateral flaccidity, it is decided to extend the incisions backward (Photo 8.1).

Marking of the regions to be lipoaspirated is carried out according to the deep plane technique (Photo 8.2).

In primary cases, according to the patient's biotype and based on the excess of supraumbilical skin and the implantation height of the navel, we will be guided by the technique to follow, which will define whether to perform an abdominoplasty or a mini-abdominoplasty.

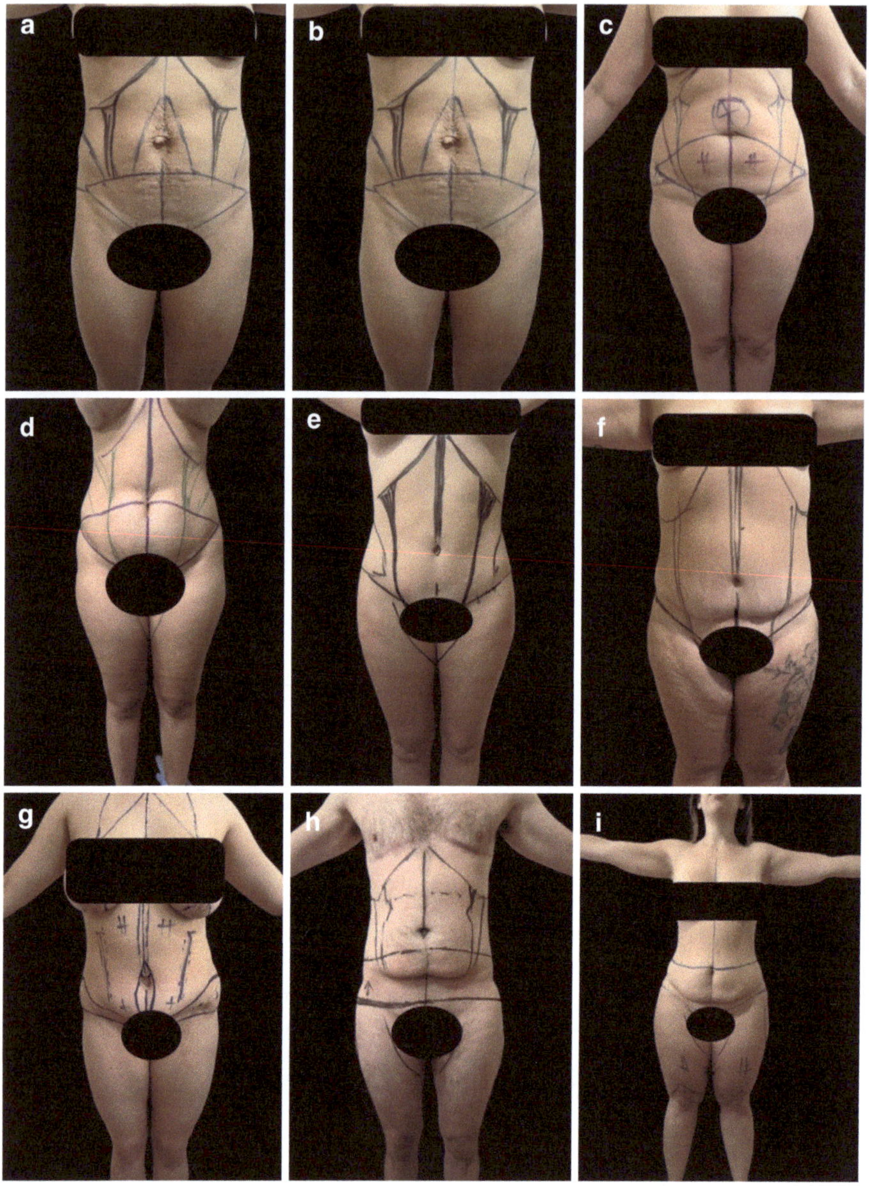

Photo 8.1 Different designs to plan abdominoplasties. Great variability is observed in the designs depending on the defect to be treated and always trying to minimize the visibility of the scars by placing them in the "bikini" area, not leaving "dog ears," as well as giving naturalness to the umbilical design

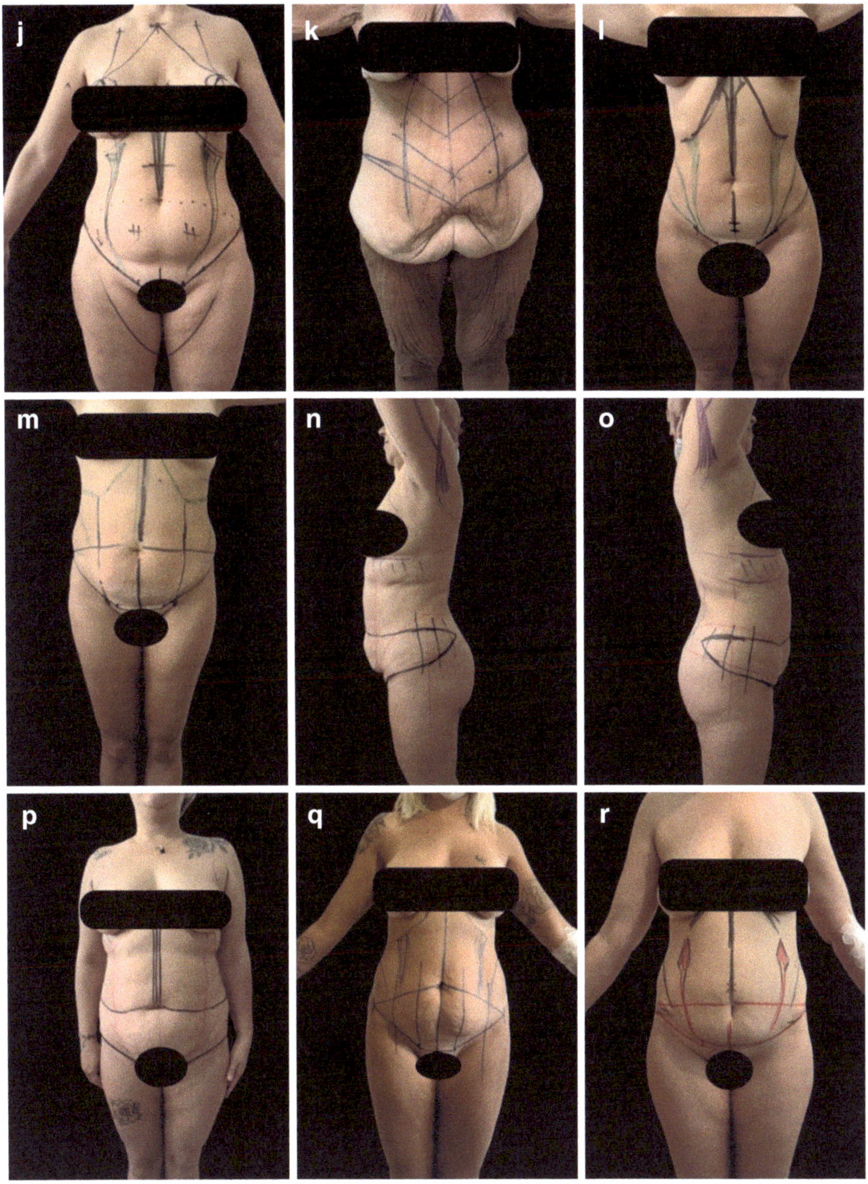

Fig. 8.1 (continued)

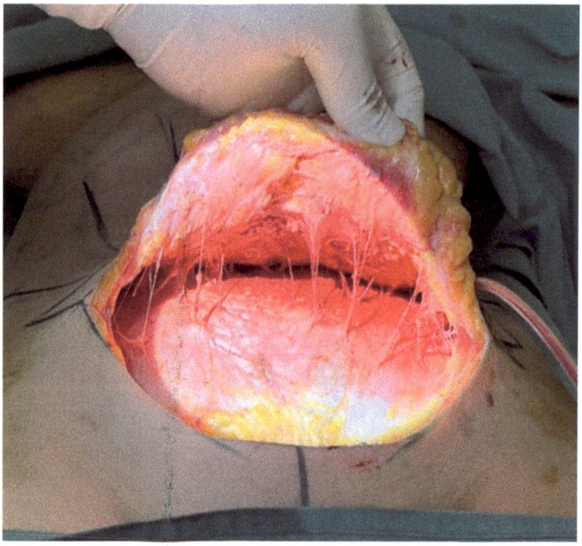

Photo 8.2 Once the deep plane liposuction technique is completed, the absence of deep fatty tissue, the fibroseptal septa, and perforating vessels joining the flap with the muscle and above the brilliance of Scarpa's fascia can be observed

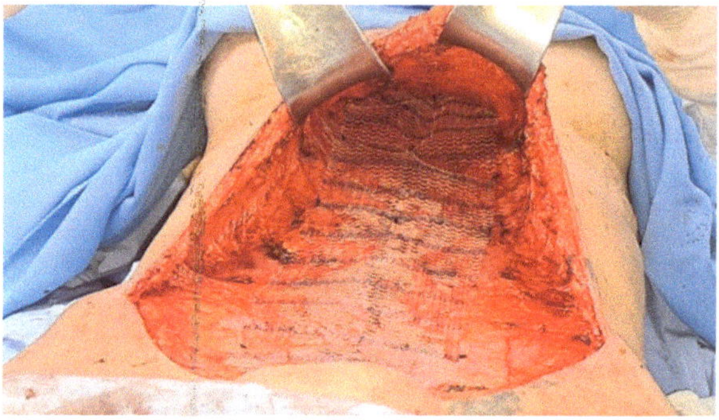

Photo 8.3 On occasions when warranted, the anterior abdominal wall is reinforced with polypropylene meshes

8.5 Choice of "Plication" and Treatment of Abdominal Muscle Weakness

In primary cases and with diastasis between 4 and 8 cm measured at the supraumbilical level, we perform anatomical plication (from the internal edge of an anterior sheath to the internal edge of the contralateral one) with a 0-gauge monoplane polydioxanone barbed suture surget after fixing the umbilical height with repairs of polypropylene points 0 (Photo 8.3).

If there is marked weakness of the anterior abdominal wall or if the patient wishes to better mark her waist, we choose to perform an extended plication taking the semilunar lines as anchorage with 1-gauge polypropylene tractor stitches and continuous suture with barbed polydioxanone suture surget gauge 0 monoplane (Photos 8.4 and 8.5).

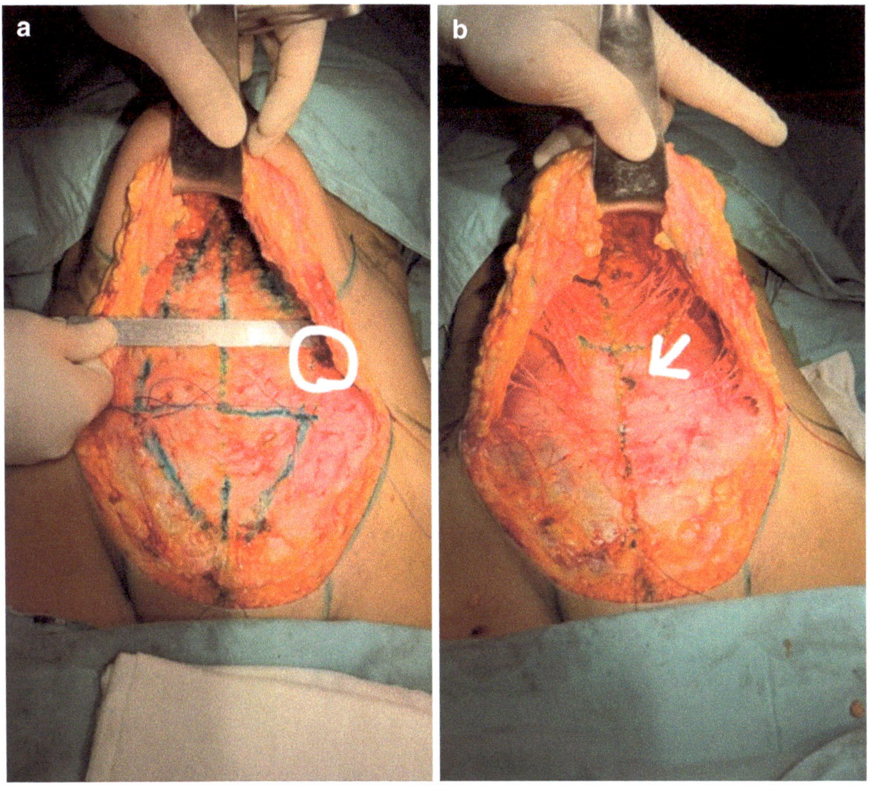

Photo 8.4 Observe the advancement of the obliques toward the midline with the muscle corset or wide plication technique

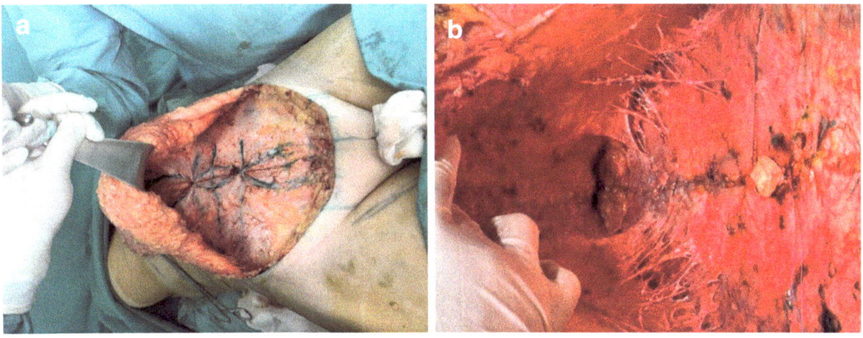

Photo 8.5 Steps of the wide or oblique plication technique. (**a**) Placement of tractor stitches, (**b**) finished barbed suture surget

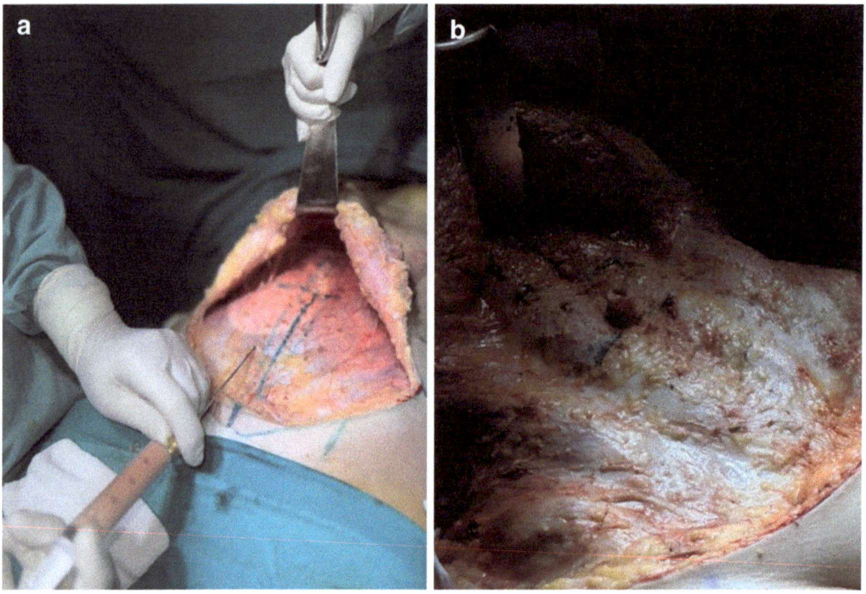

Photo 8.6 RAFT technique, using a cannula with a blunt tip (Viaro cannula), fat is infiltrated by retroinjection in the intramuscular plane of the rectus abdominis and sometimes in the anterior portion of the obliques (SPARTAN technique) to give greater definition and naturalness to the abdominoplasty

In cases of lean abdomens or desire for greater muscular marking, we use the RAFT (rectus abdominis fat transfer) technique [12] to discreetly increase the volume of the rectus abdominis muscles by infiltrating small volumes of intramuscular fat before performing an anatomical type plication taking the internal edge of both muscle sheaths with 0-gauge monoplane barbed polydioxanone suture surget (Photo 8.6).

In some secondary cases or in men where midline plication is not necessary and the objective is to thin the flap with resection of excess infraumbilical dermo-fat, we perform TULUA-type transverse plication as described by Villegas [13]. Its objective is to tighten the aponeurosis of the rectum in a vertical direction which in turn causes a displacement toward the midline of the rectus muscles (Photo 8.7).

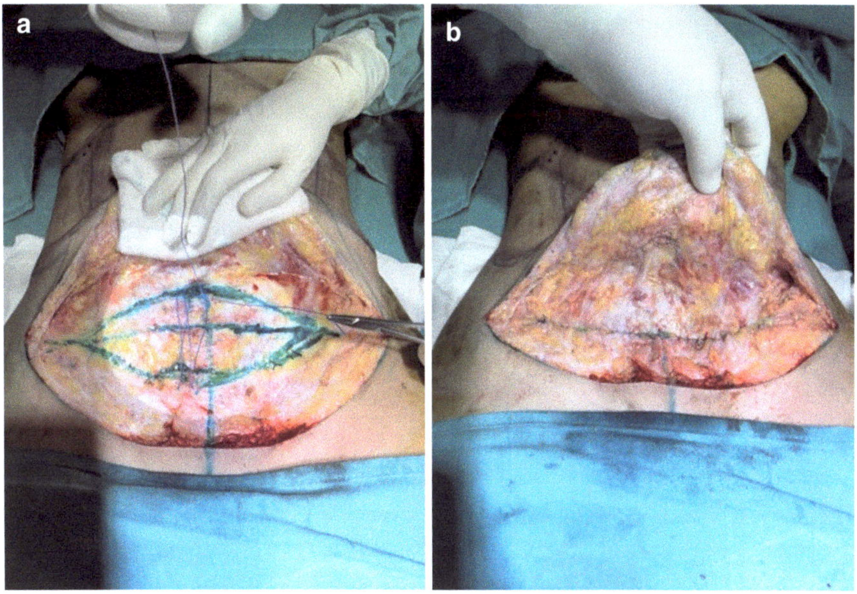

Photo 8.7 Horizontal plicature of the TULUA technique

8.6 Umbilicoplasty

To choose the type of umbilicoplasty to perform, we must first take into account whether it is a primary or secondary case, the presence of hernia defects and their impact on the umbilical shape and size, and whether the abdominal flap is going to advance caudally.

In primary cases we always fix the umbilical stem to the aponeurosis with 2-0 nylon or 2-0 polydioxanone sutures in the four cardinal points to ensure the opening of the umbilical stem without collapse, and we perform a suture with 910 0 polyglactin, from the dermis and including the Scarpa fascia of the superior flap to the deep aponeurosis with the objective of giving the flap a slope on its way toward the navel and releasing that union.

In secondary cases, we also choose to individualize the treatment of the navel, and in cases of great deformity due to umbilical hernia pathology or secondary surgical defects, as well as in all cases that we select for the TULUA technique, we can choose to perform neoumbilicoplasty, which is the most common technique used by the author the one described by Hoyos [14].

With the same objective of avoiding collapse of the umbilical opening during umbilical relocation in mini-abdominoplasties, four cardinal points are made to the stem with 2-0 polydioxanone fixed to the aponeurosis of the rectum in the midline.

8.7 Flap Resection and Refinements

The abdominal flap is lipoaspirated after infiltration with tumescent solution that is achieved by mixing saline plus adrenaline and lidocaine to ensure a vasoconstrictor effect and longer postoperative analgesia (each dilution bottle contains 1 liter of saline + 1 ampoule of adrenaline + 20 ml of 2% lidocaine) before beginning the abdominoplasty using the available technologies (HEUS, MICROAIRE), and its aggressiveness will depend on the technique chosen to reduce vascular complications of the flap and always respecting the superficial fat plane above the fascia from Scarpa, using a deep liposuction technique with 5 and 4 mm Mercedes-type cannulas, which will only be slimmed (with 4 mm and 3 mm cannulas with 3 in-line holes) in the regions where an extra negative effect is desired to greater definition of the abdomen that can be in the supraumbilical midline, semilunar lines, and iliac crest and depending on the degree of definition chosen.

The parameters of ultrasonic lipoaspiration with HEUS are chosen according to whether you want to have a greater potential retraction effect (power 70–80%) or if you prefer greater preservation of the fatty tissue to later be grafted (power 50–70%), and complementary MICROAIRE technology is used to extract fat more quickly and with less trauma to the tissues at a power between 80 and 90%.

In secondary cases and with extensive fibrosis, the parameters of both HEUS and MICROAIRE should almost always be higher due to the difficulty in dissecting the planes, as well as the surgeon's caution to avoid unwanted access to the abdominal cavity.

The dissection of the dermofat flap is performed with electrocautery at 45–50 W of power in the supraaponeurotic plane up to the xiphoid appendix, and if the TULUA technique has been selected, supraumbilical dissection is not performed, or it will be very reduced, and perforating coagulation is performed directly with electrocoagulation.

Before resecting the flaps, the patient is positioned with a slight flexion of the trunk and then proceeds to mark the flap to be removed and its lateral extension depending on what was programmed and to avoid "dog ears." Flap resection is performed after descent and release of the flap with barbed sutures as described by Baroudi [15], and in the case of TULUA, the flap resection is en block.

We routinely fix the superficial fascia of the pubic flap to the deep aponeurosis with running 910 0 polyglactin suture to prevent its rise and subsequent deformation of the pubic region.

Jackson Pratt silicone drains are placed with a reservoir system with anti-reflux valve that are externalized at the ends of the incisions so as not to cause more scars, since in the past we externalized them in the pubis, but today with the fashion of permanent hair removal of the pubis scars in this region are less accepted and with many complications (pigmentation, umbilication, among others). Refinement with more superficial liposuction is performed after the final suture.

We always perform the suture between the flaps in three planes: for the Scarpa plane, we use separate polyglactin 910 0 or 2-0 stitches depending on the patient's

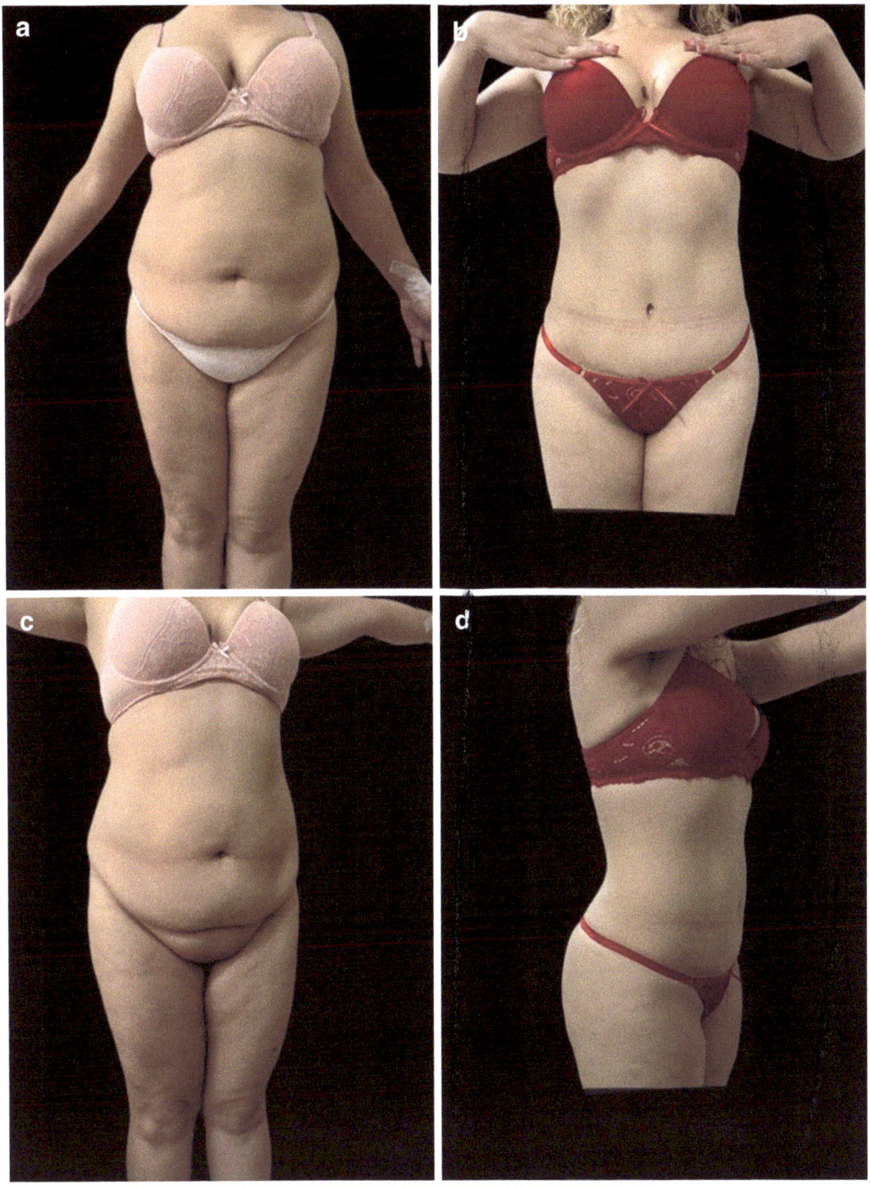

Photo 8.8 1-year postoperative control of extended abdominoplasty with liposuction of 6 liters of fat in 360° total body

build and the tension of the flaps. A second plane is performed with 2-0 polydioxanone subdermal surget, and the third plane continuous intradermal suture with 3-0 monocryl. We then perform flat curing with adhesive and micropore tape (Photo 8.8, 8.9, 8.10, 8.11, and 8.12)

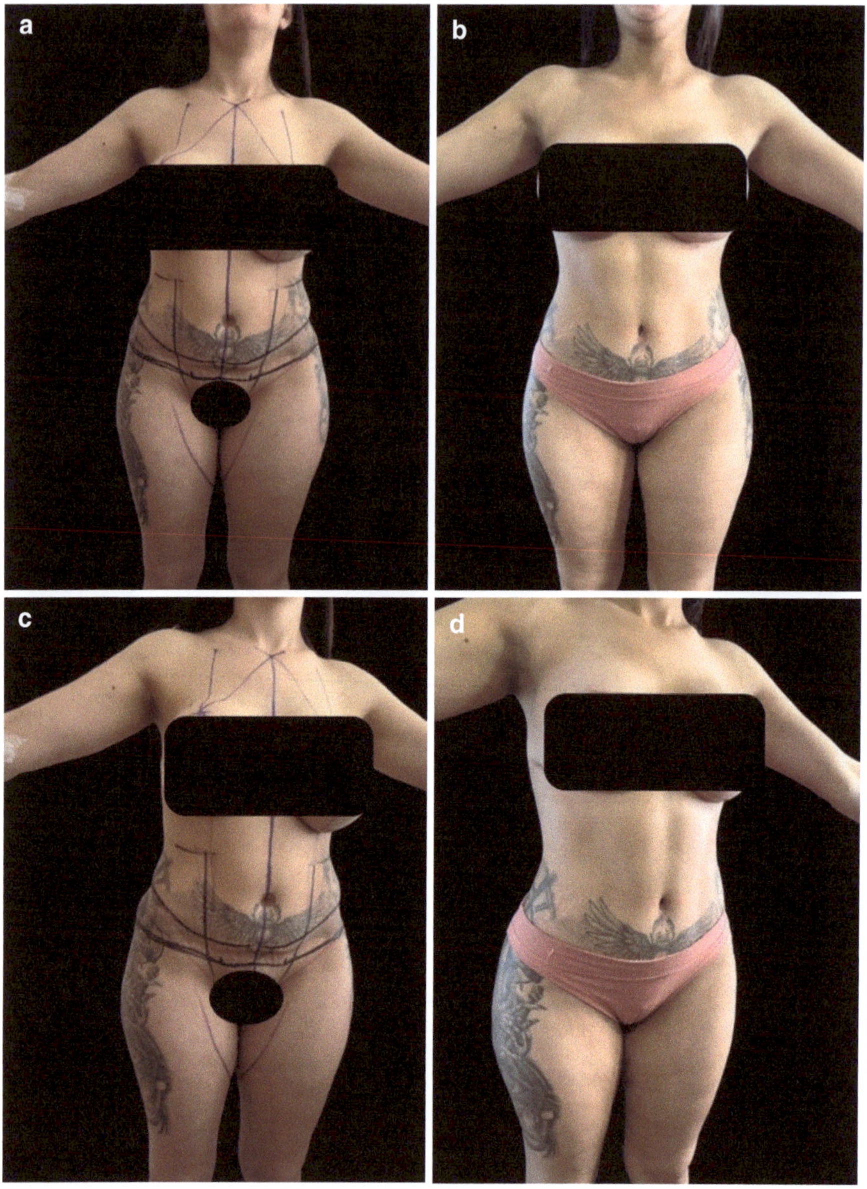

Photo 8.9 10-month follow-up of extended secondary abdominoplasty with RAFT and SPARTAN in combination with mastopexy with breast implant replacement

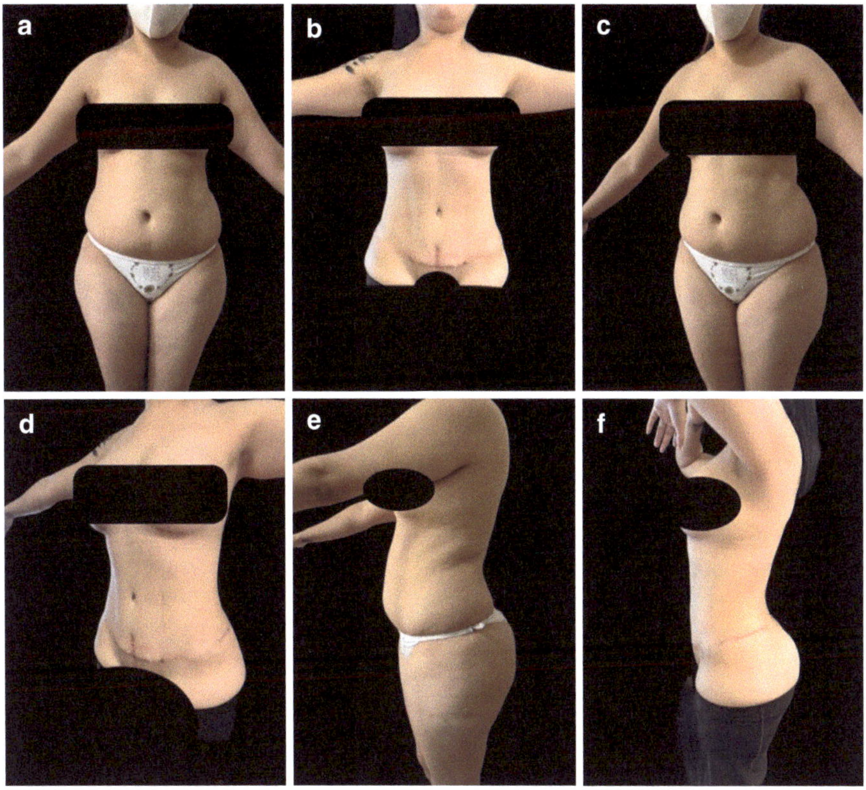

Photo 8.10 1-year postoperative control of conventional abdominoplasty with 360° lipo. Note newly consolidated scars in the anterior and lateral areas where plasties of said scars were recently performed

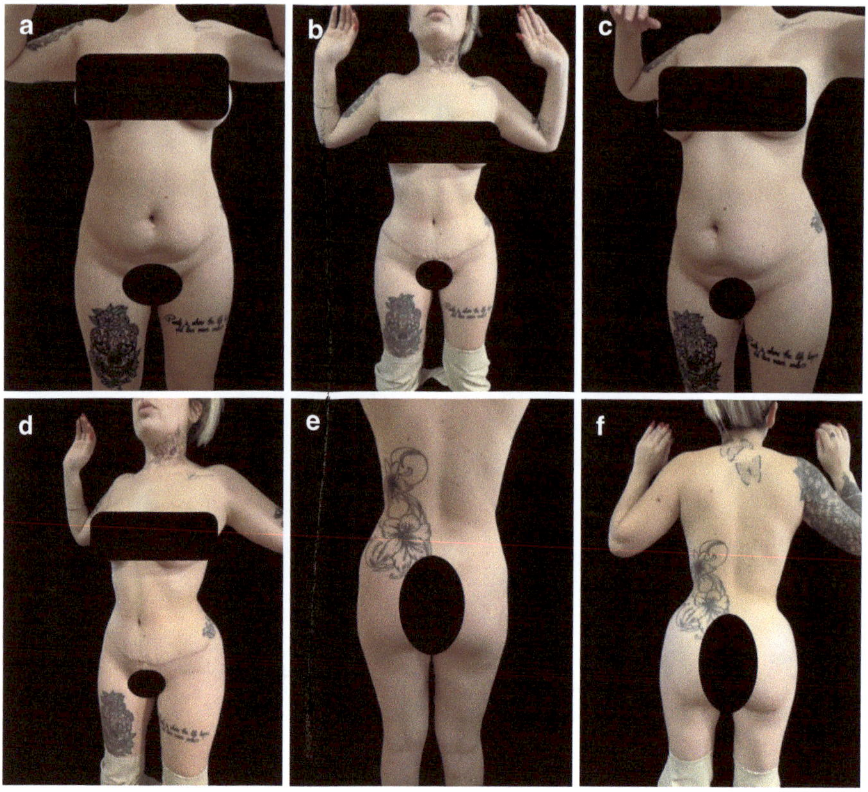

Photo 8.11 4-month postoperative control of abdominoplasty with wide corset-type plication with liposuction and gluteal augmentation with autologous fat

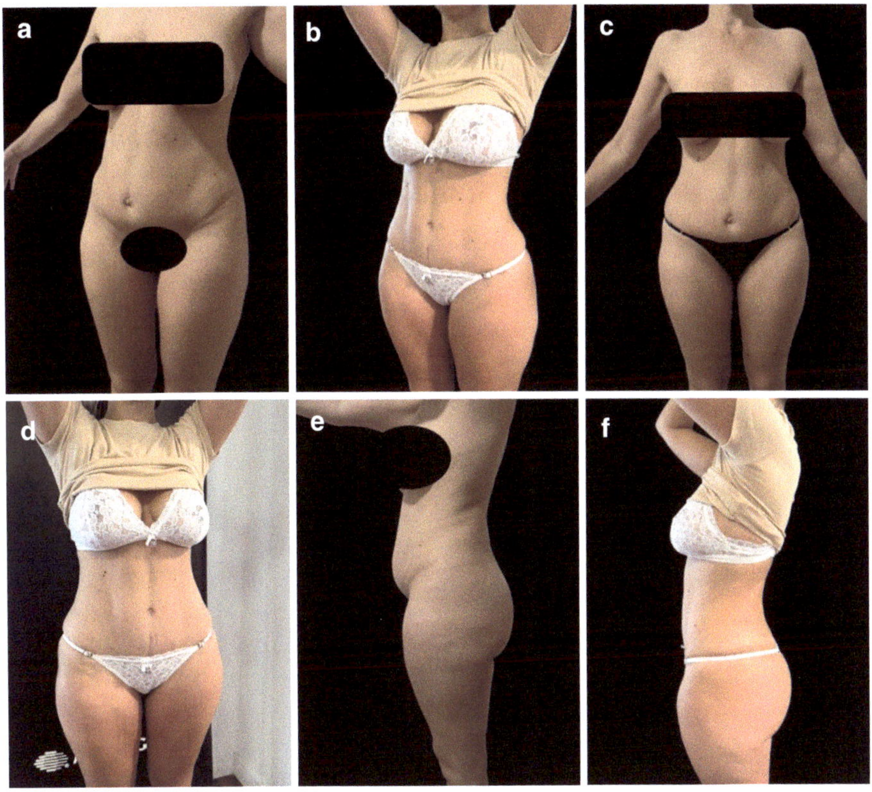

Photo 8.12 TULUA-type secondary abdominoplasty with 360° liposuction and neoumbilicus with Hoyos technique

References

1. Voloir P. Opérations plastiques aus aponévrotiques sur la paroi abdominale anterieure. Paris: Thèse; 1960. p. 25.
2. Pitanguy I. Abdominal lipectomy: an approach to it through an analysis of 300 consecutive cases. Plast Reconstr Surg. 1967;40:384–91.
3. The American Society for Aesthetic Plastic Surgery. 2018 cosmetic (aesthetic) surgery national data bank statistics. https://www.surgery.org/sites/default/files/ASAPS-Stats2018_0.pdf. Accessed 17 October 2019.
4. Cosmetic Surgery National Data Bank 2021-2022. The American Society for Aesthetic Plastic Surgery. https://cdn.theaestheticsociety.org/media/statistics/2021-TheAestheticSocietyStatistics.pdf.
5. Matarasso A. Traditional abdominoplasty. Clin Plast Surg. 2010;37:415–37.
6. Birdsell DC, Gavelin GE, Kemsley GM, Hein KS. Staying power: absorbable vs. nonabsorbable. Plast Reconstr Surg. 1981;68:742.
7. Nahas FX, Augusto SM, Ghelfond C. Nylon versus polydioxanone in the correction of rectus diastasis. Plast Reconstr Surg. 2001;107:700–6.

8. Elkhatib H, Buddhavarapu SR, Henna H, Kassem W. Abdominal musculoaponeuretic system: magnetic resonance imaging evaluation before and after vertical plication of rectus muscle diastasis in conjunction with lipoabdominoplasty. Plast Reconstr Surg. 2011;128:733e–40e.
9. Soriano M. D. Lipocontouring-back and buttocks. In: Manual of cosmetic surgery and medicine. Volume 1—body contouring procedures. Cham: Springer; 2022. p. 139–49.
10. de Redacción C. Consenso de enfermedad tromboembólica Consenso Argentino SAC. Rev Argent Cardiol. 2009;77(5):411–28.
11. Smith I, Kranke P, Murat I, Smith A, O'Sullivan G, Soreide E, et al. Perioperative fasting in adults and children: guidelines from the European Society of Anaesthesiology. Eur J Anaesthesiol. 2011;28(8):556–69.
12. Danilla S. Rectus abdominis fat transfer (RAFT) in lipoabdominoplasty: a new technique to achieve fitness body contour in patients that require tummy tuck. Aesth Plast Surg. 2017;41(6):1389–99. https://doi.org/10.1007/s00266-017-0909-9.
13. Villegas Alzate FJ. A paradigm shift for abdominoplasty: transverse hypogastric plication without supraumbilical dissection, unrestricted liposuction, neoumbilicoplasty, and low placement of the scar (TULUA). In: Aesthetic plastic surgery of the abdomen. Cham: Springer; 2016. p. 171–93.
14. Hoyos AE, Perez ME, Mogollon IR, Arcila A. H-wing neoumbilicoplasty: a new technique for advanced abdominoplasty and umbilical zones by gender. Plast Reconstr Surg. 2023;151:52–62.
15. Baroudi R, Ferreira CAA. Seroma: how to avoid it and how to treat it. Aesthet Surg J. 1998;18:439–41.

Chapter 9
Endoscopic Preaponeurotic Repair (REPA)

Derlin M. Juárez Muas

Diastasis of the rectus abdominis muscles (DRA) is a condition of the midline of the abdominal wall characterized by an abnormal separation of both rectus abdominis, evidencing a widening, thinning, and weakness of the linea alba, causing dysfunction or insufficiency of the same [1]. It is associated with a midline hernia between 93 and 98% [2].

It represents a clinical problem with an aesthetic impact of different magnitude, depending on the size of the DRA and the degree of the parietal condition.

Its diagnosis is eminently clinical, through an examination of the abdomen at rest and with a Valsalva maneuver.

The complementary diagnostic methods used are imaging studies such as abdominal wall ultrasound and computed axial tomography or magnetic resonance imaging (MRI) in cases of diagnostic doubt, to confirm or rule out associated hernias in patients with DRA or recurrent hernias, in overweight or obese patients, and in patients with multiple previous surgeries to evaluate the abdominal wall in its entirety, before deciding the surgical procedure to perform or planning the surgical tactic. The correct evaluation of the patient at the time of prehabilitation allows the choice of the correct technique.

The surgical treatment of DRA offers different options for surgical approaches, both conventionally and minimally invasive access (laparoscopic or endoscopic). This allows us to choose the most appropriate technique for each patient.

D. M. Juárez Muas (✉)
Argentine Hernia Association of Surgery, Salta, Argentina

Argentine Hernia Association, Salta, Argentina

Hispano-American hernia Society, Salta, Argentina

Public Maternal-Child Hospital, Salta, Argentina

National University of Tucumán, Tucumán, Argentine

S. Cuccomarino et al. (eds.), *New Concepts in Diastasi Recti Surgery*,
https://doi.org/10.1007/978-3-031-74947-6_9

The mini-invasive approach for the treatment of DRA is an excellent therapeutic alternative that offers different anatomical planes and multiple surgical options for the restitution of the linea alba (LA) and the repair of hernia defects.

Subcutaneous videoendoscopic access was described by Faria Corrêa MA [3] in 1995 with a 3–5 cm suprapubic approach for placement of the optic trocar and the secondary working trocar and an umbilical incision for the dermofat retractor. This author indicated the procedure for small- and medium-sized DRA, publishing a case series of 28 patients in that year. In 1998, in France, Champault [4] called video parietoscopy the performance of plication of the rectus sheath in patients with DRA associated with small midline hernias with a suprapubic and in both iliac fossae approach.

In 2015, in Spain, Bellido [5] published a modification adding a small preperitoneal polypropylene mesh to reinforce the plication when it was associated with an umbilical hernia. Subsequently, in 2016, Juárez Muas [6] presented in Tucumán, Argentina, and published in 2017 in the *Revista Hispanoamericana de Hernia* a technical modification, calling this operation preaponeurotic endoscopic repair (REPA) in which he performs a large dissection of the subcutaneous cellular tissue, creating a preaponeurotic neocavity and allowing visualization of the entire anterior wall of the abdomen. Through this technique, a restitution of the xipho-pubic LA is performed with prosthetic reinforcement with a large mesh in the preaponeurotic plane, adding the possibility of unloading or releasing the external oblique muscle, unilateral or bilateral, as needed in giant DRA (W3B) [2, 6, 7]; alternatively, the abdominal wall can be prepared with botulinum toxin infiltration 30 days prior to surgery, as presented by Juárez Muas et al. [8, 9] with the aim of achieving a suture with less tension, reducing postoperative pain in DRA greater than 10 cm, and avoiding the risk of postoperative abdominal compartment syndrome (ACS) [10]. In patients with a low risk of recurrence, who have a history of prosthesis rejection, desire for future pregnancies, or do not agree to receive a prosthesis or do not accept it, when explaining the possible complications of using a mesh, it can be performed plication alone or endoscopic repair of diastasis of the rectus abdominis muscles with plication of the LA with reinforcement of tension lines (ENDO-RTL), as published by Martín Gutiérrez et al. [11] with 6 cases with DRA of 4 cm, associated with ventral hernia in 83% and no recurrence with 8-month follow-up. A higher step in the management of DRA is the MILA (minimally invasive lipoabdominoplasty) tactic. It is an alternative and mini-invasive surgical management strategy for the treatment of patients with DRA and minimal dermofat flap, published in 2022 by Palmisano and Di Biasio [12, 13] initially as a VER (VASER-Endoscopy-Renuvion) tactic, currently known as MILA tactic. It is executed in three consecutive steps with teamwork between a plastic surgeon and a general surgeon, which allows a comprehensive treatment of the abdominal wall in those patients who require or need, apart from the anatomical-functional correction of the abdominal wall, an improvement in the aesthetic image of the body contour and abdominal skin.

9.1 Preaponeurotic Endoscopic Repair (REPA)

Preaponeurotic endoscopic repair (REPA) is a surgical option that performs a dynamic repair of the abdominal wall with closure of the hernia defect and medialization of the anterior rectus sheath of the abdomen, achieving comprehensive restitution of the linea alba (LA) from the xiphoid process to the pubis. This gesture avoids excessive tension on the reinforcing preaponeurotic mesh, providing greater mesh-tissue interface and facilitating the integration of the prosthesis in the healing process. In this way, a priori, the safety of the repair is increased and the possibility of recurrence is reduced.

REPA indication

- Interrectal separation >2.5 cm
- In symptomatic DRA
- Association of DRA with midline hernia defects
- Desires for aesthetic correction on the part of patients
- When there is no indication for dermolipectomy or the patient rejects it [1, 2, 7, 13]

We contraindicate endoscopic surgery

- Patients with a large dermofatty apron. If the flap is minimal, the MILA tactic is indicated [12, 13].
- History of open and content abdomen with healing due to secondary intention.
- History of multiple open surgeries with vicious scar.
- History of surgical site infection less than 12 months old [1, 2, 7, 13].

9.2 REPA Step by Step

On the day of surgery, in the pre-surgical admission room or in the operating room, the diastasis recti and hernia defects, if they exist, are marked (Fig. 9.1a, b).

Under general anesthesia and endotracheal intubation, the patient is placed in supine position with legs apart (Fig. 9.2a). The surgeon stands between the legs, and the assistant stands on the right or left depending on preference and comfort to manipulate the camera (Fig. 9.2b).

Classic surgical field is performed. Before starting surgery, we usually measure the xipho-pubic distance with a laparoscopic surgical forceps, especially in long-line patients or with a very acute intercostal angle, so as not to make the incision too low or distal, which will then make it difficult for us to dissect the TCS at the sub-xiphoid level and both costal margins or the beginning of the plication. A 10 mm incision is made in the suprapubic midline (Fig. 9.3a–c).

At the beginning of the dissection, the preaponeurotic space is created with scissors, Bertola or foerster clamps, which, being a ring clamp, present a greater width of dissection at the suprapubic level and both iliac fossae as wide as possible.

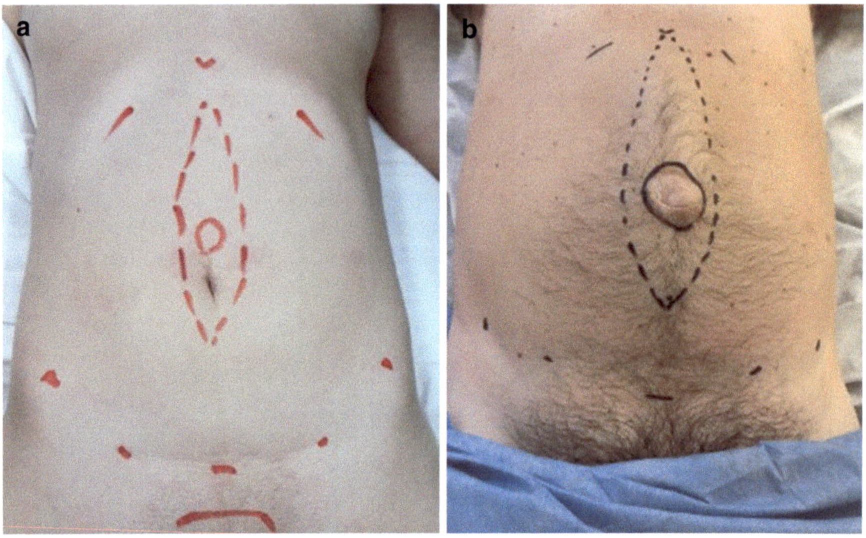

Fig. 9.1 (**a**, **b**) Marking of the DRA and hernia defects

Subsequently, a 10 mm optical trocar is placed, a fixation point can be made in the skin to avoid the loss of CO_2, or a balloon trocar can be used (Fig. 9.4a, b), and then the newly formed cavity is insufflated with CO_2 pressure between 8 and 12 mmHg. Subsequently, the 3 or 5 mm working trocars are placed in both iliac fossae under direct vision (Fig. 9.4c). The progressive increase in the space of the neocavity due to gas diffusion can be seen in the images.

The location of the trocars at the suprapubic level and in both iliac fossa allows us to create an excellent surgical field and good triangulation of the working elements. Then, the dissection of the subcutaneous cellular tissue begins along the left hemi-abdomen from the left iliac fossa upward until it exceeds the costal margin of the same name by 3 or 4 cm and laterally from the left anterior axillary line to the LA, which we call zone 1 (Fig. 9.5a); we recommend performing the dissection close to the aponeurosis to reduce the risk of thermal injury to the skin. We continue the dissection at the suprapubic level to cross over or cross the midline at the suprapubic level and go to zone 2 (right hemi-abdomen), and we perform the same surgical gestures as on the left side (Fig. 9.5b).

Once the dissection has been carried out in zones 1 and 2, we go to the midline, zone 3. At this moment, we must take special care in identifying and controlling the periumbilical perforating vessels and proceed to umbilical desinsertion with scissors or electrocautery with the use of cutting or coagulation as close to the aponeurosis (Fig. 9.5c). To facilitate this surgical gesture, we place a finger of the left or less skilled hand on the navel, which allows a better delimitation of the umbilical scar, thus avoiding thermal injury [1].

By removing the TCS and creating the neocavity, we achieved a large space (Fig. 9.6a–c) that allows us a complete exploration of the anterolateral wall of the

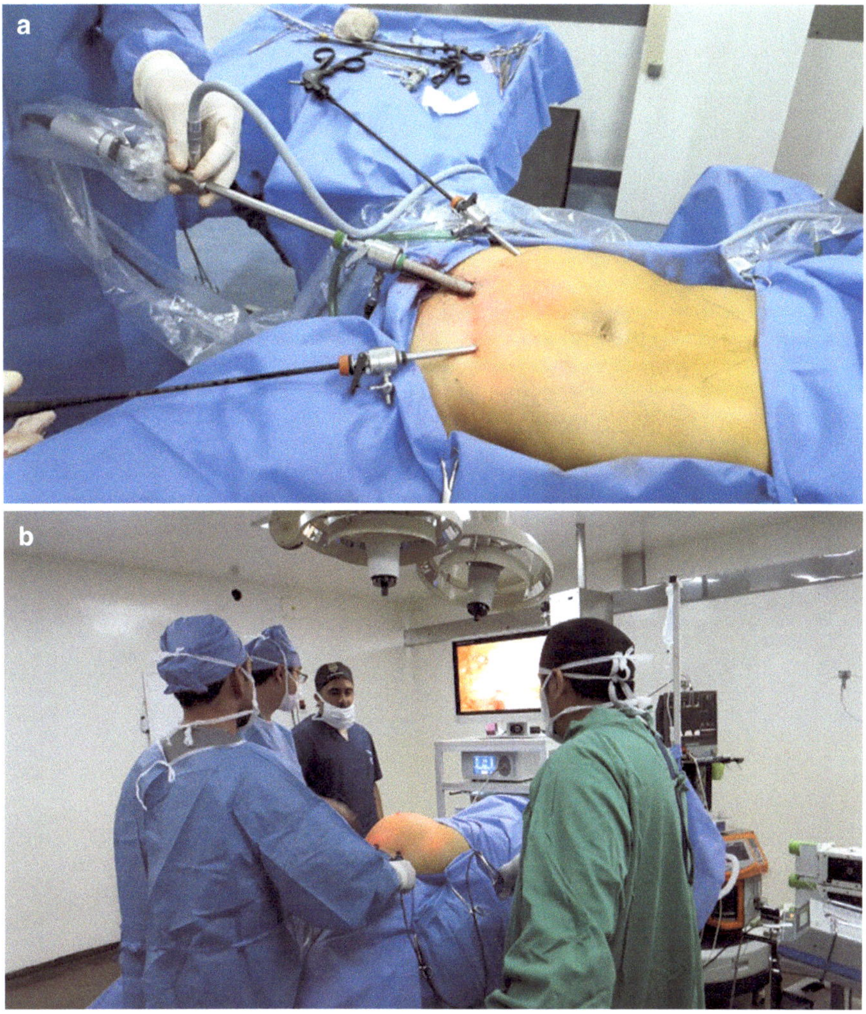

Fig. 9.2 (**a**) Patient position. (**b**) Location of surgeons

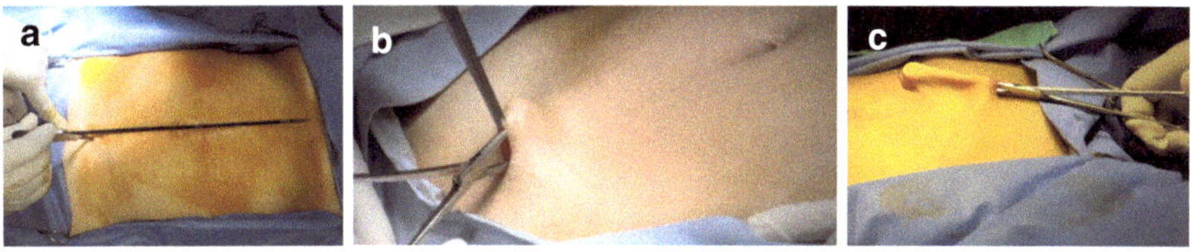

Fig. 9.3 (**a**) Measurement of xiphus-pubic distance. (**b**) Suprapubic incision. (**c**) Preaponeurotic dissection in the left iliac fossa

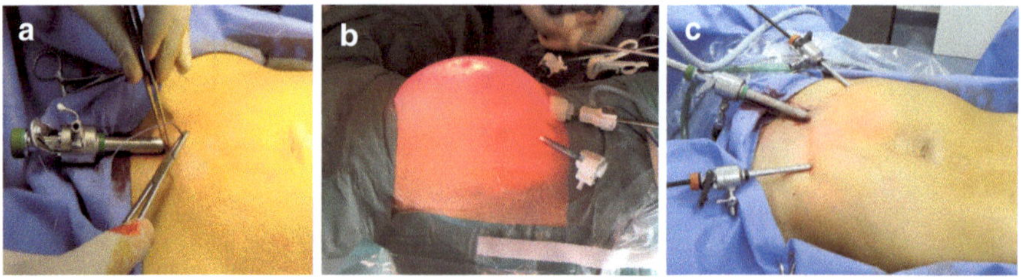

Fig. 9.4 (**a**, **b**) Suprapubic optic trocar. (**c**) Placement of working trocars

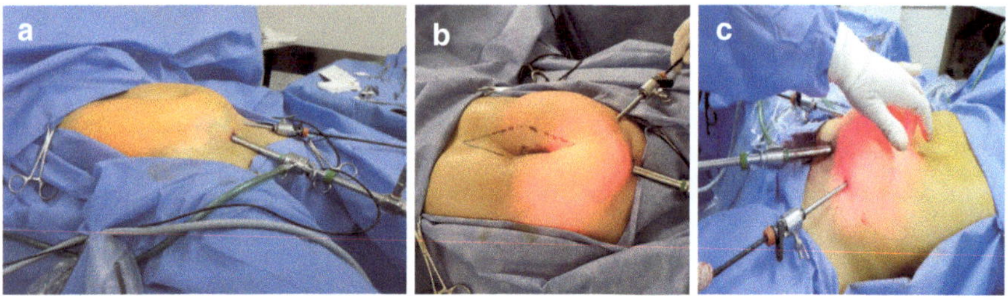

Fig. 9.5 (**a**, **b**) Dissection of zone 1 and 2. (**c**) Navel desinsertion

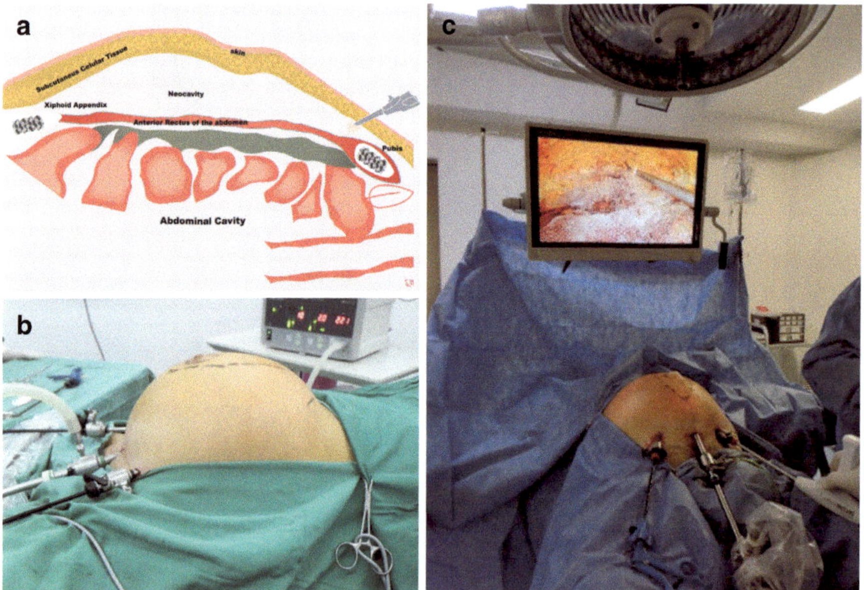

Fig. 9.6 (**a**) Neocavity diagram. (**b**, **c**) Neocavity with complete dissection of the anterolateral abdominal wall

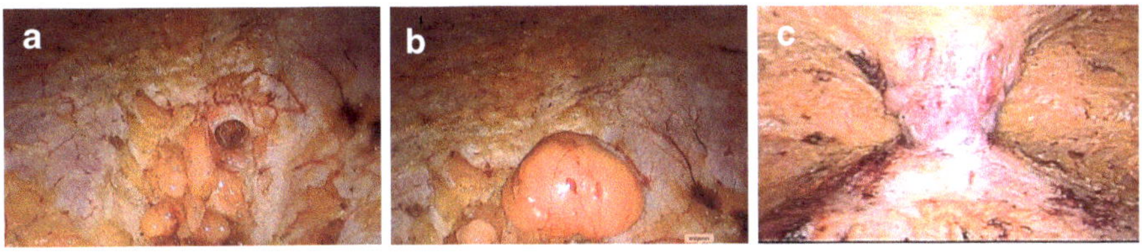

Fig. 9.7 (**a**) Epigastric hernia defect, (**b**) prehernia pseudolipoma, (**c**) sign of the erupting volcano

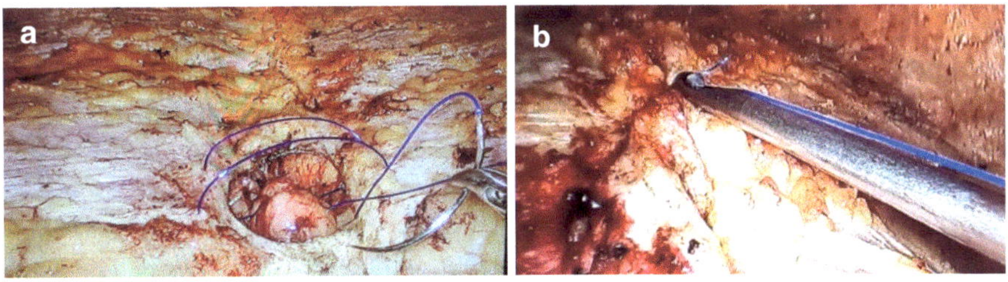

Fig. 9.8 (**a**) X point with polypropylene and (**b**) hernial ring closure

abdomen and the entire midline; with the identification of the hernia defects and the treatment of prehernia pseudolipomas, they are reintroduced into the preperitoneal space.

If the pseudolipomas are large, usually epigastric (sign of the erupting volcano (Juárez Muas et al.)), the hernial ring can be minimally expanded with a hook, which facilitates reduction (Fig. 9.7a–c). In exceptional cases it is necessary to resect them.

At this time, we are able to restore the midline by plicating the sheath of the rectus abdominis muscles. If we see the probability of tension in the suture line, it is necessary to perform muscle unloading. An incision is made in the aponeurosis of the left external oblique outside the Spiegel line as described by the Argentine Alfonso Albanese. Generally, this situation occurs when the diastasis is equal to or greater than 8 cm and can sometimes be bilateral when the interrectal separation is equal to or greater than 10 cm (DRA W 3B). Currently, we perform unloading or muscle release exceptionally, since we infiltrate the abdominal wall with 50 UR of TBA on each side with a unique application point with ultrasound guidance 30 days prior to surgery.

If the umbilical or epigastric hernia rings are larger than 2 cm, we first close them with 0-gauge polypropylene X stitches with an extracorporeal knot, or it can be with non-absorbable barbed suture (Fig. 9.8).

At this time, we are able to perform the restitution of the rectus sheath with continuous stitches with barbed polydioxanone or polybutester suture, gauge number 0 or 1 from the xiphoid process to the pubis (Fig. 9.9a, b). It can be executed by making a point and adjusting the surget by pulling it or making several points to shorten the length of the strand and facilitate its maneuverability, with the precaution of first adjusting the most cephalic points downward to achieve the same tension throughout the suture line.

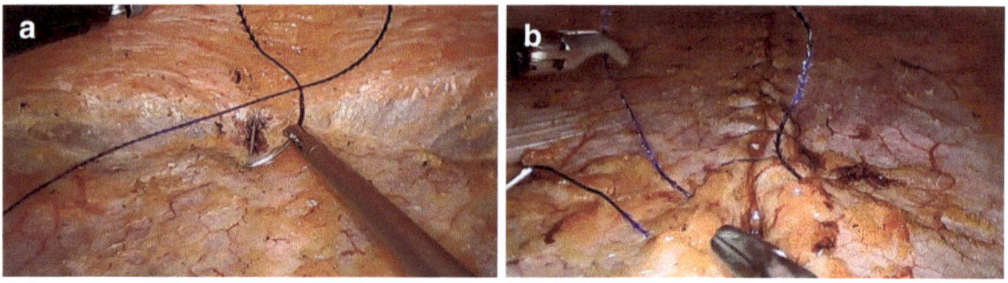

Fig. 9.9 (**a**, **b**) Plication of the sheath of the rectus muscles

Before placing the prosthesis, the neocavity is washed and aspirated with physiological solution to remove clots and devitalized TCS to reduce the risk of postoperative infection. A mesh is measured and placed in light or intermediate weight, macroporous, usually measuring 22 cm longitudinal × 15 cm transverse at the preaponeurotic level or larger transversely to cover the muscle discharge area, if it was necessary to fix it to the external flap of external oblique to refunctionalize it using the same foundation as F. Carbonell-Tatay in large eventrations. Currently, 10 cm transverse meshes are being used (Fig. 9.10a–c).

The prosthesis must be fully deployed to allow correct fixation, avoid folds, and provide better contact with the aponeurosis, which provides a greater mesh-tissue interface and facilitates the integration of the prosthesis in the healing process.

Since there is a lamellar seroma in 100% of cases as a reaction to the prosthesis, it is not advisable not to fix it. The mesh can be fixed with straps or tackers, preferably absorbable, adhesive, or absorbable stitches to reduce surgery costs (Fig. 9.11a–c).

In patients with a low risk of recurrence, who have a history of prosthesis rejection, desire for future pregnancies, or do not agree to receive a prosthesis or do not accept it when the possible complications of using a prosthesis are explained, it can be performed plication alone or endoscopic repair of diastasis of the rectus abdominis muscles with plication of the LA with reinforcement of tension lines (ENDO-RTL) published by Martín Gutiérrez et al. in Rev Hispanom de Hernia in 2023 with six cases with AKI of 4 cm. Associated with ventral hernia in 83%. There is no recurrence with 8-month follow-up.

Once the prosthesis is fixed, the navel is reinserted with 2-0 vicryl suture with intracorporeal suture or extracorporeal transcutaneous absorbable or nonabsorbable umbilical suture (Fig. 9.12a, b). It is advisable to reduce the CO_2 pressure as much as possible to determine the natural position of the navel and fix it in that location.

Hemostasis control is carried out, and suction drains are placed through the 3 or 5 mm accesses (Fig. 9.13a, b); there can be one or two according to preference: closure of optical access and fixation of drains, occlusive flat healing, and placement of tubular elastic belt in the operating room.

Fig. 9.10 (**a**, **b**) Longitudinal and transverse measurement of the mesh. (**c**) Deployment of the prosthesis

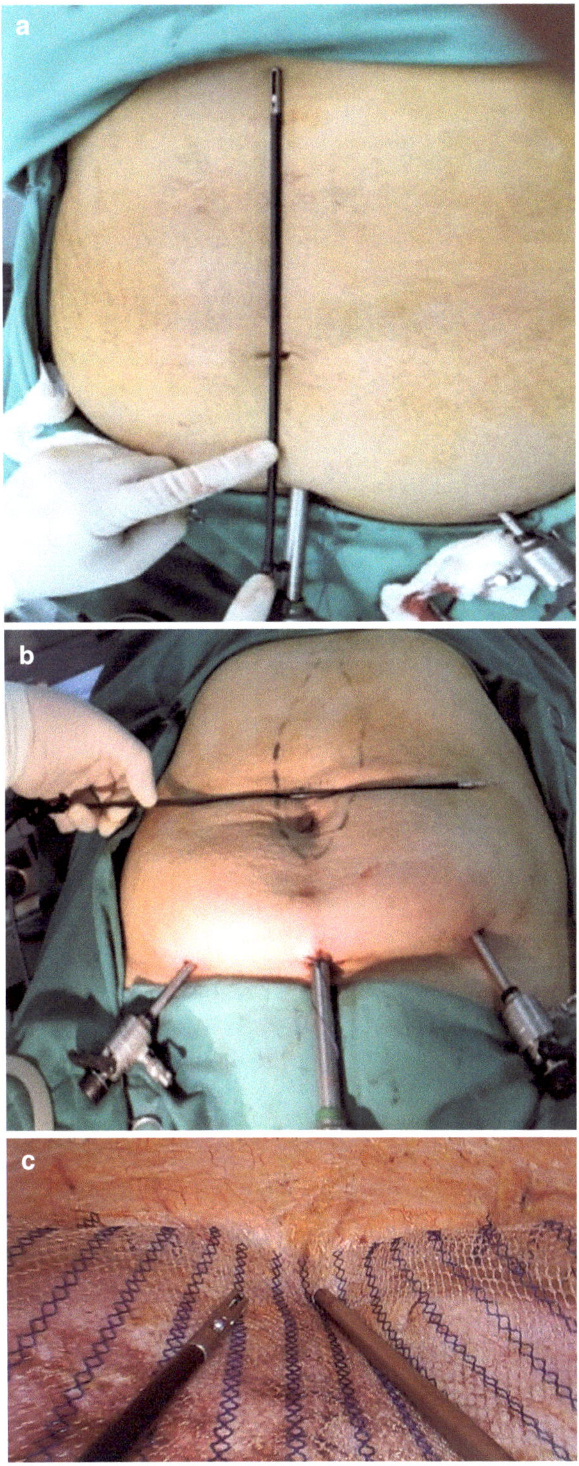

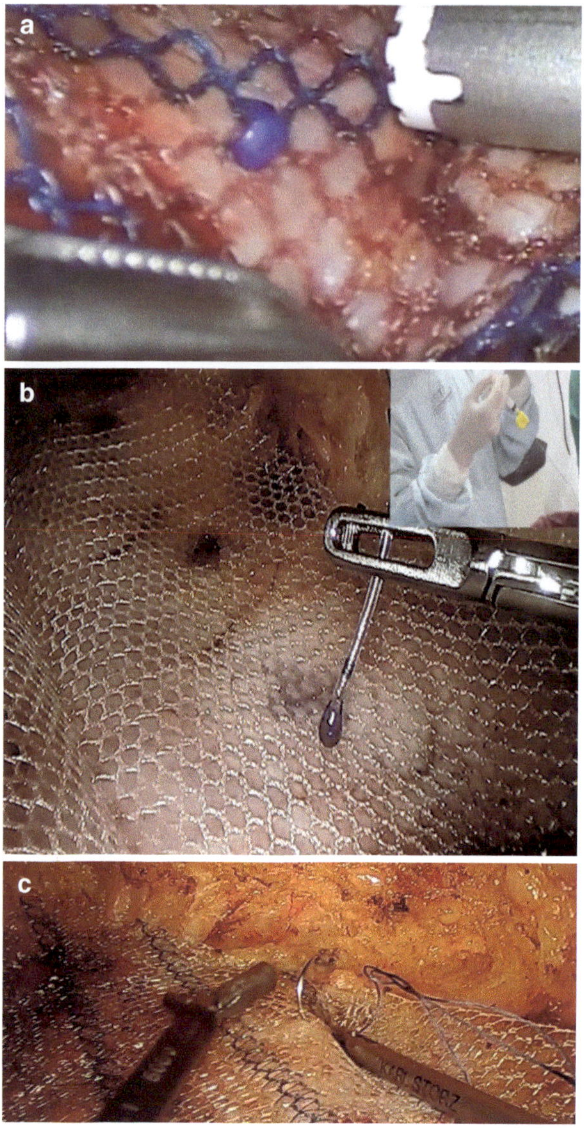

Fig. 9.11 (**a**) Fixation of the mesh with strap, (**b**) with adhesive, and (**c**) 2-0 polyglactin stitch

9.3 Control and Postoperative Care

Postoperative control is carried out daily. Oral intake begins with tolerance to liquids 4 h after surgery; if tolerated, a soft diet is progressed. We perform a daily and systematic control of the drains; they are removed when their output is equal to or less than 30 cc/24 h for 2 consecutive days. It usually happens between the fifth and seventh postoperative day. Postoperative pain control is carried out with analgesics—muscle relaxants—and local ice for 30 min every 6 h. Antibiotics are used

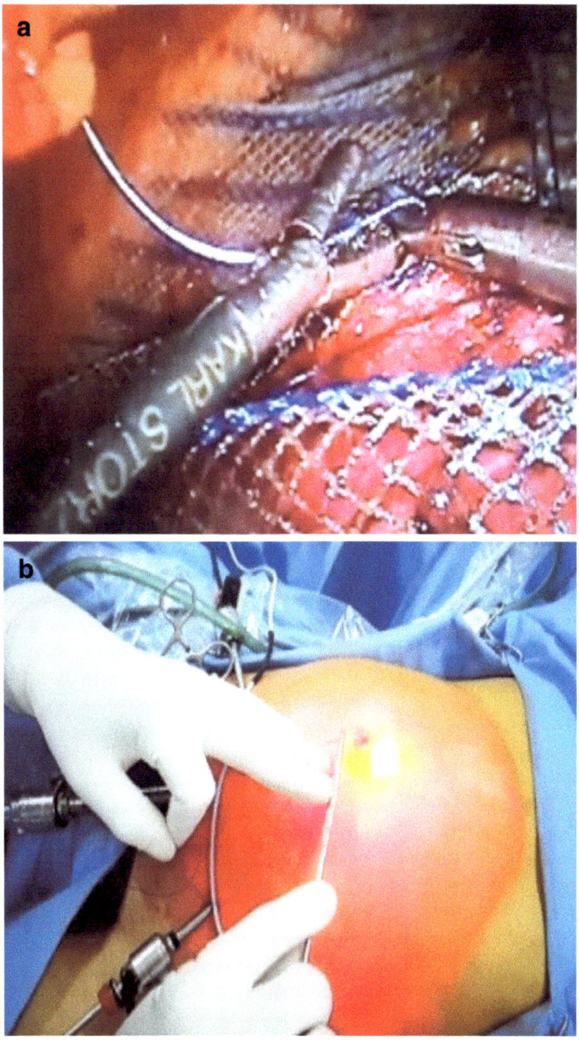

Fig. 9.12 Navel reinsertion. (**a**) Intracorporeal point and (**b**) transcutaneous point

until 48 or 72 h postoperatively. Early ambulation is initiated, according to the patient's tolerance. Permanent use of an elastic belt for 30 days is recommended to reduce postoperative seroma. Hospital discharge is indicated after 24 h depending on the level of pain; there are patients in whom the procedure can be performed as major outpatient surgery. Postoperative control follow-up is carried out at 5, 15, and 30 days and later at 6 and 12 months [1, 2, 7, 13, 14].

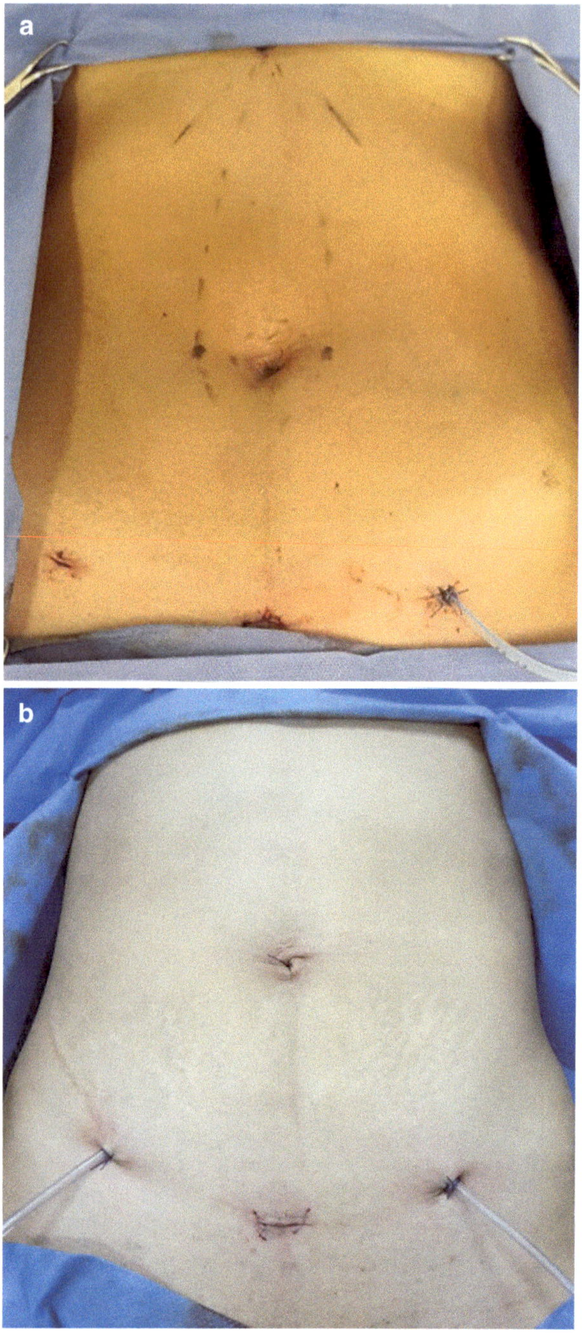

Fig. 9.13 (**a**, **b**) Subcutaneous aspiration drains

9.4 Intraoperative Adverse Events

Bleeding from perforating vessels is the most common event. Caution must be taken at the time of dissection to avoid bleeding and retraction with the possibility of causing hematoma of the rectus sheath. The second situation of probable bleeding is the moment of performing the rectus plication due to injury to a blood vessel and the trauma produced by the passage of the barbed suture.

Perforation and skin ischemia are complications due to thermal injury at the time of dissection, especially in thin patients. To avoid this situation, it is necessary to carry out the dissection close to the aponeurosis and reduce the use of excessive electrocautery to achieve hemostasis.

A rare event is the opening of the anterior aponeurosis of the rectus sheath and entering the prerectal or retrorectal space and producing a dissection in the wrong space with risk of bleeding.

A common situation is the opening of the umbilical hernia sac, which should not be considered a complication, but care must be taken to evacuate carbon dioxide at the time of plication or closure of the hernia ring to avoid postoperative omalgia [1, 2, 7, 13–15].

9.5 Postoperative Complications

Postoperative complications can be multiple, the most common being seroma (between 9 and 12%). Postoperative bleeding or abdominal wall hematoma and surgical site infection account for 1%. Sensory alteration of the abdominal wall is found in 100% of patients in the postoperative period; it recovers completely centripetally between 2 and 6 months after surgery. Recurrence of diastasis recti occurred in 0.8% [1, 2, 7, 13–15]. Postoperative complications and their prevention and long-term results will be discussed in another chapter.

References

1. Juárez MD. Hernioplastia umbilical laparoscópica asociada a diástasis de los rectos. In: Schlottmann F, Sadava EE, editors. Cirugía laparoscópica: técnica quirúrgica en cirugía general. Mexico: Medica Panamericana; 2023. p. 51–69.
2. Juárez Muas D, Palmisano EM, Pou Santonja G, González Higuera LG, Martínez Maya JD, Domínguez G, Ayala Acosta JC, Blanco M, Cuccomarino S, Cabral Castelli ML. Morbilidad a corto y largo plazo de la reparación endoscópica preaponeurótica en la diástasis de los rectos asociada o no a hernia de la línea media: estudio pros- pectivo, multicéntrico e internacional. Rev Hispanoam Hernia. 2023;11(3):111–7.
3. Faria Corrêa MA. Videoendoscopic subcutaneous techniques for aesthetic and reconstructive plastic surgery. Plast Reconstr Surg. 1995;96(2):446–53.

4. Champault G, Catheline JM, Barrat C. Chirugie vidéopariétoscopique de la paroi abdominale. Chirurgie. 1998;123:474–7.
5. Bellido Luque J, Bellido Luque A, Valdivia J, et al. Totally endoscopic surgery on diastasis recti associated with midline hernias. The advantages of a minimally invasive approach. Prospective cohort study. Hernia. 2015;19(3):493–501.
6. Juárez Muas D, Verasay G, García WM. Reparación endoscópica prefascial de la diástasis de los rectos: descripción de una nueva técnica. Rev Hispanoam Hernia. 2017;5(2):47–51.
7. Juárez MD. Preaponeurotic endoscopic repair (REPA) of diastasis recti associated or not to midline hernias. Surg Endosc. 2018. https://doi.org/10.1007/s00464-018-6450-3.
8. Muas DM, Palmisano EM, Santoja GP, Paz OR. Adjuvant botulinum toxin for endoscopic management (preaponeurotic endoscopic repair) of severe diastasis recti. Int J Abdom Wall Hernia Surg. 2021;4:45–50.
9. Ibarra HT. Toxina botulínica A: botulinum toxin type A: its importance in patients with large abdominal hernias. Rev Hispanoam Hernia. 2014;2(4):131–2. https://doi.org/10.1016/j.rehah.2014.05.003.
10. Moreno-Egea A. Abdominoplastia y reparación de hernia incisional: lo que un cirujano general debe saber. Rev Hispanoam Hernia. 2016;4(1):5–12.
11. Gutiérrez MM, Uriarte B, Pérez de Villarreal P, Hierro-Olabarria L, Moro A, Peña C, Zorraquino Á. Reparación endoscópica en la diástasis de los músculos rectos del abdomen: plicatura de la línea alba con refuerzo de líneas de tensión (ENDO-RTL). Rev Hispanoam Hernia. 2023;11(4):152–9.
12. Palmisano EM, Di Biasio G. Alternativa de manejo miniinvasivo para el tratamiento de pacientes con diástasis abdominal y colgajo dermograso mediante la táctica VER: Vaser® + endoscopia + Renuvion®. Rev Hispanoam Hernia. 2022;10(4):167–71.
13. Claus C, Palmisano EM. MILA (minimally invasive lipoabdominoplasty) for diastasis recti. Are general surgeons and plastic surgeons fighting or playing together? Rev Argent Cir. 2023;115(4):393–5.
14. Juárez Muas DM, Palmisano E, Pou Santoja G, Cuccomarino S, González Higuera G, Mayo P, Martínez Maya JD, Domínguez G, Ayala Acosta JC, Chichizola A. Reparación endoscópica preaponeurótica (REPA) como tratamiento de la diástasis de los músculos rectos asociada o no a hernias de la línea media. Estudio multicéntrico. Rev Hispanoam Hernia. 2019;7(2):59–65.
15. Cuccomarino S, Bonomo LD, Aprà F, Toscano A, Jannaci A (2021) Preaponeurotic endoscopic repair (REPA) of diastasis recti: a single surgeon's experience. Surg Endosc. https://doi.org/10.1007/s00464-021-08405.

Chapter 10
The Totally Extraperitoneal Repair [TEP]

Luis Gabriel Gonzalez Higuera, Juan David Martinez Maya, and Giovanny Vergara Osorio

10.1 Introduction

Diastasis recti is common in women over 35 who give birth to a heavy baby or have multiple pregnancies.

It is generally more noticeable after partum. It also occurs in middle-aged women and elderly men with abdominal obesity.

There are several ways to classify diastasis; the most common is Beer's, which is defined as follows:

1. Normal width of the linea alba at the level of the xiphoid <15 mm
2. Normal width of the linea alba 3 cm above the navel <22 mm
3. Normal width of the linea alba 2 cm below the navel <16 mm

Diastasis is considered severe when it exceeds 5 cm, and only when the diastasis is greater than 3 cm, but with a large defect or bulge, it is associated with a midline hernia [umbilical, epigastric, or incisional], and if it has completed treatment of

L. G. G. Higuera (✉)
National University of Colombia, Bogota DC, Colombia

Hernia and Abdominal Wall Clinic at the National University Hospital of Colombia, Bogota DC, Colombia
e-mail: luis.gonzalez@hun.edu.co

J. D. M. Maya
Salud Sura, Medellin, Antioquia, Colombia
e-mail: jdmartinez@sura.com.co

G. V. Osorio
University of Caldas, Manizales, Caldas, Colombia

High Performance Group in Abdominal Wall and Hernia Surgery at the SES University Hospital of Caldas, Manizalez, Caldas, Colombia

S. Cuccomarino et al. (eds.), *New Concepts in Diastasi Recti Surgery*,
https://doi.org/10.1007/978-3-031-74947-6_10

physiotherapy for at least 6 months without results, it can be considered a candidate for surgery.

Traditionally, diastasis recti has been considered a cosmetic but not a functional problem. Today we know that the wall dysfunction caused by it translates into several symptoms or problems such as constipation, low back pain, urinary incontinence, and other dysfunctions of the pelvic floor.

Furthermore, diastasis recti is the main risk factor for the appearance of midline hernias and also the reproduction of these hernias when the two defects are not repaired.

Currently there are a large number of surgical techniques that allow us to approach diastasis of the rectus abdominis; there are open techniques, mini-invasive open techniques, and endoscopic techniques [they do not enter the abdominal cavity].

Among endoscopic techniques, preaponeurotic repair of diastasis recti has been widely accepted among surgeons who perform abdominal wall surgeries, and based on this experience and taking advantage of the advance in minimally invasive preperitoneal and retromuscular surgery of the abdominal wall, e-TEP and e-TEP SA techniques have been positioned as a great management option for this pathology, especially when they are associated with midline hernias or with incisional hernias or with patients who have reproductions of the diastasis or hernias that have been previously repaired with previous endoscopic techniques or with abdominoplasty.

One of the advantages of using the preperitoneal or retromuscular space is that we can preserve a space for possible reproductions; we can use higher density meshes in these spaces and also not use fixation, which reduces the possibility of acute and chronic pain; the patient will also not have the possibility of foreign body sensation; a prosthesis in a preaponeurotic situation can produce the decrease in the number of post-operative seromas from the previous surgery and the decrease in the use of drains; and its aesthetic possibilities are not lost either since with techniques such as e-TEP SA, the surgical incisions remain in the same plane as the incisions of preaponeurotic repair techniques.

Thus, we consider that we have one more great alternative for patients and for abdominal wall surgeons that will require a greater need for technical preparation from the latter to dominate these techniques.

10.2 Retromuscular Repair of Rectus Abdominis Diastasis with Extended Totally Extraperitoneal View (eTEP)

Minimally invasive surgical procedures for the correction of primary hernias, ventral hernias, and diastasis of the rectus abdominis have shown great benefits such as decreased risk of infection at the surgical site, less acute postoperative pain, less probability of chronic postoperative pain, reduction in hospital stay, faster return to work activities, less postoperative medical disability, and earlier return to sports activities [1–3].

There are multiple tools, some of them innovative and with increasing acceptance, for the management of this entity clearly recognized as a disease that generates symptoms and has long-term consequences [4–7].

One possibility of surgical approach and management of diastasis of the rectus abdominis, whether associated with midline hernias or not, is the use of the preperitoneal and retromuscular space, as taught by Belyansky and Daes since 2018. This option complies with the current trend of hernia repairs to place meshes in a retromuscular position and outside the peritoneal cavity, but it is a technically demanding procedure that requires deep knowledge of the anatomy of the extraperitoneal space with emphasis on its natural limits and neurovascular packages [8].

The "eTEP access concept" is a set of maneuvers and strategies to improve the extraperitoneal space. These include retromuscular access and creation of the extraperitoneal space, section of the medial edge of the rectus sheath to effect midline crossing, and optional division of the arcuate line and the lateral limits when additional myofascial medialization is necessary to achieve midline closure [6–12].

The initial approach is done in a conventional manner on the most cephalic portion of the left anterior rectus 3–4 cm above the costal margin, the subcutaneous cell is dissected until the anterior leaf of the rectum is exposed, which is carefully incised so as not to compromise the muscle, avoid bleeding, and have a clean field; blunt dissection is made through the fibers of the rectus muscle until the posterior leaf is exposed and an ideally transparent trocar is inserted to facilitate orientation. In the first cases, we used a dissector balloon which is not mandatory but is an alternative to mention while gaining confidence with the dissection. Once the initial port has been inserted with the help of the pneumoinsufflator and the lens, we make a blunt dissection from medial to lateral until the semilunar line is identified by transillumination; once this maneuver has been carried out, the first working port can be externally located 2 cm below the flange costal; with the help of the hook with monopolar energy, we expand the space to place the second working port in the semilunar line almost at the height of the navel.

The dissection of the retrorectal space at hand is outlined by Dr. Daes in three stages: stage 1 the left retrorectum, stage 2 central dissection [midline], and stage 3 right retrorectum dissection. The central dissection is subdivided into 2a section of the ipsilateral medial edge, 2b section of the contralateral medial edge [right], and 2c midline crossing in the lower part where there is no posterior aponeurotic sheet [6–12].

With the two working ports in position, the most careful part of the dissection begins, which is the crossing of the midline. This should begin in the upper part of the retrorectus in the vicinity of the xiphoid. The hook is incised with monopolar energy at 5–10 mm from the medial edge of the linea alba; this leaves us a "rail" that has a double benefit: first it guarantees that we are not going to injure the midline to create a true hernia defect, and second it serves as a guide for this tab make the suture of the linea alba.

We advance this opening caudally to a site close to the hernial sac if there is one or until we have a working space to comfortably reach the medial edge of the contralateral rectum.

This dissection is always done in the adipose pad that is superficial to the falciform ligament so as not to generate early rupture of the peritoneum, which makes the rest of the dissection difficult.

Located on the contralateral edge, the opening of the posterior leaf of the right rectus is performed, taking the same precaution to maintain the aponeurosis "rail" of 5–10 mm as we did on the left side. A useful maneuver to locate the site to be incised is to use the monopolar hook and see the point where the muscle contraction begins and thus orient the site to begin the section of this sheet. The dissection is carried out caudally surrounding the defect; at this point there is no major difficulty with opening the peritoneum; there is already a large space created.

The next step is the closure of the peritoneal gaps and the posterior leaf, which can be performed with absorbable suture [polyglactin] to guarantee that the mesh will not come into contact with intraperitoneal structures.

Closure of the anterior leaf is performed with 0 gauge barbed suture, ideally nonabsorbable; if required for suturing convenience, 5 mm accessory ports can be used. At this point in the procedure, external compression of the wall is useful to improve the presentation of the aponeurosis "rails" to be sutured and the lateralization of the table.

Once satisfactory closure of the anterior wall is achieved, a prosthesis is inserted after measuring the space. The recommended prosthesis is of intermediate weight, macroporous. It is not required to fix it; it must be guaranteed that there are no folds of it when exsufflated, and selectively if required, an 18 Fr. gauge closed drainage is left that is removed in the shortest possible time.

10.3 Retromuscular Repair of Rectus Abdominis Diastasis with Fully Extraperitoneal Extended View via Suprapubic Approach [eTEP-SA]

A new possibility of surgical management of rectus abdominis diastasis using the preperitoneal and retromuscular space may be approaching it from the lower part of the abdomen or suprapubic [eTEP-SA] which has demonstrated in its publications technical and ergonomic advantages, as well as excellent cosmetic results and reduction in costs and operating time, compared to the classic technique, in selected cases [9].

eTEP-SA is a new minimally invasive surgical option for hernia repair with an extraperitoneal approach, primary closure of the defects, and mesh implantation in a retromuscular position, modifying the surgical technique known as eTEP for the approach to ventral hernias, as well as hernia midline primaries associated or not with diastasis recti abdominis [6, 9].

This approach consists of placing the patient in the French position, flexion of the hips and arms next to the body. Three trocars are implanted under direct vision in the suprapubic area, one of them 10 mm and the other two 5 mm, until reaching the central preperitoneal or Retzius space, followed by a dissection of the arch of Douglas and separating it from the parietal peritoneum in its central part. The medial edge of both sheaths of the rectus abdominis is sectioned until an adequate overhang is achieved in the cephalad direction or to the xiphoid according to the specific needs of the patient; subsequently, the following steps are performed: closure of the ventral defects, plication of the rectus abdominis fascia and mesh implantation into the retromuscular space, aspiration of the pneumo from the extraperitoneal space, removal of trocars under direct vision and closure by planes [9].

In reference to the technical details of the eTEP-SA, many of the current surgical principles are maintained, such as performing the procedure ideally by minimally invasive surgery, dissection of the retrorectal or retromuscular plane with closure of the hernia defects, adequate mesh by-pass and restitution of the linea alba which improves the cosmetic appearance, muscle mechanics, and function of the abdominal wall. When there is presence of diastasis of the rectus abdominis, the plication can be performed with a much more ergonomic positioning of the surgeon's hands, in addition to closing the defects of the parietal peritoneum, thus avoiding exposure of the mesh to the intra-abdominal organs, reducing future complications such as the generation of adhesions, obstruction, and intestinal fistulas.

The eTEP-SA requires fewer ports, with only three trocars, compared to the classic Rives-Stoppa eTEP technique where between four and five are usually required, with incisions in higher areas of the abdomen and therefore more visible. It must be taken into account that the position of the trocars in the eTEP-SA places the incisions in a less visible area, an aspect that becomes highly relevant from a cosmetic point of view while performing a more ergonomic surgery for the team surgical with therapeutic purpose and functional impact [6, 9].

The eTEP-SA publications have shown very satisfactory results such as shorter surgical time, perception of greater ergonomics of the surgeon during the procedure, fast postoperative recovery, and excellent cosmetic results with fewer surgical scars and in less exposed abdominal areas compared to the eTEP classic technique for the correction of ventral hernias. With the use of only three ports, it implies a lower cost for performing this approach, associated with a low rate of complications, being also compatible and also improving comfort in performing other surgical techniques such as eTEP with release of the transversus abdominis [TAR] by laparo-endoscopic route, preserving the principles of hernia defect closure, a wide coverage of the mesh in the retromuscular space, or the pretransverse space without requirements for fixation or use of routine drains [9].

References

1. Majumder A. Clinical anatomy and physiology of the abdominal wall. In: Novitsky Y, editor. Hernia surgery: current principles. Cham: Springer; 2016. p. 1–13.
2. LeBlanc KA, Booth WV. Laparoscopic repair of incisional hernias using expanded polytetrafluoroethylene: preliminary findings. Surg Laparosc Endosc. 1993;3:39–41.
3. Heniford BT, Park A, Ramshaw BJ, Voeller G. Laparoscopic repair of ventral hernias: nine years' experience with 850 consecutive hernias. Ann Surg. 2003;238(3):391–400.
4. Daes J. La técnica totalmente extraperitoneal de vista extendida (e-TEP) para la reparación de la hernia inguinal. Cirugía Endoscópica. 2011;12(3):118–22.
5. Daes J. The enhanced view-totally extraperitoneal technique for repair of inguinal hernia. Surg Endosc. 2012;26:3693–4.
6. Belyansky I, Daes J, Radu VG, Balasubramanian R, Reza Zahiri H, Weltz AS, et al. A novel approach using the enhanced-view totally extraperitoneal (eTEP) technique for laparoscopic retromuscular hernia repair. Surg Endosc. 2018;32(3):1525–32.
7. Quezada N, Milenko G, Besser N, Jacubovsky I, Achurra P, Crovari F. Enhanced-view totally extraperitoneal (e-TEP) approach for the treatment of abdominal wall hernias: mid:term results. Surg Endosc. 2021;36(1):632–9.
8. Daes J, Belyansky I. Anatomical considerations and tips for laparoscopic and robotic-assisted enhanced-view totally extraperitoneal rives-stoppa repair for midline hernia. J Am Coll Surg. 2021;233(2):e1–e11. https://doi.org/10.1016/j.jamcollsurg.2021.05.007.
9. Vergara Osorio G, González Higuera LG, Buriticá Vélez JE. eTEP-SA: nueva alternativa como variación al abordaje e-TEP clásico en reparaciones de hernias ventrales por abordaje suprapúbico. Rev Hispanoam Hernia. 2023;11(1):4–12.
10. Juárez Muas DM. Preaponeurotic endoscopic repair (REPA) of diastasis recti associated or not to midline hernias. Surg Endosc. 2019;33(6):1777–82. https://doi.org/10.1007/s00464-018-6450-3.
11. Zorraquino González A. Guía clínica de la diástasis de los músculos rectos del abdomen y pequeños defectos de la linea alba. Rev Hispanoam Hernia. 2021;9(2):118–25. https://doi.org/10.20960/rhn.00446.
12. Juárez Muas DM, Palmisano E, Pou Santoja G, Cuccomarino S, González Higuera G, Mayo P, Martínez Maya JD, Domínguez G, Ayala Acosta JC, Chichizola A. Reparación endoscópica preaponeurótica (REPA) como tratamiento de la diástasis de los músculos rectos asociada o no a hernias de la línea media. Estudio multicéntrico. Rev Hispanoam Hernia. 2019;7(2):59–65.

Chapter 11
Robot Repair

Pedro Trauczynski

11.1 Introduction

The robotic minimally invasive surgical approach for diastasis recti (DR) has brought significant benefits for patients and surgeons [1, 2]. For patients, it entails improved recovery, less postoperative pain, better aesthetic results, shorter hospital stay, and early return to daily activities and [3–5] for surgeons better ergonomics and lesser learning curve [5, 6]. Over the past 10 years, there has been a significant evolution in abdominal wall surgery due to a better understanding of abdominal wall anatomy and its anatomical and functional relationships (abdominal core) [6–8]. Consequently, various new techniques for correction of abdominal wall defects are now part of the therapeutic arsenal of surgeons who focus on abdominal wall surgery [9–11]. Surgeons can work in different muscle planes and compartments (onlay, sublay, underlay, intraperitoneal), close defects, or weaknesses in abdominal wall without tension and place increasingly larger meshes in the retromuscular plane. Consequently, surgeons were able to proportionate better functional outcomes, with fewer recurrence rates and lower postoperative complications [3–11].

Surgical treatment for diastasis recti has made significant progress with the combination of these new concepts of abdominal core and advances in minimally invasive robotic technology [12, 13]. Until recently, diastasis recti plication required large incisions, resulting in poor aesthetic outcomes and higher postoperative morbidity [13]. However, to harness the benefits of minimally invasive approaches and the new understandings of abdominal wall anatomy, surgeons face a primary constraint, which is the technical and ergonomic difficulty in performing these procedures laparoscopically, especially concerning suturing the abdominal wall, as in the case of diastasis recti. In this context, the use of robotic platforms has come to

P. Trauczynski (✉)
ACSC Santa Isabel Hospital, Blumenau, SC, Brazil

S. Cuccomarino et al. (eds.), *New Concepts in Diastasi Recti Surgery*,
https://doi.org/10.1007/978-3-031-74947-6_11

provide better ergonomics to the surgeon, enabling more precise procedures, improved dissection, and, most importantly, better closure of the abdominal wall. This is one of the main reasons for the significant growth of robotic surgery in general surgery worldwide, currently being the specialty that most utilizes the platform in terms of total number of procedures. The advantages include enhanced 3D visualization, the possibility of image inversion, and, most importantly, the 360-degree articulation of the instruments, enabling suturing even in non-ergonomic conditions, which allows surgeons to work in all compartments of the abdominal wall. In this chapter, we will discuss the main robotic platforms available on the market today, future perspectives, challenges, and their use in the main surgical techniques for the treatment of diastasis recti.

11.2 Robotic Platforms

Since FDA approval in 2000, four generations of the INTUITIVE Robotic surgical platform have been introduced to the market. Recently, a fifth generation received FDA approval. More than 12 million procedures were realized, and almost 8000 platforms are installed worldwide. For the last 20 years, it was the only platform available on the market. With the patent expiration in 2019, new platforms are now available for clinical use, which will make robotic surgery even more accessible, bringing the advantages of its technology to a larger number of patients and surgeons. The British robotic platform CMR-VERSIUS has been experiencing rapid growth, with surgeons' clinical experience advancing in various areas, including complex abdominal wall cases. In addition to these, we have the MEDTRONIC HUGO RAS platform, already approved for clinical use in abdominal wall surgery in some countries. Another example is the Senhance system by TransEnterix, already performing hernia procedures in animal models and close to entering the market.

Certainly, we will soon have an even greater variety of new platforms worldwide. This will lead to greater technology expansion and cost reduction, resulting in increased access to robotic surgery. In the context of the abdominal wall, robotic platforms are expected to improve the surgeon's ergonomics and the precision of suturing on the anterior wall, which are technically more challenging to perform by conventional laparoscopy. With the development of surgical expertise, we realize that robotic surgery gives us surgeons not only better suturing but better dissection and greater precision due to fine movements and 360-degree instrument articulation. Additionally, there is improved visualization of anatomical structures and planes for dissection through augmented three-dimensional static images controlled by the surgeon. The major barrier to greater technology adoption still lies in economic factors and access to platforms due to the high acquisition costs and use of non-permanent materials.

The challenge in applying new robotic platforms, specifically in the abdominal wall, is still related to collisions that may occur between robotic arms or with the patient's table, due to the angles required for suturing on the anterior abdominal wall.

11.3 Abdominal Wall Anatomy Compartments—Abdominal Core

We divide the surgical dissection, mesh positioning, and closure of hernia defects and diastasis recti plication into onlay, sublay, underlay, and intraperitoneal approaches. There are specific details when working in each one of these compartments. To work at the onlay (premuscular) space is technically easier for dissection and suturing but has a higher incidence of surgical wound complications, such as seroma, hematomas, and surgical site infections. The diastasis plication is technically easier because we suture the abdominal wall inferiorly (downward). The sublay and underlay spaces are more explored by experienced abdominal wall surgeons but, however, are technically more challenging to dissect and to close.

Precise anatomical knowledge of the abdominal wall is essential to work in these spaces, avoiding injuries to neurovascular bundles in the semilunar line, which can lead to permanent complications and catastrophic deformities of the abdominal wall. When working in these spaces, there is a lower incidence of surgical wound complications, such as seroma, hematoma, and infection. Also, in this space, due to the medial advancement of the abdominal rectus muscles, we can close larger defects with less tension in the abdominal wall. If necessary, we can also place retro-muscular meshes for greater reinforcement, especially when associated with several hernia repairs. The diastasis recti plication is technically more challenging because surgeons are basically suturing on the roof.

11.4 Choosing the Ideal Surgical Technique

Each patient must be individually assessed for a proper and individualized surgical planning. Factors to consider in choosing the best individualized operative technique include the following:

- Size of the diastasis recti
- Association of diastasis recti with abdominal wall hernias
- Patient characteristics and expectations regarding surgery
- Association of surgery with aesthetic procedures (liposuction and skin retraction techniques) or associated intra-abdominal procedures.

11.5 Surgical Techniques

11.5.1 Preaponeurotic (SCOLA/REPA/ELAR, etc.)

There are different nomenclatures for the same procedure. It involves the same surgical principle: diastasis recti plication in the preaponeurotic compartment. The use of robotic platforms seems to further facilitate dissection due to 3D static magnified imaging and the 360-degree movements of the instrument. But it mainly facilitates the plication of the medial edges of the rectus muscles/anterior sheath with closure of the linea alba. This allows a precise suturing even for surgeons with low experience in advanced minimally invasive suturing. Among the techniques we will present, this seems to be the one that brings the least advantages with robotic use and can also be safely performed with conventional laparoscopy. We tend to perform increasingly central and restricted dissections to reduce the risk of seroma formation and skin devascularization.

11.5.1.1 Operative Technique

Surgery is performed with the patient under general anesthesia. Neither urinary nor nasogastric catheters are routinely used. Antibiotic prophylaxis is done during anesthetic induction.

11.5.1.2 Patient's and Robotic Position

Patient is placed in a supine position with slight spine extension. Robotic platform positioning depends on what platform the surgeon uses. For intuitive platforms the robot is positioned 90 degrees lateral to thc patient from any side (Xi platform) (Fig. 11.1) and 45 degrees to the patient's elbow also from any side at Si and X platform (Fig. 11.2). For CMR/Versius platform, the robot arms are positioned between the patient's legs (Fig. 11.3).

The technical steps are as follows:

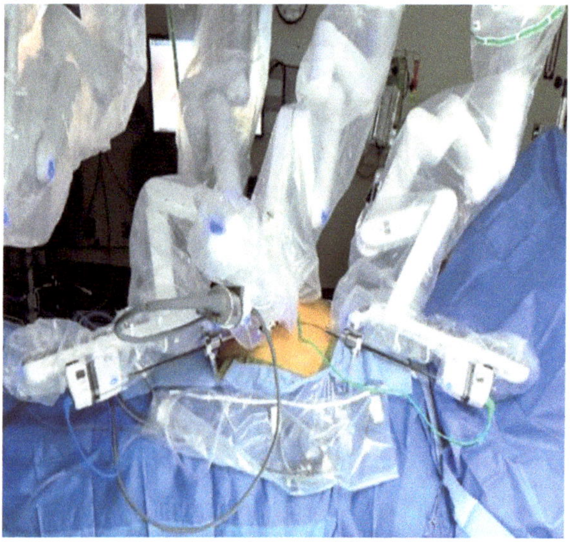

Fig. 11.1 Side docking 90 degrees Da Vinci

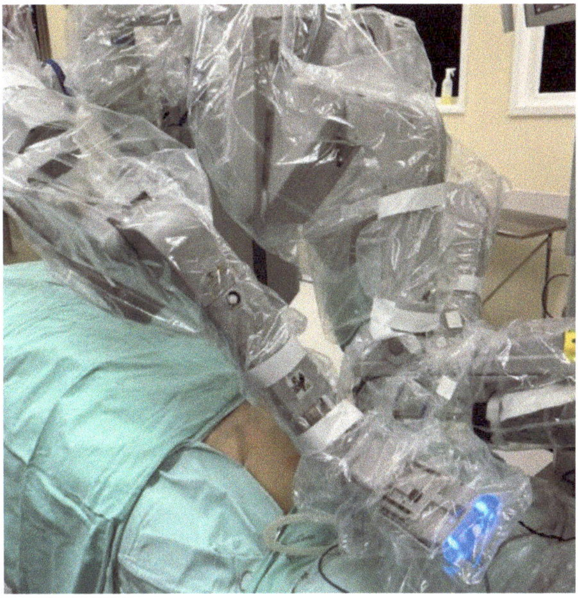

Fig. 11.2 45 degrees at the patient's elbow Da Vinci

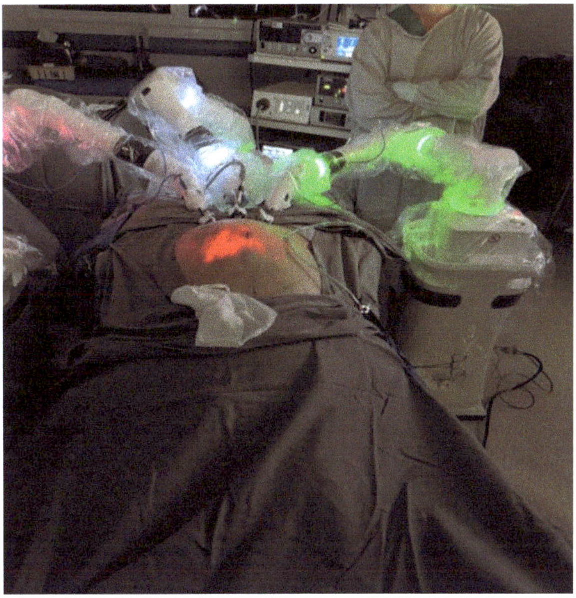

Fig. 11.3 Docking CMR Versius

1. Eight millimeters suprapubic incisions, initial preaponeurotic dissection using retractors and monopolar cautery, and placement of the trocars spaced 6–8 cm apart. We usually dissect superiorly and laterally 4–5 cm prior to trocar positioning (Fig. 11.4).

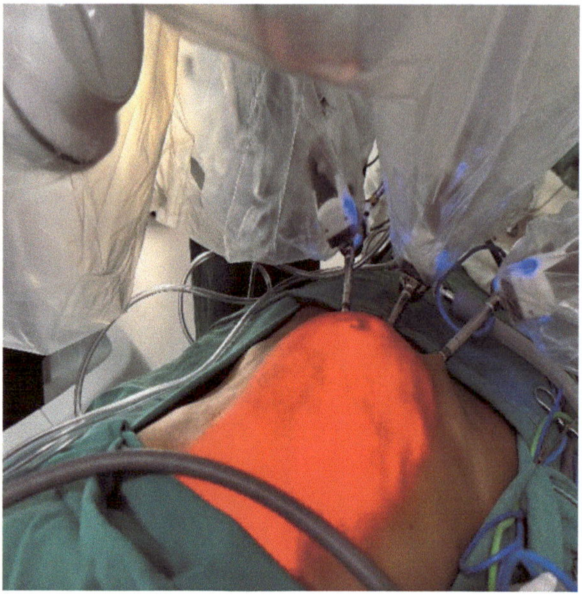

Fig. 11.4 Trocars positioning Da Vinci

2. The subcutaneous tissue is separated from the anterior sheath of the rectus abdominis muscles with limited dissection to the rectus sheath, with the maximum lateral limits being the semilunar lines. CO2 insufflation pressure is maintained at 8–10 mmHg which helps dissection and at these levels prevents subcutaneous emphysema and/or hypercapnia. Release of the umbilical stump and dissection of any hernia sac (if present) are done only after lateral dissection advance, because of the risk of creation of pneumoperitoneum, decreasing operative field (Fig. 11.5). The upper limit of dissection is the costal arches and the xiphoid appendix (Fig. 11.6).
3. Suturing for diastasis recti plication is done in the medial edges of the recti with a distance of 0.5 cm apart, ideally with two suture lines for tension distribution. We preferably use barbed non-absorbable or long-lasting sutures (Fig. 11.7) (STRATAFIX Symmetric PDS 0 18"or VLoc PBT 1 18″). Mesh positioning is indicated only when midline hernias higher than 1.0–1.5 cm are associated.
4. Positioning and fixation of the umbilicus stalk are done at aponeurosis with one or two simple sutures. Placement of a drain is essential once seroma is the most common complication. Drain removal usually is done when the volume is less than 30 ml/day.

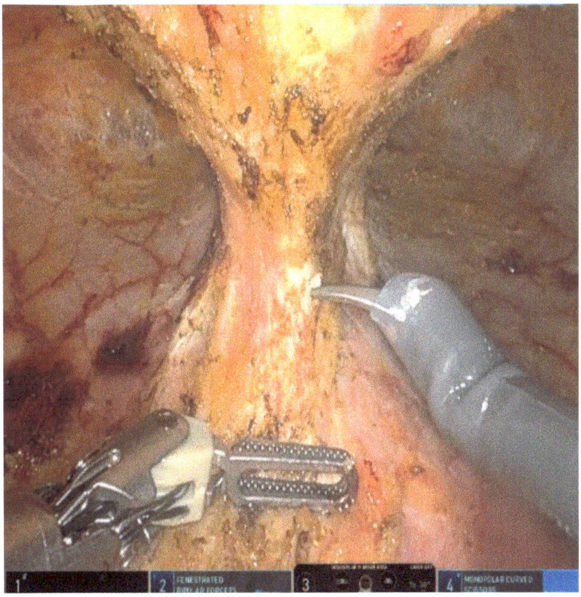

Fig. 11.5 Lateral dissection and umbilical stump at place

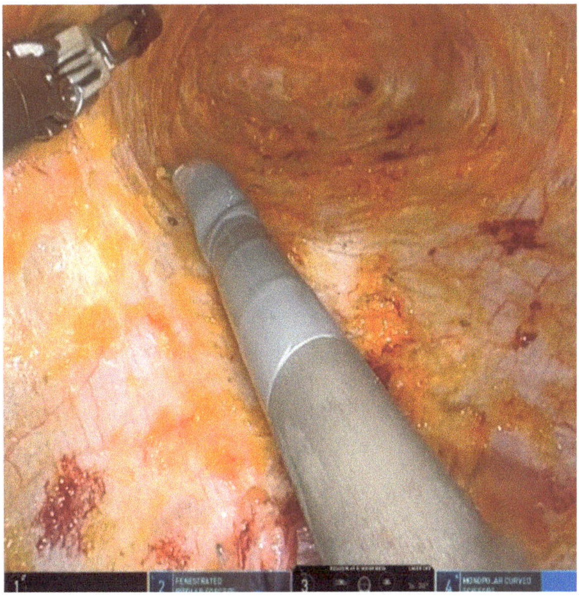

Fig. 11.6 Onlay dissection (premuscular)

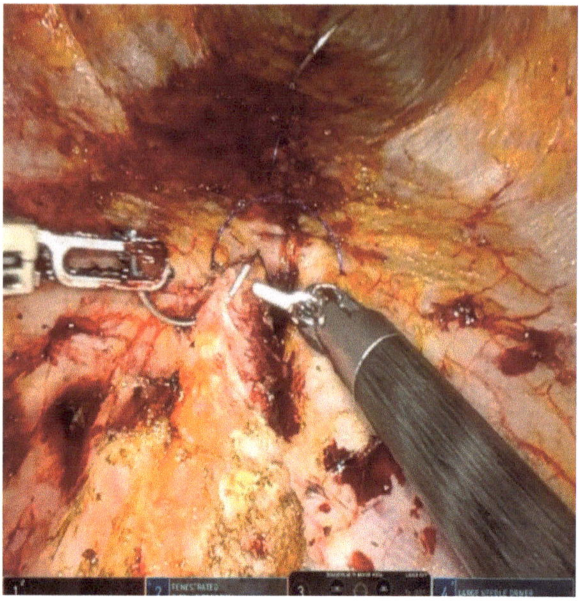

Fig. 11.7 Diastasis recti plication

11.5.2 *Retro-muscular (R-ETEP, TARUP)*

In this technique, we access the retro-muscular space, between the rectus abdominis muscle and the posterior sheath of the rectus (sublay). Thus, we do not dissect the subcutaneous tissue, thereby reducing surgical wound complications. Dissection can be performed using a dissector balloon (Spacemaker) (Fig. 11.8) or manually with finger dissection followed by the use of robotic or laparoscopic optics and instruments (Fig. 11.9). The rectus diastasis plication is done upward at the "roof" of the abdominal wall in the retro-muscular compartment. The use of the robotic platform in this surgery greatly facilitates retro-muscular dissection but is mainly fundamental for the plication suture of the edges of the abdominal recti. The 3D vision, 360-degree movements, and quality of energy of the platform reduce surgical time and bleeding and significantly improve surgeon ergonomics and facilitate the learning curve.

11.5.2.1 Operative Technique

Surgery is performed with the patient under general anesthesia. Urinary catheter is usually used, reducing the risk for bladder injury at the infrapubic preperitoneal area of dissection. Nasogastric tubes are not routinely used. Antibiotic prophylaxis is done during anesthetic induction.

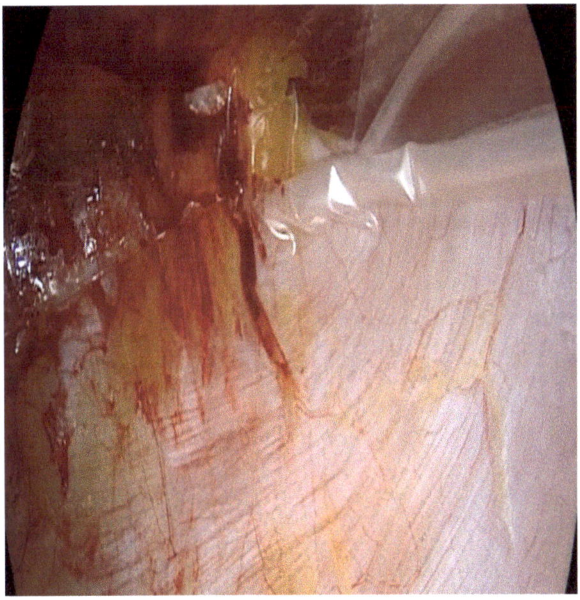

Fig. 11.8 Dissector balloon dissection retro-muscular

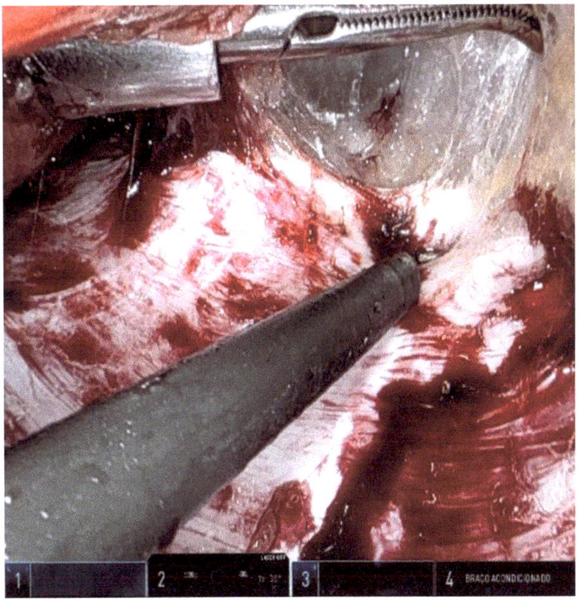

Fig. 11.9 Optic and laparoscopic retro-muscular dissection

11.5.2.2 Patient's and Robotic Position

Patient is placed in a supine position with moderate spine extension. Arms are placed along the body and positioned slightly inferior to the posterior axillar line (Fig. 11.10). Robotic platform positioning is done laterally at a 90-degree angle

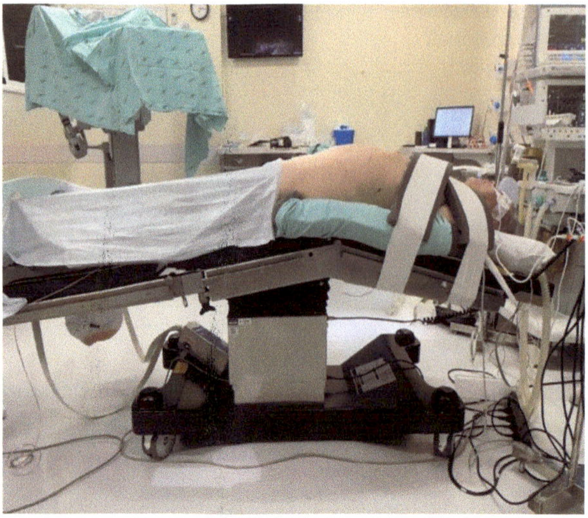

Fig. 11.10 Patient positioning R-Etep

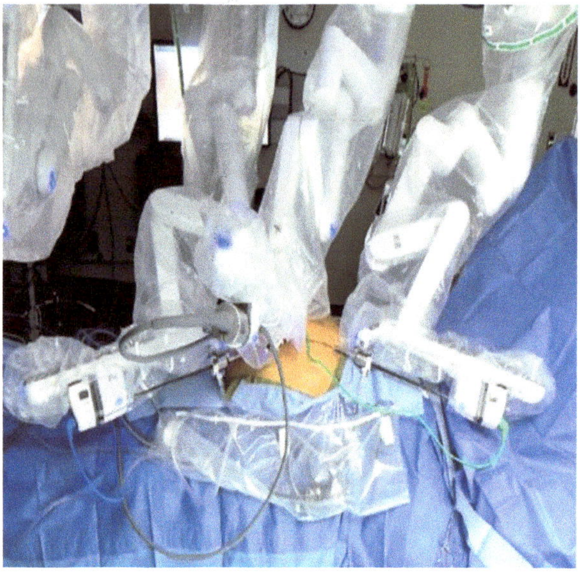

Fig. 11.11 Side docking 45 degrees Da Vinci—intuitive

with the patient (Fig. 11.11) at any side. For the CMR/Versius platform, the robot arms are also positioned aside the patient at a 90-degree angle (Fig. 11.12).

The technical steps are as follows:

1. Pre-costal or subcostal incision of 8 mm slightly medial to the semilunar line and dissection of the retro-muscular space using retractors, finger, and gauze blunt dissection or directly with optical trocar/dissector balloon (Fig. 11.13).

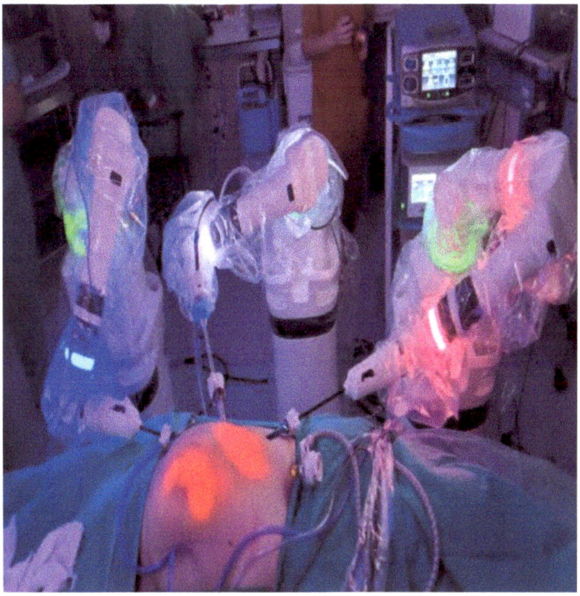

Fig. 11.12 Side docking Versius

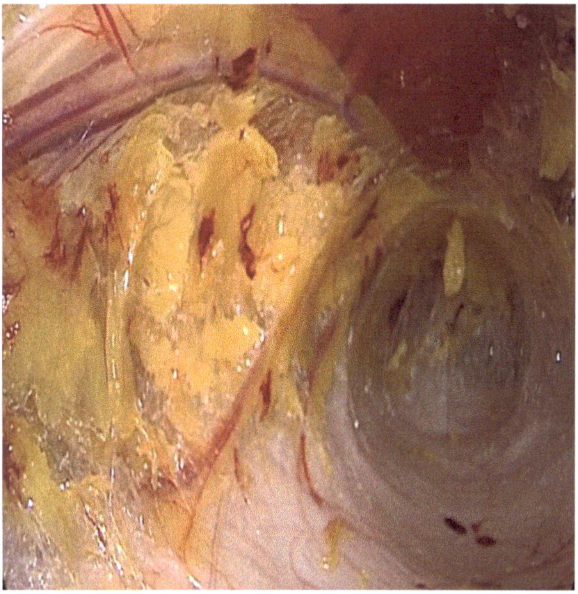

Fig. 11.13 Retro-muscular dissection

2. Dissection of the retro-muscular space using optics or dissector balloon (Spacemaker). The lateral limit of dissection is the semilunar line (neurovascular bundles), and the medial limit is the linea alba (Fig. 11.14).
3. Placement of the three robotic trocars at the lateral edge of the recti with minimal spacing of 6–8 cm is done after initial dissection of the retro-muscular space

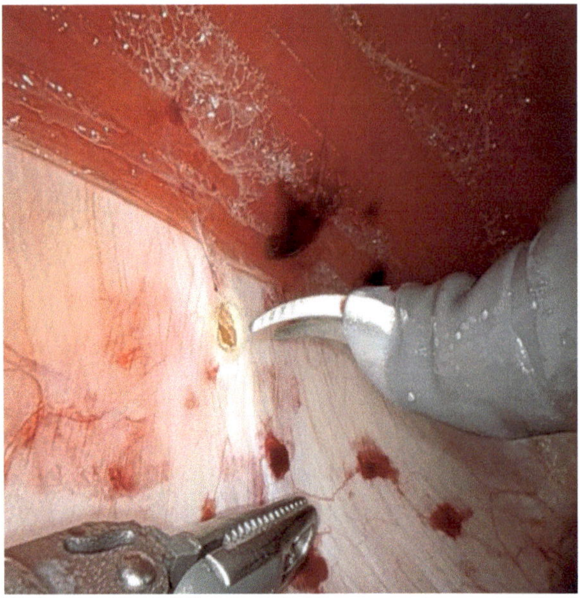

Fig. 11.14 Medial Limit—Linea Alba

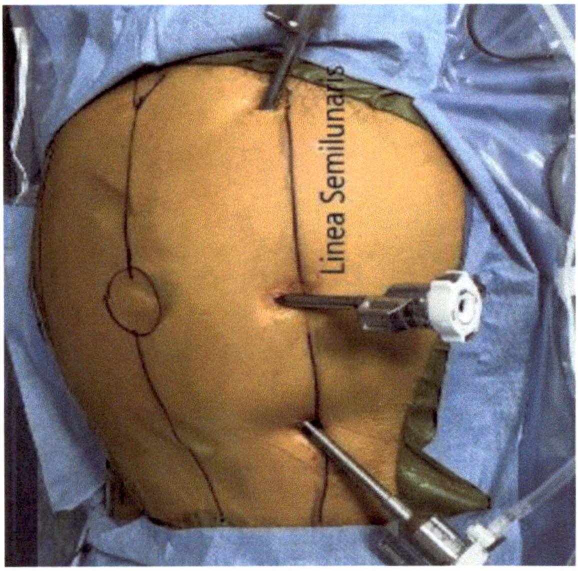

Fig. 11.15 R-Etep trocars

with the dissection balloon or initially with laparoscopic instruments through the robotic trocars. The lower trocar must be positioned at least 2 cm away from the anterior superior iliac spine to avoid arm collision with the bony structure and cause limitation of the movements of the robotic arm. Robotic docking (Fig. 11.15).

4. After robotic docking we continue with the complete dissection of the retro-muscular space laterally reaching the semilunar line and medially the linea alba. We perform the opening of the posterior sheath in the midline with a minimum margin of 5 mm to the rectus muscle (Fig. 11.16), identifying the diastasis in the linea alba until finding the contralateral rectus abdominis muscle (Fig. 11.17). This 5 mm margin facilitates suturing of the anterior abdominal wall afterward.
5. Opening of the posterior sheath of the contralateral rectus abdominis muscle with a 5 mm margin (Fig. 11.18) and creation of the contralateral retro-muscular space until the semilunar line and neurovascular bundles are reached (Fig. 11.19).
6. Diastasis recti plication by approximating the edges of the posterior sheath with continuous suture using barbed non-absorbable or long-lasting suture (STRATAFIX Symmetric PDS 0 18"or VLoc PBT 1 18″) (Fig. 11.20). More than one suture line can be performed for better tension distribution. Robotic platforms give an extra advantage at this time with the image inversion resource (Fig. 11.21). Recently we are placing a suture inverting the diastasis, preventing the palpable anterior "ridge" after posterior plication. This "ridge" tends to solve after 3–4 weeks postoperatively.
7. If there is any peritoneal injury in the midline or posterior sheath, closure of the holes is indicated. Drainage of the space is optional according to the surgeon's personal experience, preventing hematoma formation.

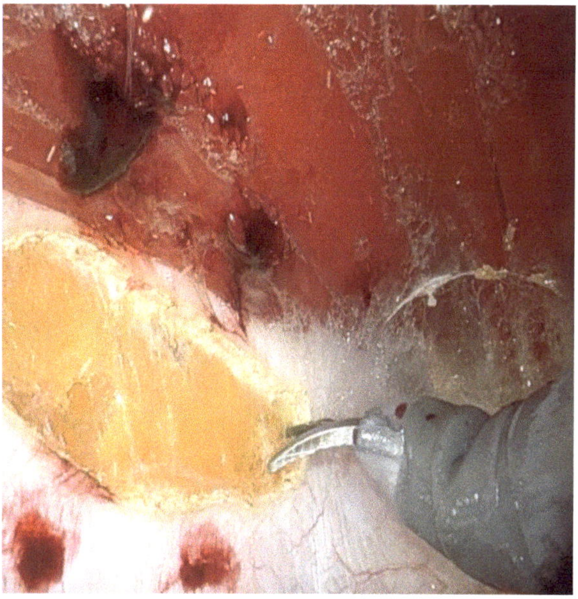

Fig. 11.16 Cross-over—5 mm margin

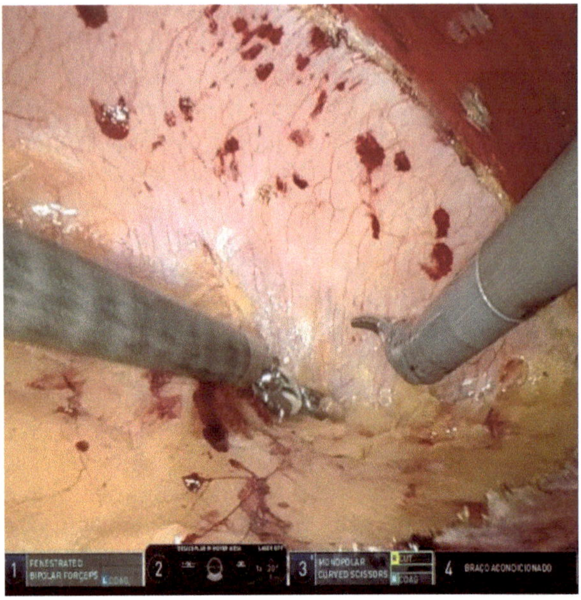

Fig. 11.17 Contralateral rectus muscle

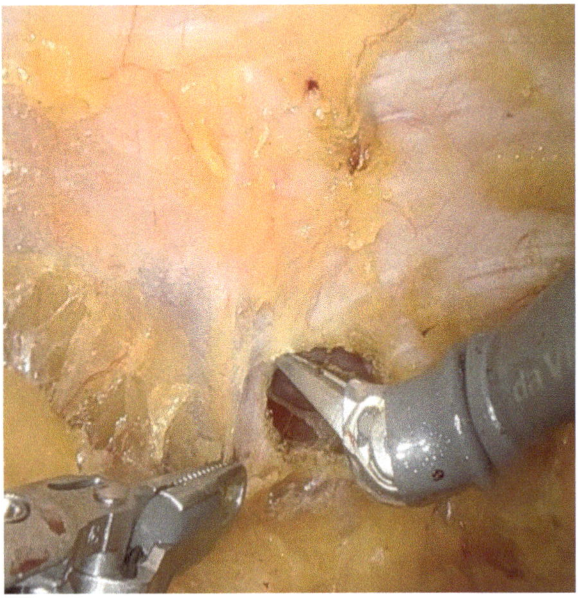

Fig. 11.18 Contralateral posterior sheath—5 mm margin

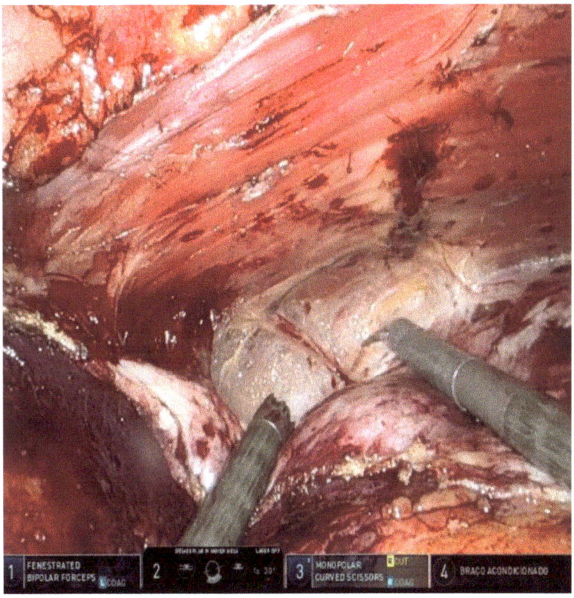

Fig. 11.19 Contralateral neurovascular bundles—lateral margin

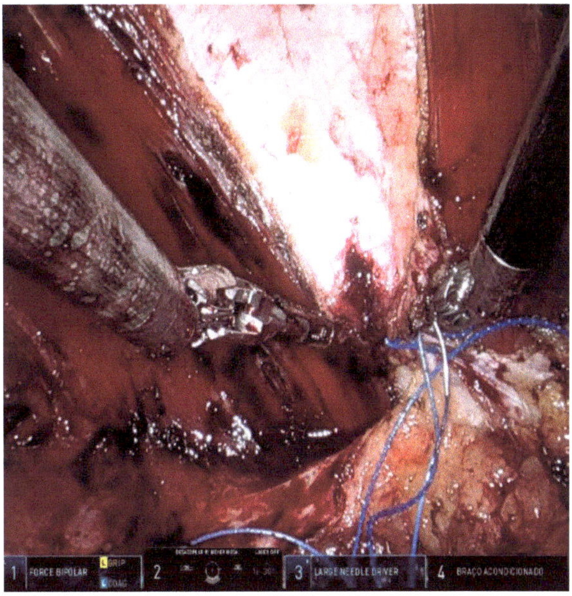

Fig. 11.20 Diastasis recti plication

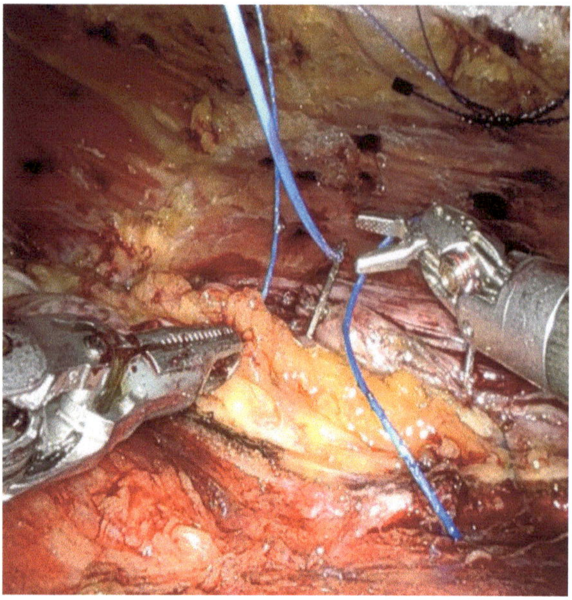

Fig. 11.21 Image inversion facilitating suture

11.5.3 Trans-Abdominal Preperitoneal/Intraperitoneal (R-TAPP/R-TARRD/R-LIRA/R-TES)

There are several nomenclatures and technical variations to correct diastasis recti in the underlay or intraperitoneal compartment. In this technique, the approximation of the diastasis recti is also done upward in the "roof" of the abdominal wall, intraperitoneal, or trans-abdominal preperitoneal. Robotic technology greatly facilitates this type of suturing, improving the technical quality of the plication and surgeon ergonomics. Several authors have described different approaches for this type of surgery. These vary in trans-abdominal accesses, with dissection of peritoneal flaps (R-TAPP/R-TARRD/R-TES) or completely intraperitoneal with (R-LIRA) or without opening the posterior sheath of the rectus and plication. In this technique, the subcutaneous tissue is also not dissected, reducing surgical wound complications. It seems to be a good option, especially in smaller supraumbilical diastasis in association with more aggressive liposuction with the use of skin retraction devices (Renuvion/Body Tite/Argoplasma/Morpheus), as there may be a higher risk of skin ischemia described by some authors in these cases. To facilitate the technical description, we will focus on the access our team has expertise, where we perform intraperitoneal plication.

11.5.3.1 Operative Technique

Surgery is performed with the patient under general anesthesia. Urinary catheter is inserted, reducing the risk for bladder injury as we place trocars at a suprapubic position. Nasogastric tubes are not routinely used. Antibiotic prophylaxis is done during anesthetic induction.

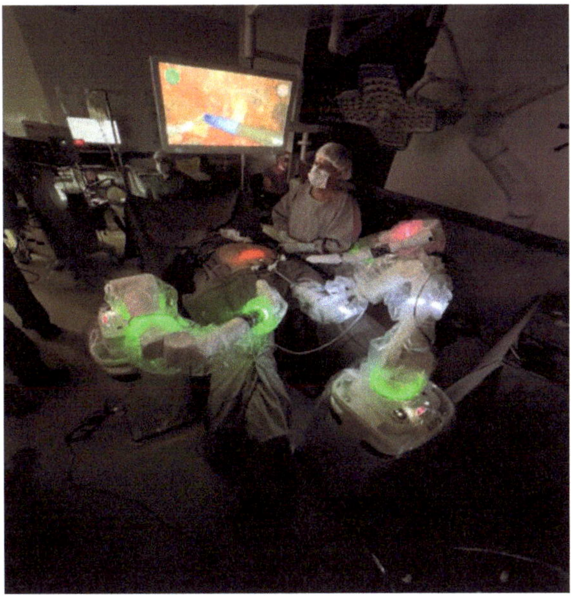

Fig. 11.22 Versius in between legs docking

11.5.3.2 Patient's and Robotic Position

Patient is placed in supine position with slight spine extension. Robotic platform positioning depends on what platform we are using. For CMR/Versius platform, the robot arms are positioned between the patient's legs (Fig. 11.22). For Intuitive platforms the robot is positioned 90 degrees lateral to the patient from any side (Xi platform) (Fig. 11.23) and 45 degrees to the patient's elbow also from any side (Fig. 11.24).

The technical steps are as follows:

1. Placement of a subcostal Veress needle (in the Palmer's point) and pneumoperitoneum.
2. Placement of suprapubic 8 mm robotic ports spaced 6–8 cm apart. Surgeon should be careful when visualizing epigastric vessels for positioning lateral trocars. Robotic docking (Fig. 11.25).
3. We always perform an inventory of the cavity and adhesiolysis if needed, and then we divide and "pull down" the falciform and round ligament to better expose the medial edges of the rectus, posterior sheath, and xiphoid appendix (Figs. 11.26 and 11.27).
4. Diastasis recti plication is done with continuous suture using barbed nonabsorbable or long-lasting suture (STRATAFIX Symmetric PDS 0 18"or VLoc PBT 1 18″). Suturing is done every 5 mm, and we can use two suture lines to reduce tension and improve approximation (Figs. 11.28 and 11.29). External compression by the assistant of the medial rectal edge to be involved in the suture can facilitate. Also, reducing intra-abdominal pressure with a pneumoperitoneum of 8–10 mmHg can facilitate. Drains are not usually indicated.

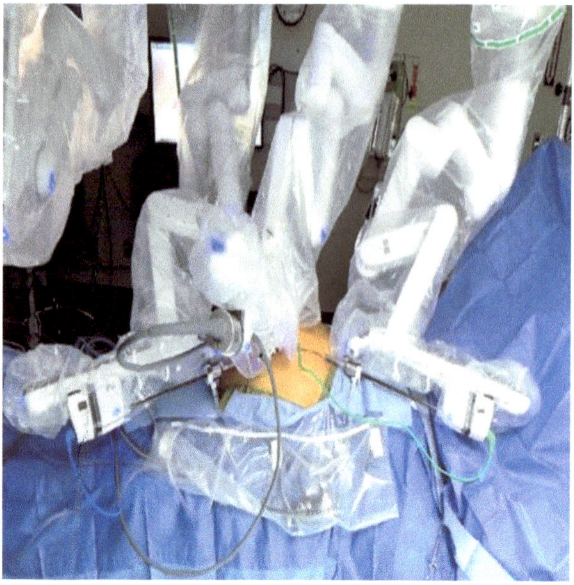

Fig. 11.23 Da Vinci Xi 90 degrees side docking

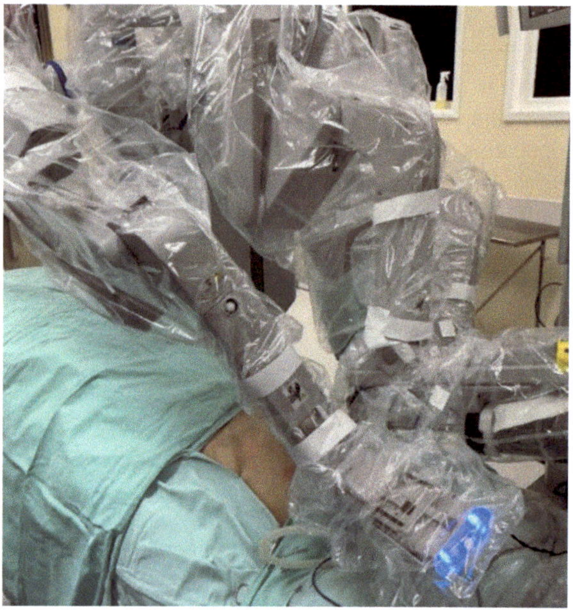

Fig. 11.24 Da Vinci Si 45 degrees from elbow's docking

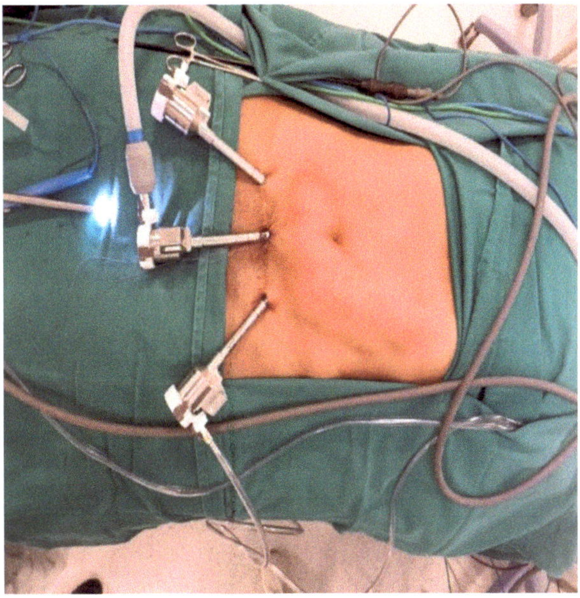

Fig. 11.25 Trocars position

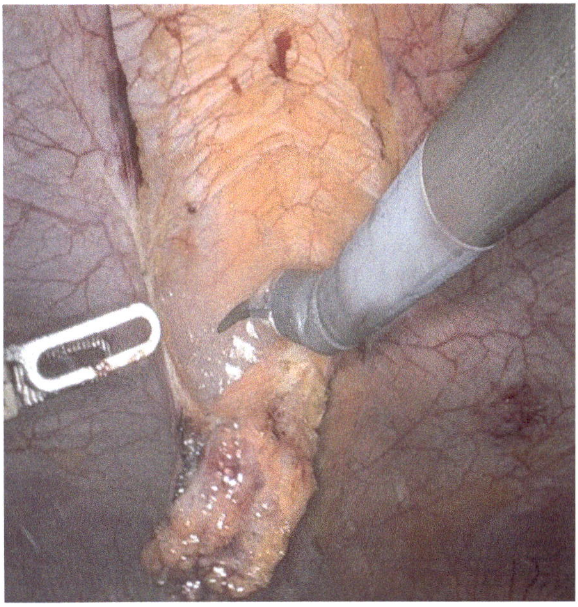

Fig. 11.26 Falciform ligament pulling down—Da Vinci

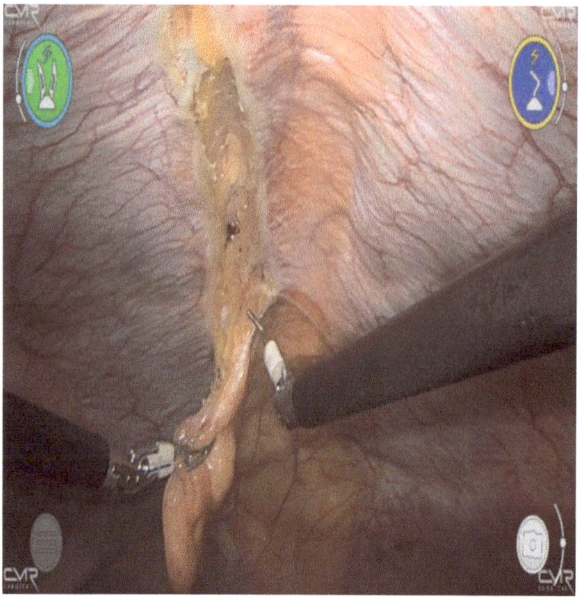

Fig. 11.27 Falciform ligament pulling down—Versius

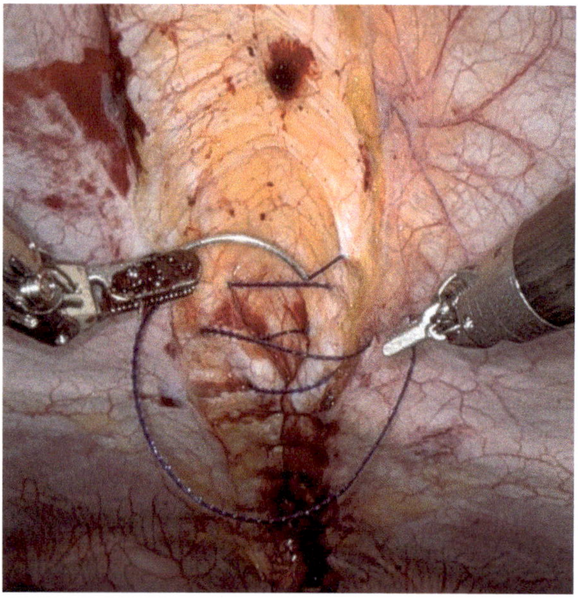

Fig. 11.28 Diastasis recti plication

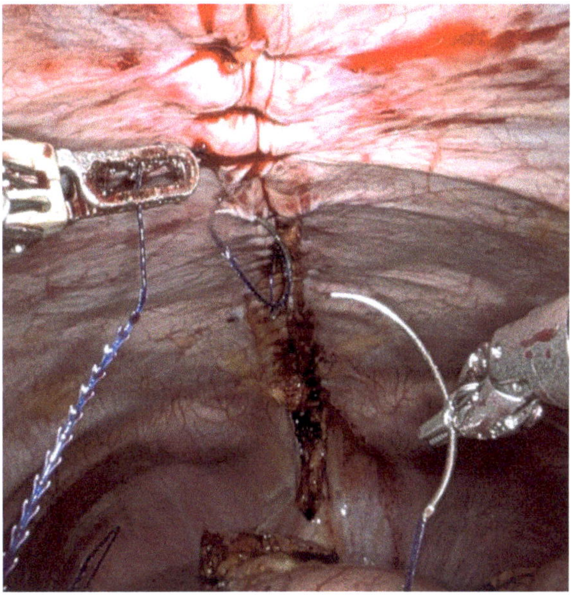

Fig. 11.29 Diastasis recti plication final

11.6 Conclusions

Advancements in understanding abdominal wall anatomy and the concept of abdominal core and its spaces and anatomical relationships, combined with the development of dedicated abdominal wall surgeons and technological advances, are certainly the main factors associated with the growth of surgery for diastasis recti [6, 12]. Currently, it is known that the indications for diastasis recti plication are not merely aesthetic but also functional, leading to an improvement in the patient's quality of life in the short and long term [1, 2]. Minimally invasive techniques, whether laparoscopic or robotic surgery, have brought numerous benefits to patients and surgeons and are now being considered the gold standard techniques [3–10].

The use of robotic platforms, especially in the abdominal wall, seems to bring even more benefits compared to other surgical specialties. It allows the surgeon to perform the ideal and tailored surgery for each patient, without the technical and ergonomic barriers that accompany conventional laparoscopy. For these reasons, the robotic approach for abdominal wall surgery may be one of the areas with the greatest applicability and growth in the next few years.

However, the main barrier to broader adoption and dissemination of this technology is still due to the high costs of platforms and associated supplies [14, 15]. With new platforms entering the market, new pricing policies, and an increasing number of qualified surgeons, coupled with the growing demand by patients with surgical indications, the robotic approach for the treatment of diastasis recti will be consolidated.

References

1. Parker MA, Millar LA, Dugan SA. Diastasis rectus abdominis and lumbo-pelvic pain and dysfunction-are they related? J Women's Health Phys Ther. 2009;33(2):15–22.
2. Fiori F, Ferrara F, Gobatti D, Gentile D, Stella M. Surgical treatment of diastasis recti: the importance of an overall view of the problem. Hernia. 2021;25(4):871–82. https://doi.org/10.1007/s10029-020-02252-0. Epub 2020 Jun 20.
3. Bellido Luque J, Bellido Luque A, Valdivia J, Suarez Grau JM, Gómez Menchero J, García Moreno J, Guadalajara Jurado J. Totally endoscopic surgery on diastasis recti associated with midline hernias. The advantages of a minimally invasive approach. Prospective cohort study. Hernia. 2015;19(3):493–501.
4. Core GB, Mizgala CL, Bowen JC, Vasconez LO. Endoscopic abdominoplasty with repair of diastasis recti and abdominal wall hernia. Clin Plast Surg. 1995;22(4):707–22.
5. Aitken G, Gallego EJ. A novel robotic approach for the repair of Abdominal Wall hernias with concomitant diastasis recti: outcomes and long-term follow-up. Surg Laparosc Endosc Percutan Tech. 2023;33(2):137–40. https://doi.org/10.1097/SLE.0000000000001155.
6. Mazzola Poli de Figueiredo S, Tastaldi L, Mao RD, Lu R. Management of diastasis recti during ventral hernia repair: an analysis of the abdominal core health quality collaborative. Hernia. 2024;28(4):1063–8. https://doi.org/10.1007/s10029-023-02753-8. Epub ahead of print.
7. Corrêa MA. Videoendoscopic subcutaneous techniques for aesthetic and reconstructive plastic surgery. Plast Reconstr Surg. 1995;96(2):446–53.
8. Belyansky I, Daes J, Radu VG, Balasubramanian R, Reza Zahiri H, Weltz AS, Sibia US, Park A, Novitsky Y. A novel approach using the enhanced-view totally extraperitoneal (eTEP) technique for laparoscopic retromuscular hernia repair. Surg Endosc. 2018;32(3):1525–32. https://doi.org/10.1007/s00464-017-5840-2.
9. Claus CMP, Malcher F, Cavazzola LT, Furtado M, Morrell A, Azevedo M, Meirelles LG, Santos H, Garcia R. Subcutaneous onlay laparoscopic approach (SCOLA) for ventral hernia and rectus abdominis diastasis repair: technical description and initial results. Arq Bras Cir Dig. 2018;31(4):e1399. https://doi.org/10.1590/0102-672020180001e1399.
10. Juárez Muas DM. Preaponeurotic endoscopic repair (REPA) of diastasis recti associated or not to midline hernias. Surg Endosc. 2019;33(6):1777–82. https://doi.org/10.1007/s00464-018-6450-3.
11. Malcher F, Lima DL, Lima RNCL, Cavazzola LT, Claus C, Dong CT, Sreeramoju P. Endoscopic onlay repair for ventral hernia and rectus abdominis diastasis repair: why so many different names for the same procedure? A qualitative systematic review. Surg Endosc. 2021;35(10):5414–21. https://doi.org/10.1007/s00464-021-08560-5.
12. Forester E, Sadiq A. Comparative analysis of the efficacy and functionality of abdominoplasty versus minimally invasive techniques in the surgical treatment of diastasis rectus abdominis in postpartum women. Surg Endosc. 2023;37(12):9052–61. https://doi.org/10.1007/s00464-023-10540-w. Epub 2023 Nov 10.
13. ElHawary H, Abdelhamid K, Meng F, Janis JE. A comprehensive, evidence-based literature review of the surgical treatment of rectus diastasis. Plast Reconstr Surg. 2020;146(5):1151–64. https://doi.org/10.1097/PRS.0000000000007252.
14. Morrell ALG, Morrell-Junior AC, Morrell AG, Mendes JMF, Tustumi F, DE-Oliveira-E-Silva LG, Morrell A. The history of robotic surgery and its evolution: when illusion becomes reality. Rev Col Bras Cir. 2021;48:e20202798. https://doi.org/10.1590/0100-6991e-20202798.
15. Lima DL, Pinto RD, Trauczynski P, Liu J, Cavazzola LT. Feasibility of image inversion for ventral hernia repair using the Versius system. J Laparoendosc Adv Surg Tech A. 2024;34(2):144–6. https://doi.org/10.1089/lap.2023.0404. Epub 2023 Dec 6.

Chapter 12
Repair of Large Diastasis Recti

Derlin M. Juárez Muas and Ezequiel M. Palmisano

The diastasis of the rectus abdominis muscles (DRA) is a frequent entity; it is observed in both sexes, with a higher prevalence in women after pregnancy and puerperium, leaving as a permanent condition between 15% and 32% [1, 2]. According to the Classification of Rectus Diastasis proposed by the German Hernia Society (DHG) and the International Endohernia Society (IEHS) [3], the diastasis, in relation to its size, can be small (W1), medium (W2), or severe (W3); this last group of patients, reported in 6% of cases, is mainly represented by multiparous women [2] and by patients with rapid and wide weight fluctuations and is associated with linea alba hernias in 100% of cases (umbilical, epigastric, and/or incisional) [2, 4]. This anatomo-functional alteration of the abdominal wall conditions a clinical and cosmetic problem, describing manifestations, such as dorso-lumbar pains (68%), digestive disorders (constipation), and alterations of the pelvic floor associated with urogynecological pathologies (60%) [4–6].

Juarez Muas et al. in 2021 suggested to carry out a subdivision in the group of patients with Dra W3, in Dra W3 a to the 5–8 cm (Fig. 12.1a), and Dra W3 b to Dra > 8 cm (Fig. 12.1b because in this subgroup there is a serious weakness of the entire abdominal wall and urogynecological alterations of the pelvic floor and of respiratory mechanics) [7]. In some cases, muscle weakness is evidenced throughout the abdominal wall (defeated abdomen) when DR is of great magnitude, as

D. M. Juárez Muas (✉)
Argentine Hernia Association of Surgery, Salta, Argentina

Argentine Hernia Association, Salta, Argentina

Hispano-American Hernia Society, Salta, Argentina

Public Maternal-Child Hospital, Salta, Argentina

National University of Tucumán, Tucumán, Argentine

E. M. Palmisano
Italian University Institute of Rosario (IUNIR), Rosario, Argentina

S. Cuccomarino et al. (eds.), *New Concepts in Diastasi Recti Surgery*,
https://doi.org/10.1007/978-3-031-74947-6_12

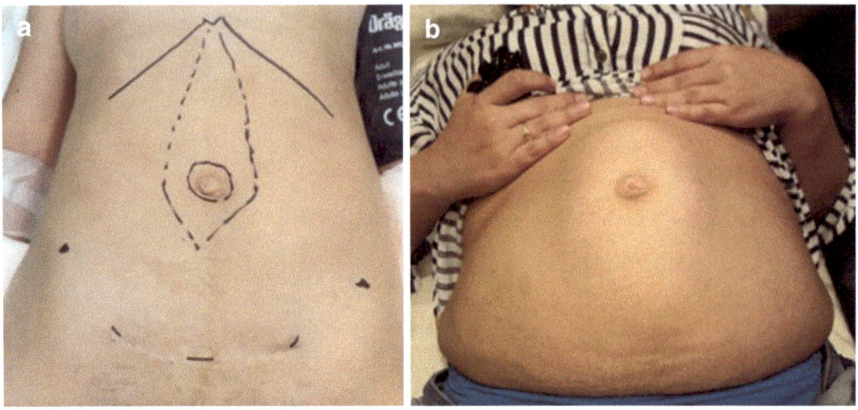

Fig. 12.1 (a) Patient with diastasis recti abdominis (DRA) W3 A and (b) DRA W3 B

evidence of a hypotonia of the abdominal core, many times, simulating a pregnancy (Fig. 12.2a, b), considerably affecting the quality of life [4–7].

The repair of the DRA W3 associated with hernias of the midline is a challenging situation for the surgeon, because the alba line is very thinned and large, usually associated with multiple hernia defects. This predisposes to the opening of the peritoneum and/or aponeurosis and entry to the abdominal cavity. This generates a difficulty in the restitution of the midline at the time of performing the suture, with a high risk of developing a tension closure and favoring a tear of the rectum sheath, an acute eventration contained between the mesh and the abdominal wall, exposure of abdominal viscera, or a postoperative abdominal compartment syndrome [4, 7].

When carrying out a dynamic parietal repair, it is taken for granted that a closure of the defect will be carried out, and the wall will be refunctionalized with the "medialization" of the rectus abdominis muscles.

For this, it is so important the aponeurotic sheath, since the restructured wall works as primary support and prevents excessive tension on the mesh, allowing greater mesh-tissue interface, facilitating its integration into the cicatrization process, reducing the possibility of recurrence [7, 8].

In this selected group of patients, the correct diagnosis through physical examination and computed axial tomography is of great importance. Preoperative planning and preparation are the key points to optimize the outcome of surgery, allow adequate recovery in the shortest possible time, and minimize the risk of postoperative complications and hospitalization times [1–4, 7–12].

Therefore, abdominopelvic physiotherapy acquires great importance in preoperative management and postoperative muscle recovery. If carried out by trained physiotherapists and kinesiologists, correct preparation of the abdominal wall (anterior and posterior) and the pelvic floor can be achieved by strengthening the abdominal core through the use of isometric abdominal exercises, hypopressive exercises (postural and respiratory) which strengthen the transversus muscle, and neuromuscular electrostimulation in one or more muscles. These actions allow a re-education

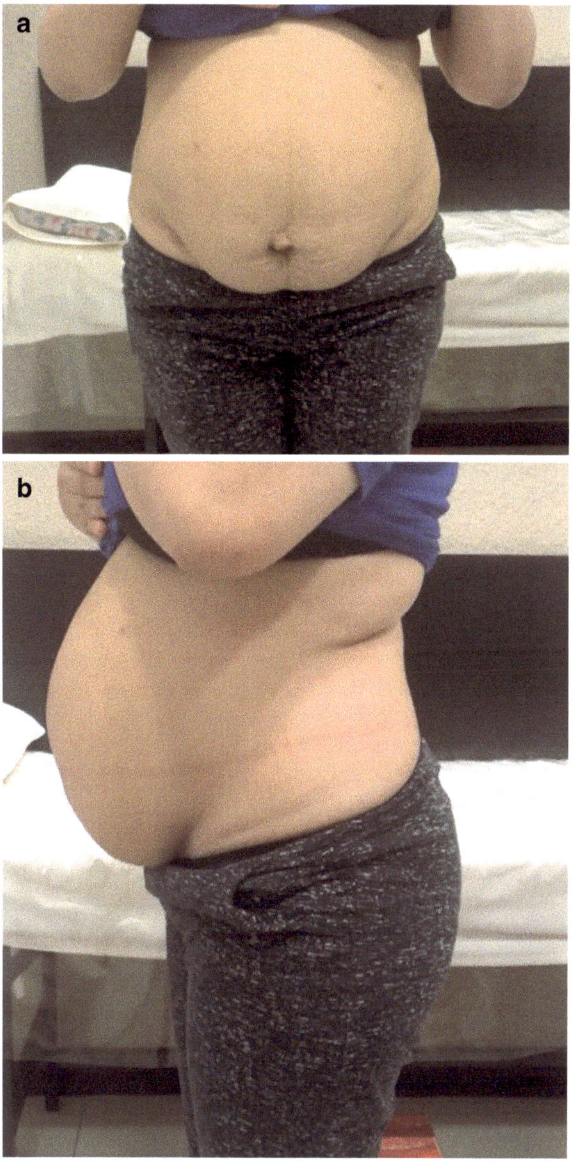

Fig. 12.2 (**a** and **b**) Patient with a defeated abdomen with DRA of 13 cm

of the abdominal wall and pelvic floor, since DRA is frequently associated with stress urinary incontinence [13]. All this allows muscle strengthening and rehabilitation of the abdominal wall, with an excellent anatomical, functional, and aesthetic result. Another work carried out by kinesiologists is manual lymphatic drainage, which improves lymphatic and superficial vascular microcirculation, which reduces the sensation of swelling and improves skin sensitivity with greater well-being for patients. It provides better healing and a reduction of the seroma in the postoperative period, leading patients to cope better with the postoperative period, facilitating their return to usual activities in the shortest possible time [5, 6]. After adequate evaluation, selection, and preparation of the patient for approximately 8 weeks, the surgical indication and type of surgical approach are decided. In patients with DRA and with significant dermoadipose flap or apron belly 1 year after giving birth, abdominoplasty and classic dermolipectomy are recommended for the evident aesthetic benefit [5, 14], but it must be clarified that there is a selected group of patients for whom abdominoplasty surgery is indicated but who refuse this option due to extensive scarring and surgical aggressiveness. If the flap is small and the patient wishes to change the image of her body contour, the MILA tactic would be the indication [15, 16].

In patients with large diastasis without skin flaps or who refuse open surgery, we recommend the REPA technique [2, 5, 6, 17]. The main objective is to give priority to the anatomical and functional restoration of the midline and the repair of hernia defects; this does not make the aesthetic aspect any less important. According to the Classification of Diastasis Recti of the German Hernia Society (DHG) and the International Endohernia Society (IEHS) [3], interrectal distance greater than 5 cm is defined as severe DR, without discriminating against DRA with a transverse diameter greater than 8 cm, as we have mentioned above. In the latter, closure of the midline without tension is practically impossible, requiring in these cases the support of neoadjuvant techniques such as TBA or the release of the external oblique muscle (uni- or bilateral) in order to perform a tension-free suture. In rectus diastases greater than 8 cm (DRA W3 B), if botulinum toxin has not been previously applied, a unilateral or bilateral muscle discharge is to be considered. It will depend on the size of the DRA, whether it is primary or recurrent, the laxity or stiffness of the abdominal wall, and the caliber of the suture used, since there are patients with 8 cm DRA and with a loose abdominal wall and if we use a No. 0 or 1 barbed suture for plication of the rectus muscles, muscle discharge may not be necessary. In DRA W3 A (5–8 cm), there are usually not many inconveniences to perform plication of the rectus muscles [7].

Preoperative preparation of the abdominal wall is carried out with botulinum toxin type A (TBA), and the minimally invasive endoscopic technique (REPA) becomes an excellent option for the management of DRA (W3) associated with midline hernia. The TBA infiltration technique is carried out in a scheduled and outpatient session. It is performed in a triangular area between the costal margin and the iliac crest (Fig. 12.3a). This area has the highest density of neuromuscular unions of the broad muscles of the abdomen; at this level and in correspondence with the mid-axillary line, 1 point is marked for each side (Fig. 12.3b). The 100 RU of TBA was diluted in 4 cc of saline and applied 2 cc, 50 RU on each side (100 RU in total) under ultrasound guidance (Fig. 12.3c), 30 days before surgery [7].

Patients undergo a surgical examination 15 days after application, to evaluate the effect of the TBA and plan the operation between 30 and 45 days after the infiltration. Both at rest and in Valsalva, flaccid paralysis of the large abdominal muscles is evident, effects similar to those observed by Ibarra-Hurtado et al. [7–12].

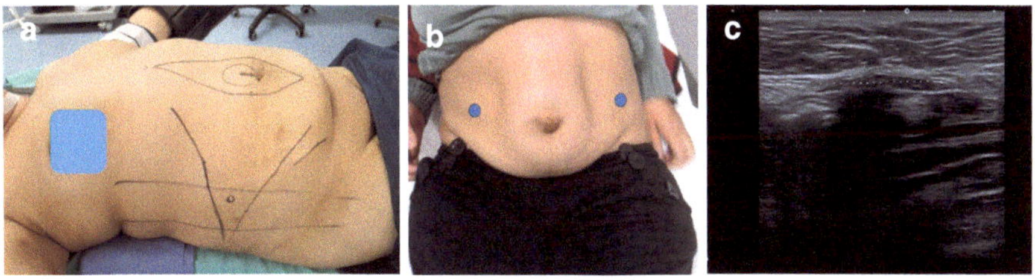

Fig. 12.3 (**a**) Marking of the TBA application site. (**b**) TBA application point. (**c**) Identification of the needle and TBA solution in the muscular plane under ultrasound guidance

The use of TBA has been shown to produce a temporary (between 6 and 8 months) flaccid paralysis in the abdominal muscles, which promotes midline suturing with less tension in most large defects [9, 10], allowing in selected cases to add component separation techniques as needed [10, 18].

In patients who have not received abdominal wall preparation with TBA, due to poor availability of the patient, refusal of the patient or because the size of the DRA was underestimated, and at the time of performing the plication of the rectus muscles, a suture with evident tension, it is advisable to make relief incisions in the external oblique muscle lateral to the semilunar line, according to the Albanese technique (Fig. 12.4a, b) [2, 5–7, 12]. The muscle discharge can be uni- or bilateral, depending on the extent of the interrectal separation, as supported by J. Daes [18–20], with the aim of obtaining a tension-free midline restitution. This maneuver is irreversible and causes a risk of abdominal wall pseudohernia (swelling at the incision site due to muscle weakness).

Once the dissection of the subcutaneous cellular tissue (SCT) is completed, if the patient has neoadjuvant treatment with TBA or a muscle release has been performed, it continues as a classic REPA [2, 5, 6, 18–20]. If hernia defects are larger than 2 cm, they must be repaired with a non-absorbable suture separately from the plication. We then proceed with the reconstruction of the linea alba using a continuous suture at the level of the internal edge of the aponeurosis of the sheath of the rectus muscles, from the xiphoid process to the pubis with an absorbable barbed suture of absorbable polydioxanone or non-polybutester 0 or 1 (Fig. 12.5a).

On several occasions, it was necessary to remove the optic trocar to complete the suture line at the suprapubic level (Fig. 12.5b).

We believe that midline reconstruction should be performed along its entire length, from the xiphoid appendix to the pubis, and not sectorized, especially in patients with predominance of DRA at the epigastric or periumbilical level, which allows for complete refunctionalization of the abdominal wall. We believe it is a fundamental principle to re-establish the biomechanics of the abdominal wall in its entirety and not in sectors [7, 9, 10].

Before positioning the prosthesis, the neocavity is washed with saline solution to remove clots and devitalized subcutaneous cells to reduce the risk of postoperative infection [2, 5–7, 17, 18, 20].

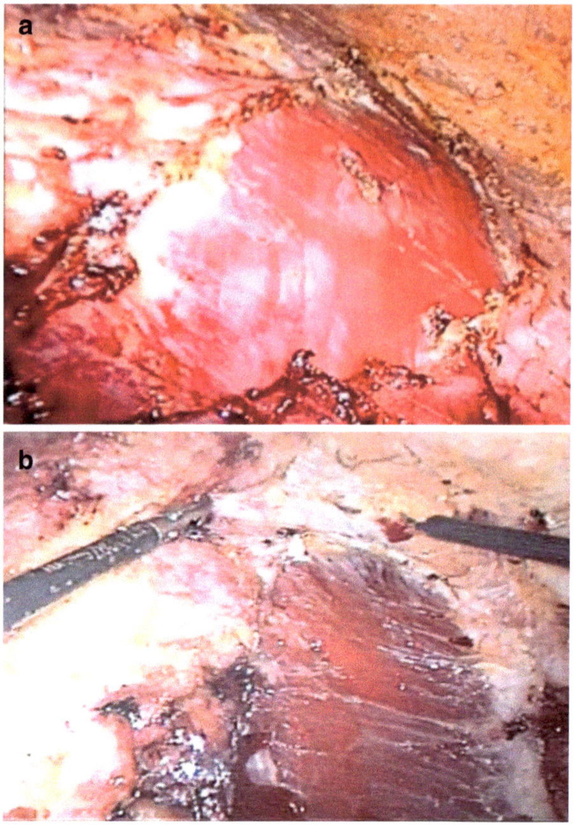

Fig. 12.4 (**a** and **b**) Unloading of the left external oblique

Once the midline has been restored, the abdominal wall is strengthened, especially at the plication level, using light or intermediate weight polypropylene (PP) prostheses, of the classic type or self-fixing, which give greater security to the suture line [7]. The size of the mesh to be used must have an overlap of 5 cm depending on the transverse diameter of the preplication DRA (Fig. 12.6a–c). It is important to handle the prosthesis correctly, avoid contact with the skin, and use antibiotic prophylaxis pre-incision and, in the first 24 h after surgery, to reduce the risk of infection of the surgical site or prosthesis [2, 5, 18].

Fixation of the prosthesis can be performed with absorbable sutures, glues, and absorbable tacks depending on preference or availability, as described in the chapter on endoscopic preaponeurotic repair (REPA).

The use of different fixation materials has no influence on postoperative pain, complications such as seroma, infection, or recurrence of diastasis recti or hernia defects.

If muscle release has been performed, the mesh must cover the entire exposed area of the internal oblique muscle, and its fixation must be carried out on the external edge or flap of the external oblique muscle to refunctionalize it, according to the F. Carbonell-Tatay technique for the large laparoceles [2, 5, 7, 18, 20].

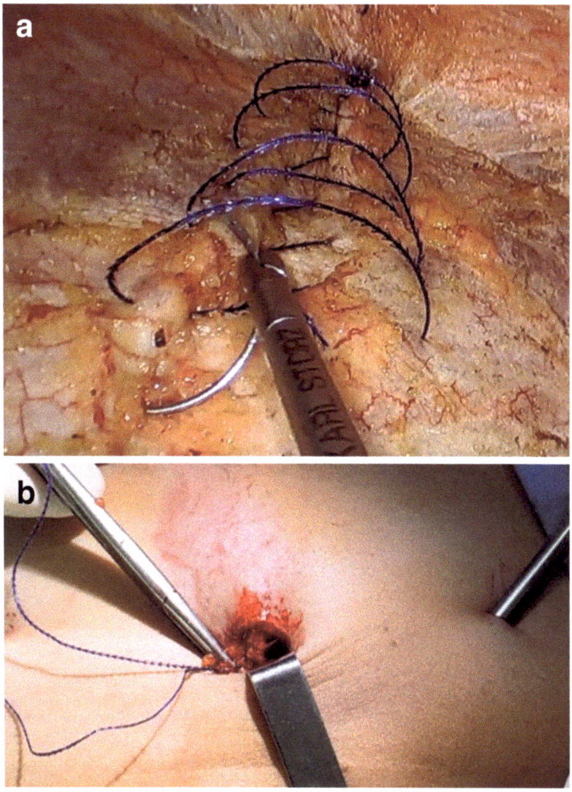

Fig. 12.5 (**a**) Restitution of the midline with barbed polydioxanone suture. (**b**) Completion of plication with extracorporeal suture

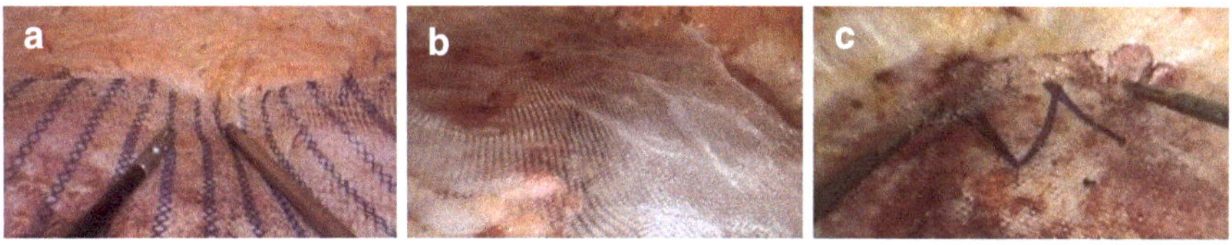

Fig. 12.6 (**a** and **b**) Intermediate density PP meshes and (**c**) self-fixing mesh

Negative pressure suction drains are routinely placed, one or two drains through the iliac portals depending on preference (Fig. 12.7a, b). They are withdrawn when the charge is less than 30 cc/24 h for 2 consecutive days.

Management of W3 B DRA represents a challenge for the surgeons who perform it. Adequate preoperative management by kinesiologists and relaxation of the abdominal wall induced by the application of TBA allow medialization of the rectus muscles without tension. TBA facilitates endoscopic suturing and avoids muscle unloading incisions, an irreversible condition with potential risk of bulging in the postoperative period. It also allows minimizing the risk of postoperative abdominal compartment syndrome and better management of analgesia after surgery by

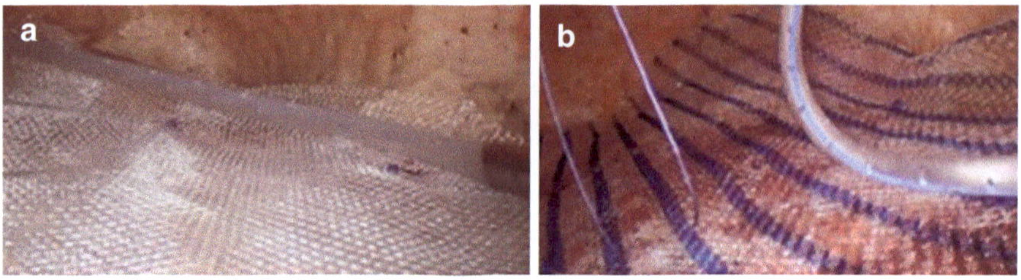

Fig. 12.7 (**a** and **b**) Systematic use of aspiration drains

reducing the level of pain [7, 10, 17–19] and minimizing hospital stay. Furthermore, it allows for an early return to work.

Postoperative seroma and hematomas are the most frequent complications in the endoscopic approach. This topic is developed extensively in the corresponding chapter. The only study reporting TBA preparation of the abdominal wall in large DRA showed no complications or recurrence after 1 year of follow-up [7].

References

1. Mota P, Pascoal AG, Sancho F, et al. Test-retest and intrarater reliability of 2-dimensional ultrasound measurements of distance between rectus abdominis in women. J Orthop Sports Phys Ther. 2012;42(11):940–6.
2. Juárez Muas DM, Palmisano E, Pou Santoja G, Cuccomarino S, González Higuera G, Mayo P, Martínez Maya JD, Domínguez G, Ayala Acosta JC, Chichizola A. Repa- ración endoscópica preaponeurótica (REPA) como tratamiento de la diástasis de los músculos rectos asociada o no a hernias de la línea media. Estudio multicéntrico. Rev Hispanoam Hernia. 2019;7(2):59–65. https://doi.org/10.20960/rhh.194.
3. Reinpold W, Köckerling F, Bittner R, Conze J, Fortelny R, Koch A, Kukleta J, Kuthe A, Lorenz R, Stechemesser B. Classification of rectus diastasis—a proposal by the German Hernia Society (DHG) and the International Endohernia Society (IEHS). Front Surg. 2019;6:1. https://doi.org/10.3389/fsurg.2019.00001.
4. Moreno-Egea A. Abdominoplastia y reparación de hernia incisional: lo que un cirujano general debe saber. Rev Hispanoam Hernia. 2016;4(1):5–12.
5. Juárez MD. Preaponeurotic endoscopic repair (REPA) of diastasis recti associated or not to midline hernias. Surg Endosc. 2019;33(6):1777–82. https://doi.org/10.1007/s00464-018-6450-3.
6. Juárez Muas D, Verasay G, García WM. Reparación endoscópica prefascial de la diástasis de los rectos: descripción de una nueva técnica. Rev Hispanoam Hernia. 2017;5(2):47–51.
7. Muas DM, Palmisano EM, Santoja GP, Paz OR. Adjuvant botulinum toxin for endoscopic management (preaponeurotic endoscopic repair) of severe diastasis recti. Int J Abdom Wall Hernia Surg. 2021;4:45–50.
8. Chávez-Tostado K, Cárdenas-Lailson L, Pérez-Trigos H. Resultado de la aplicación preoperatoria de toxina botulínica A en el tratamiento de hernias incisionales gigantes. Rev hispanoam hernia. 2014;2(4):145–51.
9. Palmisano E, Mustone O, Pou Santoja G, Juárez Muas D, Blanco M. Infiltración preoperatoria con toxina botulínica serotipo A en la preparación de hernias ventralescon defectos de tamaño de 10–15 cm: estudio multicéntrico. Rev hispanoam hernia. 2020;8(4):162–7. https://doi.org/10.20960/rhh.00257.

10. Hernández López A, Villalobos RE. Infiltración de toxina botulínica en la preparación preoperatoria de las hernias con defectos de 10 cm (y hasta 15 cm). Rev hispanoam hernia. 2016;4(2):43–9.
11. Ibarra-Hurtado TR, Nuño-Guzmán CM, Echeagaray-Herrera JE, Robles-Vélez E, de Jesús G-JJ. Use of botulinum toxin type a before abdominal wall hernia reconstruction. World J Surg. 2009;33(12):2553–6. https://doi.org/10.1007/s00268-009-0203-3.
12. Ibarra HT. Toxina botulínica A: su importancia en pacientes con grandes hernias abdominales. Rev hispanoam hernia. 2014;2(4):131–2. https://doi.org/10.1016/j.rehah.2014.05.003.
13. Sánchez Sánchez B. Efectividad de la gimnasia abdominal hipopresiva frente al entrenamiento perineal clásico en el fortalecimiento del suelo pélvico de la mujer: Revisión sistemática. Alcal de Henares: Universidad de Alcal., Facultad de Fisioterapia, Departamento de Fisioterapia; 2012.
14. Brandi CD, Pinto LM. Dermolipectomía asociada a defectos de la pared abdominal. Enciclopedia Cirugía Digestiva; 2016. p. 1–15. www.sacd.org.ar.
15. Palmisano EM, Di Biasio G. Alternativa de manejo miniinvasivo para el tratamiento de pacientes con diástasis abdominal y colgajo dermograso mediante la táctica VER: Vaser® + endoscopia + Renuvion®. Rev Hispanoam Hernia. 2022;10(4):167–71.
16. Claus C, Palmisano EM. MILA (Minimally invasive lipoabdominoplasty) for diastasis recti. Are general surgeons and plastic surgeons fighting or playing together? Rev Argent Cir. 2023;115(4):393–5. https://revista.aac.org.ar/index.php/RevArgentCirug/article/view/637.
17. Juárez Muas D, Cuccomarino S. Reparación Endoscópica Preaponeurótica (REPA). Munual Práctico de Cirugía endoscópica de Pared Abdominal. Ezequiel Palmisano y Col. 1° ed. Ed. Autores de Argentina. Bs. As. 2020. 14:159–70.
18. Juárez Muas D, Palmisano EM, Pou Santonja G, González Higuera LG, Martínez Maya JD, Domínguez G, Ayala Acosta JC, Blanco M, Cuccomarino S, Cabral Castelli ML. Morbilidad a corto y largo plazo de la reparación endoscópica preaponeurótica en la diástasis de los rectos asociada o no a hernia de la línea media: estudio pros- pectivo, multicéntrico e internacional. Rev Hispanoam Hernia. 2023;11(3):111–7.
19. Daes J. Endoscopic subcutaneous approach to component separation. J Am Coll Surg. 2014;218:1–4.
20. Juárez Muas D. (2023). Hernioplastia umbilical laparoscópica asociada a diástasis de los rectos. Schlottmann F—Sadava EE. Cirugía Laparoscópica: Técnica Quirúrgica en Cirugía General. Editorial Medica Panamericana. 51–69.

Chapter 13
Anesthetic Techniques and Postoperative Pain Control

Antonio Toscano

13.1 Introduction

Postoperative pain is a frequently underestimated complication after diastasis recti abdominis (DRA) repair, significantly influencing surgical outcome and patient satisfaction. Several studies describe that pain management significantly decreases in complications with a verifiable reduction of hospitalization days [1, 2].

Therefore, postoperative pain management is essential not only for individual patients, but chronification of underestimated postoperative pain represents an economic burden, with enormous potential for optimization.

In the case of abdominoplasty, the pain derives from a somatic component, resulting from the surgical incision, and from a visceral component. Abnormal abdominal skin sensation (hyposensitivity or hypersensitivity) is common, and there is a risk of developing persistent neuropathic pain [3]; in fact, single case reports describe the existence of neuropathic pain syndromes of the iliohypogastric and lateral femoral cutaneous nerve after abdominoplasty [4].

The mechanisms include direct injury caused by a scalpel or suture and indirect injury such as nerve entrapment in scar tissue. Nerves within the surgical field include the iliohypogastric nerve with its lateral and anterior cutaneous branches, the intercostal nerves with its anterior and lateral cutaneous branches, the lateral femoral cutaneous nerve, and the ilioinguinal nerve. The main reason for pain is likely to be a lesion of the anterior cutaneous branches of the iliohypogastric, intercostal, and subcostal nerves, whereas a few patients have sensory abnormalities suggestive of a lesion of the lateral femoral cutaneous nerve or the ilioinguinal nerve.

A. Toscano (✉)
Department of Anesthesia, Critical Care and Emergency, Città della Salute e della Scienza Hospital, Turin, Italy
e-mail: atoscano@cittadellasalute.to.it

S. Cuccomarino et al. (eds.), *New Concepts in Diastasi Recti Surgery*,
https://doi.org/10.1007/978-3-031-74947-6_13

Even in the case of modern minimally invasive techniques, postoperative pain after surgical DRA repair is often difficult to control; in fact it is multifactorial and derives from the preapopneumoexpansion, the musculofascial plane dissection conducted bilaterally about 2 cm over the costal margin superiorly and along the anterior axillary line laterally, the disconnection of the umbilicus, the rectus muscles' plication, and the fixing of the prosthesis.

13.2 Postoperative Pain Control

Opioids have long been used for postoperative pain management after abdominal wall reconstruction surgery, but they are associated with multiple adverse effects including sedation, respiratory depression, delirium, nausea, vomiting, and ileus [5]. For this reason, the Enhanced Recovery After Surgery (ERAS) guidelines for perioperative care in elective abdominal and pelvic surgery recommend a multimodal opioid-sparing analgesia; this approach facilitates early mobilization and return of bowel function [6].

13.3 Neuraxial Anesthesia

Neuraxial anesthesia, mainly spinal and epidural analgesia, has been proposed to achieve a better postoperative pain control for abdominal surgery.

A mid-thoracic epidural (TEA), T7-10, is recommended for DRA surgery performed through open abdominal surgery. It should be commenced before surgery and continued intraoperatively and ideally for 48–72 h postoperatively [7]. TEA has been shown to be better than systemic opioids in several RCTs for open abdominal surgery [8, 9]. Additional benefits include reduction in the surgical catabolic response, insulin resistance, protein loss, and time to return of bowel function [10]. Unfortunately TEA is burdened by the risk of hypotension with possible fluid overload and urinary retention and failure rates of up to 33.6% [10, 11] and, above all, the risk of spinal epidural hematoma (SEH). SEH is an accumulation of blood in the loose areolar tissue between the vertebrae and the dura of the spinal canal. Typically, the hematoma is asymptomatic, but in rare cases it will compress the spinal cord, with potentially devastating neurological consequences.

The incidence of major complications after neuraxial anesthesia, such as SEH or abscess, is more common than estimated in the past decades, and TEA (compared with spinal anesthesia) is associated with a greater incidence of hematoma and a much greater incidence of abscess [12].

The incidence of SEH after neuraxial anesthesia has historically been approximated to be less than 1 in 150,000 epidural placements and less than 1 in 220,000 spinal anesthetics. However, recent epidemiologic surveys suggest that the frequency is increasing and may be as high as 1 in 3000 in some patient populations [13].

It follows that the American Society of Regional Anesthesia and Pain Medicine (ASRA) is still recommending a conservative approach to neuraxial techniques and other deep blockades, especially in the patient receiving antithrombotic or thrombolytic therapy [13]. For all these reasons, we do not recommend neuraxial anesthesia for postoperative pain control after surgical repair of DRA.

13.4 Abdominal Wall Blocks

Abdominal wall blocks, also called fascial plane blocks, rely on the spread of local anesthetic (LA) within musculofascial planes to anesthetize multiple small nerves or plexuses, rather than targeting specific nerve structures. The nerve itself is not targeted, and the needle is not directed toward the neural axis; therefore, the risks of serious complications such as neural injury and neuraxial hematoma can be prevented or at least reduced.

These blocks are technically straightforward and relatively safe and reduce pain and opioid requirements in many clinical settings. In addition, they are also considered safe in patients receiving anticoagulants and antithrombotic drugs [14].

The popularity of abdominal wall blocks has increased in the last decade, thanks to the introduction of simple yet effective techniques such as the transversus abdominis plane (TAP) block and the widespread availability of ultrasound imaging, accompanied by an explosion in the scientific literature [15].

A variety of fascial plane blocks can be performed to provide anesthesia and/or analgesia for surgical repair of DRA, all performed by injection of LA into fascial planes through which intercostal nerves run. They include the following:

- Transversus abdominis plane (TAP) block
- Rectus sheath block (RSB)
- Quadratus lumborum (QL) plane blocks
- Erector Spinae Plane (ESP) block

Absolute contraindications to abdominal wall blocks include the following:

- Patient refusal
- True local anesthetic allergy
- Risk of local anesthetic toxicity; in other words, the patient has already received the maximum recommended local anesthesia dose
- Local infection at the procedure site

Below discuss the innervation of the abdomen, indications, techniques, and drugs used for some of these blocks and complications specific to each block.

13.4.1 Abdominal Wall Innervation

Numerous nerves traverse the anterolateral abdominal wall to serve regions of the abdominal wall, pelvis, and perineum.

The sensory supply of the skin, muscles, and parietal peritoneum of the anterolateral abdominal wall is derived from ventral rami of the thoracoabdominal intercostal nerves (from T7 to T11), the subcostal nerve (T12), and the L1 spinal nerve. The ilioinguinal (II) and iliohypogastric (IH) nerves arise from the lumbar plexus (L1) and provide sensory cutaneous innervation in the groin, upper hip, and thigh. Cutaneous branches of all of these nerves travel variably through the transversus abdominis (TA) and internal oblique (IO) muscles and course within the transversus abdominis plane (TAP). At the lateral edge of the rectus muscle near the linea semilunaris, the anterior cutaneous branches gather posterior to the rectus muscle, pierce through the muscle, and terminate at the umbilicus and anterior abdominal wall.

The fascial layers in the abdomen are essential to the performance of the abdominal nerve blocks.

The fascial plane is filled with adipose cells, collagen, and elastic fibers of loose connective tissue and a hydrated glycosaminoglycan matrix. It contains vessels and nerves. This plane is readily distended by the hydraulic pressure of the fluid injection (hydrodissection phenomenon).

The planes between the TA and IO muscles, between the rectus muscle and its sheath, and between the transversalis fascia and quadratus lumborum muscle are target sites for deposition of LA.

The peritoneum and bowel lie deep to the rectus sheath and the IO muscle and must be avoided during block placement.

The triangle of Petit, or lower lumbar triangle, refers to the section of the abdominal wall bounded by the iliac crest, the posterior margin of the external oblique muscle, and the lateral margin of the latissimus dorsi muscle. The floor of the triangle is formed by the IO muscle, and the TA muscle inserts on the inner lip of the iliac crest.

13.4.2 Transversus Abdominis Plane (TAP) Block

The transversus abdominis plane (TAP) block is a fascial plane block performed by injecting LA in the plane between transversus abdominis (TA) and internal oblique (IO) muscles or, in the case of subcostal TAP block, between the TA muscle and the posterior sheath of the rectus abdominis (RA) muscles, providing analgesia of the skin, muscles, and parietal peritoneum of the anterior abdominal wall by blocking the anterior branches of the spinal nerves from T7 to L1 [16]. These nerves are anesthetized by the deposition of large volumes of dilute LA (20–40 ml per side) across the transversus abdominis fascial plane.

It's a block technically easy to perform, relatively safe, and best used as adjuncts to multimodal analgesic regimens.

Cadaver studies confirmed that the dermatomal extension, duration, and consequent analgesic efficacy of the tap block are closely related to the type of approach with which it is performed, as well as the concentration and volumes used [17]. The TAP block can be performed with blind or ultrasound-guided technique. In the blind technique, described by Rafi et al. [18], the passage of the two fascial planes (external oblique/internal oblique muscles and internal oblique/transverse muscles) produces a loss of resistance. Although the blind technique, in expert hands, is characterized by a low incidence of complications, the use of ultrasound (US) allows real-time vision of the needle, the target anatomical structures, and the correct diffusion of the AL. The US-guided TAP block, described by Hebbard [19], allows positioning of the needle tip and injection of AL into the transversus abdominis plane.

13.4.2.1 Sonoanatomy and Approaches

The sonoanatomy of the abdominal wall, in the classic approach between the costal margin and the iliac crest on the midaxillary line, is characterized by three muscle layers separated by a hyperechoic band: external oblique (EO), internal oblique (IO), and transversus abdominis (TA) muscles (Fig. 13.1).

The goal of the block is to place the tip of the needle between the OI and TA muscles and inject the AL into the fascial plane between the two muscles (Fig. 13.2).

Four approaches of ultrasound-guided TAP block are described:

- In the **subcostal approach**, a linear transducer is placed in an oblique orientation along the lower margin of the rib cage. Scanning toward the midline will reveal

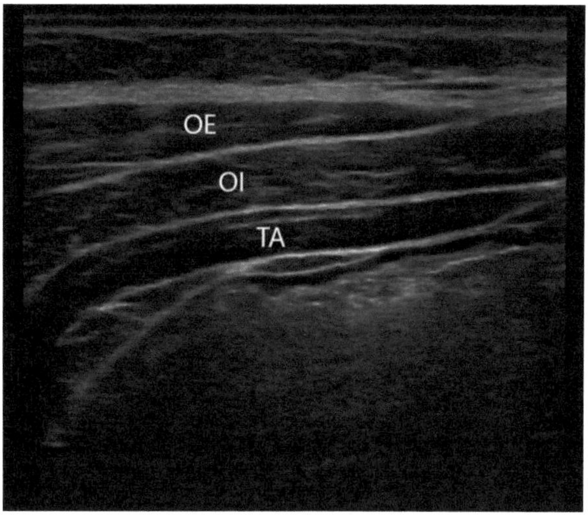

Fig. 13.1 External oblique (EO), internal oblique (IO), and transversus abdominis (TA) muscles

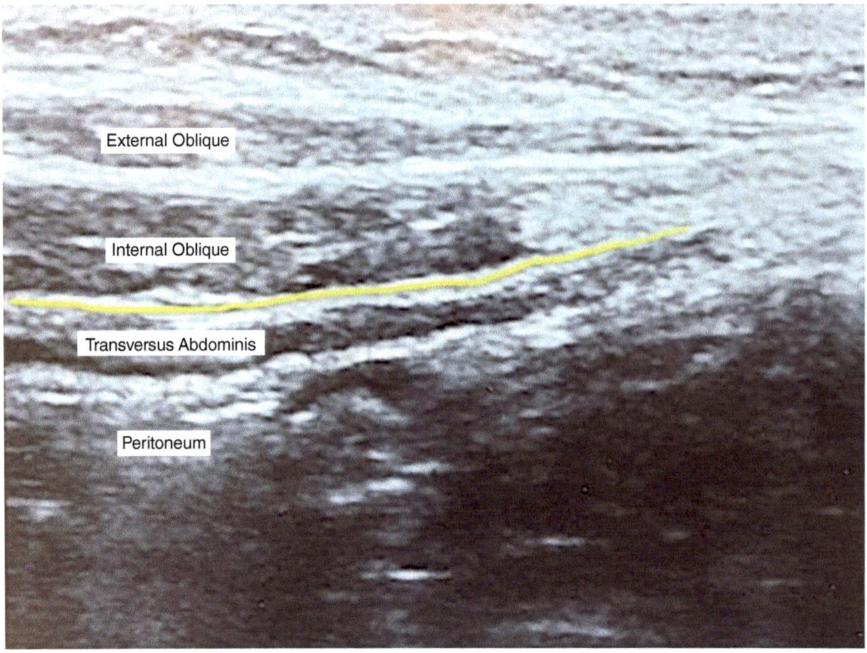

Fig. 13.2 The yellow line indicates the transversus abdominal plane (TAP), the target of the block

the oval-shaped rectus abdominis muscle. The aponeurosis of the EO, IO, and transversus abdominis should be seen immediately lateral to the rectus abdominis muscle. The needle should be directed into the fascial plane between the posterior sheath of the rectus abdominis muscle and the muscle of the transversus abdominis. Correct injection will reveal separation of the fascial plane with clear formation of a hypoechoic, oval-shaped collection of LA. Target nerves for the subcostal TAP are the anterior cutaneous branches originating from T6 to T9, innervating the upper abdomen just below the xiphoid and parallel to the costal margin.

- For **lateral or midaxillary approach**, the high-frequency linear probe is positioned in the midaxillary line, between the subcostal margin and the iliac crest. The three layers of abdominal wall muscles are visualized: external and internal obliques, as well as the transversus abdominis muscle. A needle is inserted in-plane from anterior to posterior and directed to the transversus abdominis plane in between the internal oblique and transversus abdominis muscles. Target nerves for the lateral TAP are the anterior cutaneous branches from T10 to T12 and, to a lesser extent, L1.
- For the **posterior TAP nerve block**, the linear transducer is placed in the axial plane in the midaxillary line and moved posteriorly to the most posterior limit of the TAP between the internal oblique and transversus abdominis muscles. The target is the most posterior end of the TAP. The needle is inserted in the midaxil-

lary line and advanced posteriorly until it reaches the posterior end of the TAP. Target nerves for the posterior approach are similar to that of the lateral approach but may also include the lateral cutaneous branches. Since the lateral cutaneous branches may be blocked, incisional analgesia can extend lateral to the anterior axillary line, resulting in coverage of most of the truncal surface below the umbilicus.

- A combination of these two approaches (subcostal and lateral TAP) is termed the **four-quadrant TAP or bilateral dual-TAP block** and has been purported to provide analgesia to most of the anterior abdominal wall.

Choice of approach should be determined on a case-by-case basis, considering the surgery, anticipated incisions, and patient demographics and comorbidities.

Based on preliminary studies, the pattern of spread also seems to differ between approaches. In a volunteer study, Carney et al. [17] observed (with magnetic resonance imaging) that levobupivacaine-gadolinium injected with the lateral and subcostal approaches remained in the transversus abdominis plane compartment. In contrast, the mixture reached the quadratus lumborum muscle and T5-L1 paravertebral spaces with the posterior approach. The authors demonstrated that lateral and subcostal approaches result in predominantly anterior diffusion within the TAP with little posterior spread; on the contrary, the posterior approach allows a predominantly posterior diffusion of the solution reaching the paravertebral space from T5 to L1.

Before 2014, no randomized trial had compared the subcostal, lateral, and posterior approaches head to head in clinical settings, and much of the knowledge was inferred from cadaveric [20] and volunteer [17, 21] investigations as well as meta-analyses [22]. For instance, in a cadaveric study (n = 13), Milan et al. [20] injected 40 ml of dye under direct vision in the subcostal, lateral, and posterior transversus abdominis plane compartments. These authors then traced the area of dye spread onto clear plastic, which was then photographed. The authors found that the spread was greatest for the subcostal approach (85 cm^2) followed by its posterior (78 cm^2) and lateral (59 cm^2) counterparts, with statistical significance reached for the difference between subcostal and lateral approaches. These findings echoed the results of a 2010 volunteer study by Lee et al. [21], who reported a higher number of dermatomes (4 vs. 3) anesthetized with the subcostal compared to the lateral approach.

For complete analgesic coverage of the abdominal wall from T6-T7 to L1, it is always necessary to perform a double approach in order to obtain greater extension of the block. Borglum et al. [23] suggest a four-point bilateral approach (the four-quadrant TAP or bilateral dual-TAP block): bilateral subcostal approach associated with bilateral lateral approach, to allow analgesia above and below the umbilical.

In scientific literature there are few articles on the use of wall blocks for diastasis surgery.

The subcostal approach has been considered effective in managing postoperative pain after REPA surgery [24], but other combinations should still be evaluated in future studies.

In a retrospective observational study [24], Toscano et al. evaluated the efficacy of bilateral subcostal TAP block on postoperative pain relief in the first 48 postoperative hours following REPA. A multimodal analgesia consisting of subcostal TAP + acetaminophen ensured good postoperative analgesia reducing total opioid consumption and side effects compared to a postoperative analgesia based exclusively on iv opioid.

13.4.2.2 Ultrasound Technique of TAP Block

The operator will place the ultrasound monitor in front of him on the opposite side to the chosen side and must adopt the most comfortable position to allow adequate needle-probe alignment. With the patient in a supine position and after careful disinfection of the skin, a high-frequency linear probe (6–18 MHz) will be used, with variable orientation depending on the type of approach used. The three muscle layers are then identified, separated by a hyperechoic band: OE, OI (generally the most represented), and TA (the thinnest).

The peritoneal cavity and peritoneum are located beneath the TA. If the identification of the three muscle layers is difficult, it may be useful to preliminarily visualize the peritoneum and, starting from the bottom upwards, find the first hyperechoic line above the peritoneum which corresponds to the target interfascial plane of the block. When optimal visualization is obtained, the needle is inserted with an in-plane technique through the OE and OI muscles. Once the first resistance encountered (fascial plane between the OE and OI muscles) the tip of the needle, proceed until it reaches the TAP, perceived as a second loss of resistance. After aspiration, 2–3 ml of saline solution will be injected (hydrodissection) causing the opening of the interfascial plane, confirming the correct position. Subsequently, the AL solution will be injected.

Table 13.1 shows the dosages and volumes of LA used for TAP block in the adult patient. The use of new molecules such as liposomal bupivacaine can increase the duration of the block [25].

In the literature, several adjuvants (i.e., dexamethasone, alpha-2 agonists, magnesium, opioids), added to the local anesthetic mixture, have been investigated to prolong the duration of transversus abdominis plane blocks: dexmedetomidine (0.5–1 mcg/kg), clonidine (1 ug/kg per side), and dexamethasone (4–8 mg) can increase the duration of transversus abdominis plane blocks by almost 10 h, 4 h, and 3 h, respectively [26].

The TAP block, if performed by expert operators and with an ultrasound-guided technique, represents a simple technique with a low incidence of complications.

Table 13.1 Dosage and volumes for TAP block

Dosages and volumes of local anesthetic (LA) for TAP block		
Volume of LA	Mixture of LA	Dosage
0.3–0.6 ml/kg for side (20–40 ml for side)	Ropivacaine or levobupivacaine 0.25% or 0.375%	Ropivacaine 3 mg/kg, levobupivacaine 2.5 mg/kg

Although rare, some are described in scientific literature: liver trauma [27], intestinal lesions, hematoma, infection at the injection site, and local anesthetic systemic toxicity (LAST) [26]. Interestingly, if the needle tip is positioned just between the transversus abdominis muscle and the transversalis fascia (without puncturing the peritoneum), local anesthetic injection could result in transient femoral nerve blockade because the fascia iliaca constitutes the posterolateral continuation of the transversalis fascia [28].

13.4.3 Rectus Sheath Block

The rectus sheath block (RSB) is used for analgesia after umbilical or incisional hernia repairs and other midline surgical incisions. First described in 1899 by Schleich, it was initially used for abdominal wall muscle relaxation during laparotomy before the introduction of neuromuscular block. Originally, the block was performed using a blind, loss-of-resistance technique. The accuracy and safety of a RSB are now greatly increased through the utilization of ultrasound guidance and echogenic needles [29, 30].

The block's targets are the terminal branches of the T_{9-11} intercostal nerves which run between IO and TAM to penetrate the posterior wall of rectus abdominis muscle (RAM) and end in an anterior cutaneous branch supplying the skin of the umbilical area [15, 31].

The injection of LA into the posterior fascia of the RAM ensures somatic anesthesia of the central part of the anterior abdominal wall, unlike the TAP block which, as we have already said, ensures somatic analgesia of the anterolateral portion of the abdomen.

Studies done by Purdy et al. [32], Bashandy et al. [33], Smith et al. [34], and Allene [35] showed that RSB is effective in reducing the severity of postoperative pain score and analgesic consumption and increases time to first analgesic request.

In the Enhanced Recovery After Surgery (ERAS) era, the abdominal wall blocks, such as TAP block or RSB, are considered a valid alternative to intravenous opioids in the management of postoperative pain after DRA surgery.

Blocking the anterior cutaneous branches of the intercostal nerves, the RSB provides analgesia to the anteromedial abdominal wall and periumbilical area (spinal dermatomes T9, T10, and T11), while the lateral or subcostal TAPB anesthetizes intercostal nerves T10-T12 or T6-T9, respectively.

The combination of bilateral ultrasound RSB and TAP block, through different and synergistic mechanisms of action, may provide more effective analgesia. This combined approach, which takes advantage of the overlap of two fascial plane blocks, allowed to provide a multi-dermatomal sensory block of the anterior and lateral abdominal wall through a synergistic effect.

If two interfascial blocks are associated, care must be taken not to exceed the maximum recommended dose of local anesthetic.

13.4.3.1 Sonoanatomy and Ultrasound-Guided Technique

The goal of the rectus sheath block is to deposit LA between the RAM and the posterior rectus sheath (PRS) (Fig. 13.3).

With the patient in the supine position, the ultrasound transducer should be placed in a transverse orientation above the umbilicus, centered approximately 1 cm from the midline. The RAM and posterior rectus sheath should be identified (as a thick, spindle-like shaped muscle with a hyperechoic fascial covering deep to the muscle). The needle (a 50–100 mm, 21–22-gauge echogenic nerve block needle) is inserted using an in-plane technique and directed from medial to lateral as this trajectory may reduce the risk of iatrogenic visceral injury. Once the needle tip is advanced posterior to the RAM and anterior to the posterior sheath, a small aliquot of saline is administered to hydrodissection and confirm needle tip placement prior to the injection of local anesthetic (Fig. 13.4).

Bilateral catheters may be placed for a continuous block; in this case the catheter is advanced 5–6 cm into the space.

In midline laparotomy, ultrasound-guided RSB is considered clinically more useful than TAP block because it can completely anesthetize the area of the midline incision in the rectus abdominis muscle, but in the DRA surgery, we recommend using it in association with another abdominal wall block such as the TAP block.

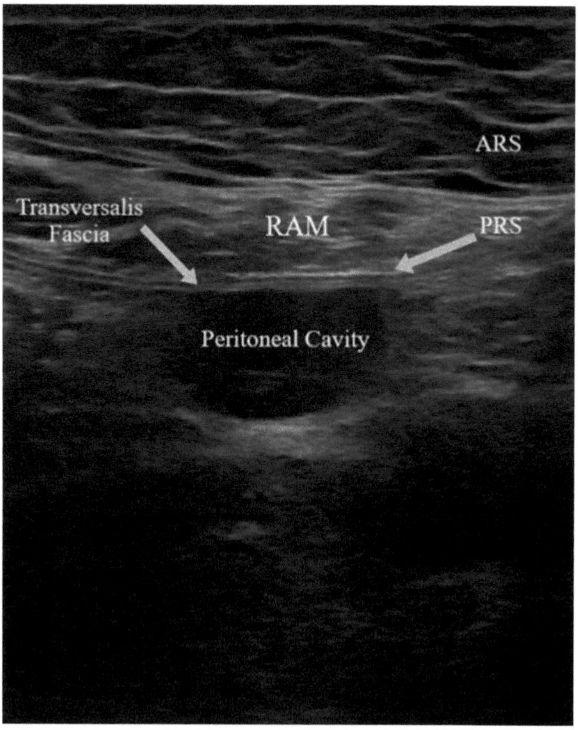

Fig. 13.3 Rectus sheath block sonoanatomy. *RAM* rectus anterior muscle, *ARS* anterior rectus sheath, *PRS* posterior rectus sheath

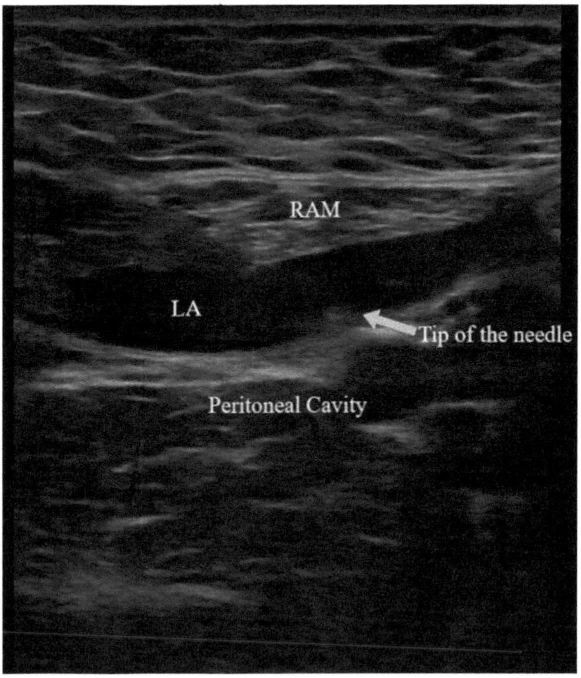

Fig. 13.4 Post-injection ultrasound imaging: This image illustrates the local anesthetic injected in the space between RAM and PRS. *RAM* rectus anterior muscle, *AL* local anesthetic, *PRS* posterior rectus sheath

There are adverse events related to RSB including preperitoneal injection (when a needle was located beyond the transversalis fascia), intraperitoneal injection, vascular injury, bowel injury, and LAST [36].

Care should be taken to identify the superior epigastric artery with color Doppler when possible (Fig. 13.5).

Avoidance of needle advancement into the deep aspect of the RAM near its midpoint should minimize the risk of potential vascular trauma. Medial to lateral needle insertion may minimize the risk of intraperitoneal needle advancement and possible visceral injury, but deep needle placement within the mid rectus muscle might risk injury to the epigastric artery.

Table 13.2 shows the dosages and volumes of LA used for RSB in the adult patient.

With regard to the addition of adjuvants to the anesthetic mixture, dosages and prolongation times are the same as those indicated in paragraph 13.4.2.2.

13.4.4 Quadratus Lumborum Block

Ultrasound-guided quadratus lumborum block is a recently described fascial plane block where local anesthetic is injected adjacent to the quadratus lumborum muscle with the goal of anesthetizing the thoracolumbar nerves.

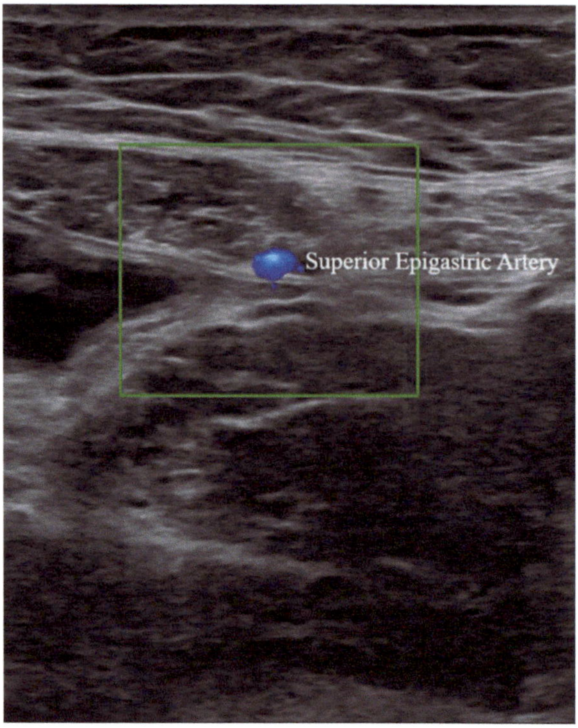

Fig. 13.5 Superior epigastric artery in the deep part of the RAM. *RAM* rectus anterior muscle

Table 13.2 Dosage and volumes for rectus sheath block (RSB)

Dosages and volumes of local anesthetic (LA) for RSB		
Volume of LA	Mixture of LA	Dosage
15–20 ml for side	Ropivacaine or levobupivacaine 0.25% or 0.375%	Ropivacaine 3 mg/kg, levobupivacaine 2.5 mg/kg

It is a block of the posterior abdominal wall that requires the injection of LA into the thoracolumbar fascia (TLF), which is a posterior extension of the abdominal wall muscle fascia and encompasses the back muscles (quadratus lumborum [QL], psoas major, and the erector spinae muscles). The TLF extends posteriorly to connect with the lumbar paravertebral region. It has three layers—anterior, middle, and posterior—based on its relation to the back muscles it encapsulates. The TLF extends from the lumbar spine to the thoracic spine in a craniocaudal direction [37].

The QL muscle is part of the posterior abdominal wall dorsal to the iliopsoas muscle. It originates from the medial half of the iliac crest and inserts into the lower medial border of the 12th rib. It has four small tendinous insertions to the apices of the transverse processes of the upper four lumbar vertebrae. The ventral rami of the spinal nerve roots (including the subcostal and iliohypogastric nerves) pass between the QL and its anterior fascia. The quadratus lumborum and psoas major muscles traverse posterior to the lateral and medial arcuate ligaments of the diaphragm, respectively. Posterior to the quadratus lumborum muscle lies the erector spinae muscle. The quadratus lumborum muscle is surrounded by a fibrous composite of aponeurotic and fascial tissue: the TLF.

The TLF contains mechanoreceptors, nociceptors, and sympathetic fibers. The spread of local anesthetic to the paravertebral space and inhibition of these sympathetic fibers are believed to be responsible for the visceral pain coverage provided by this block [38].

Variants of this block have been described, each involving a different injection site relative to the quadratus lumborum muscle. **QL1 or lateral QLB** refers to the deposition of LA lateral to the QL muscle. **QL2 or posterior QLB** refers to injection posterior to the QL muscle (anterior to the TLF separating QL muscle from erector spinae and latissimus dorsi muscles). **QL3 or anterior QLB** refers to injection anterior to the QL muscle at the level of the L4 vertebral body. To acquire the ultrasound view for this block, the clinician should obtain the "shamrock sign," which consists of the transverse process of L4 as the "stem" and psoas major, QL, and erector spinae as "3 cloves of the shamrock" [39]. **QL4 or intramuscular QL block** involves the injection into the muscle itself.

13.4.4.1 Sonoanatomy and Ultrasound-Guided Technique

The lateral decubitus position is preferred over the supine position as it gives more exposure to the neuroaxial structures and more stability in handling the ultrasound probe and needle. If possible, the hip is abducted and laterally flexed toward the same side of the block to contract the QL muscle. After sterile prepping and draping, a curvilinear low-frequency (2–6 MHz) transducer is often required, facilitating tissue penetration of ultrasound and to visualize the three lateral abdominal muscle layers, the QL muscle, and the anatomy of the adjoining lumbar paravertebral area. This also may be a better option when a transmuscular approach is intended. The orientation marker is directed laterally for a transverse scan. It is possible to perform the QL block in the supine position; however, visualization of the lumbar paravertebral area may be impaired.

Scanning is usually started at the midaxillary line between the iliac crest and subcostal margin, moving the probe posteriorly until tapering of the three abdominal muscle layers and appearance of fascia transversalis and QL muscle is observed. The fascia transversalis usually appears as a hyperechoic layer, which forms a safe landmark to separate the muscle layers from the perinephric fat and the abdominal contents below the level of the lower pole of the kidney. Sometimes the bowel, kidney, and perinephric fat movements with breathing can be visualized underneath, making it helpful to make it a more definite landmark.

Because identifying the quadratus lumborum muscle is critical to performing quadratus lumborum block, it is important to note the following landmarks and relationships: the aponeuroses of the abdominal wall muscles (external oblique, internal oblique, transversus abdominis) are located posterolateral to the quadratus lumborum muscle; the quadratus lumborum muscle is often hypoechoic relative to psoas major muscle, which is found anteromedially, and the lumbar transverse processes are apparent with their hyperechoic curved appearance.

Scanning also can be performed positioning the transducer posteriorly 4–5 cm lateral to the lumbar spinous process at the L2–L4 level with the objective of imaging the quadratus lumborum and erector spinae muscles, together with a transverse process forming the "shamrock sign" [39, 40].

Absolute contraindications include local infection, allergy to local anesthetics, and a known bleeding diathesis because it is a deep block. Relative contraindications include anatomical abnormalities, hemodynamic instability, and known neurologic disorders.

Adverse events related to QLB include LA distribution to the lumbar plexus and prolonged motor block, delaying mobilization and hospital discharge. Lower limb weakness has been reported after use of all quadratus lumborum block approaches [41, 42]. Hypotension has been reported, which may be related to LA spread to the paravertebral space [43]. Because of the doses used and the vascularity of the area, LAST is a potential risk [44] although peak concentrations of LA are lower after quadratus lumborum blocks than transversus abdominis plane blocks [45].

Being considered a deep block, it has the same contraindications as neuraxial anesthesia and cannot be performed in patients taking antiaggregating and anticoagulant drugs.

The LA dosage recommended in the QLB is comparable to that of the TAP block approaches with the recommendation to decrease the concentration of the drug in favor of the volume.

Table 13.3 shows the dosages and volumes of LA used for QLB in the adult patient.

13.4.5 *Erector Spinae Plane Block*

The ESP block was first described by Forero in 2016 "as a successful interfascial plane block for thoracic neuropathic pain" and is considered a relatively recent addition to the field of regional anesthesia and pain management [46].

The ESP block involves the injection of LA into the interfascial plane located between the erector spinae muscles and the tip of the transverse vertebral process. It is a very versatile fascial plane block, used for many types of surgery (cardiac, thoracic, vascular, abdominal, urological, gynecological) [47–50] which provides visceral and somatic analgesia for abdominal surgery and, although not yet tested for the specific surgery of DRA repair, strongly recommended by the authors.

Table 13.3 Dosage and volumes for quadratus lumborum block (QLB)

Dosages and volumes of local anesthetic (LA) for QLB		
Volume of LA	Mixture of LA	Dosage
0.3–0.6 ml/kg for side (20–30 ml for side)	Ropivacaine 0.25% or levobupivacaine 0.125%–0.25%	Ropivacaine 2–3 mg/kg, levobupivacaine 2.5 mg/kg

In fact pain during abdominal surgery consists of somatic (related to the body wall and musculoskeletal structures) and visceral pain (related to internal organs). Somatic pain contains 70–75% of the pain, lasts 72 h after open surgery, and is arising from the anterior abdominal wall. Visceral pain lasts for 24–36 h; it is intense but short-term. Opioids are very effective in the treatment of visceral pain but not so effective for somatic pain and are related to side effects in the postoperative period [51]. ESP block is able to cover both the visceral and somatic components of intra- and postoperative pain and has been shown its value and efficacy in acute as well as in chronic pain management.

Since its first description, ESP block has gained attention and stimulated an interesting debate over its mechanism of action [52]. To date, thanks to several cadaveric studies and magnetic resonance imaging, we know that ESP block has been found to provide both somatic and visceral analgesia. This suggests that it can be effective for managing pain originating from different sources [53, 54].

In fact, it has been observed that the local anesthetic injected into the fascial plane between the erector spinae muscles and the transverse vertebral processes can spread through channels in the intertransverse connective tissues reaching ventral and dorsal ramus of the spinal nerve along with the sympathetic ramus communicans at the intervertebral foramen level.

Moreover, the involvement of lateral cutaneous branches of intercostal nerves contributes to the block's analgesic effect.

Scharztmann et al. [55], using magnetic resonance imaging (MRI), provide valuable insights into the spread and clinical effects of the erector spinae plane (ESP) block injectate.

The MRI study demonstrated that the injectate used in the ESPB consistently spread to several anatomical areas. These areas included the erector spinae muscles (which are the target of the block), neural foramina (openings through which spinal nerves exit the spinal column), and the intercostal space (the space between the ribs). A recent meta-analysis of randomized trials [56] confirmed that ESP block provides more beneficial analgesic efficacy than TAP block in adult abdominal surgery.

In particular, compared with TAP block, ESP block significantly reduced pain scores at 6, 12, and 24 h and 24-h opioid consumption and prolonged the time to first rescue analgesia postsurgically. Furthermore, subgroup analysis showed that ESPB significantly reduced pain scores at various time points and opioid consumption within 24 h after laparoscopic cholecystectomy, percutaneous nephrolithotomy, and bariatric surgery.

The distribution of the erector spinae muscle (ESM) from the neck to the lumbar region makes the ESP block a versatile regional anesthesia technique. Its ability to deliver analgesia in a large area of the trunk and abdomen has indeed contributed to its popularity in various surgical procedures. Here are some reasons why ESP block has gained popularity.

13.4.5.1 Sonoatomy and Ultrasound-Guided Technique

The ESP block can be performed in different positions, depending on the clinical situation and the preferences and expertise of the healthcare provider.

It can be performed with the patient in a sitting position, prior to general anesthesia, or it can also be performed with the patient in a lateral position. This may be done either before or after the induction of general anesthesia, depending on the clinical circumstances and the anesthesia team's preferences. A linear probe is generally placed in a sagittal view at the level of T10-T12 spinous process, 2–3 cm laterally from the midline in order to identify the transverse process, the trapezius, rhomboideus, and erector spinae muscles (Fig. 13.6a). The needle is then inserted via an in-plane approach, and LA is injected in the caudal to cranial direction into the interfascial plane between the erector spinae muscle and the transverse process (Fig. 13.6a).

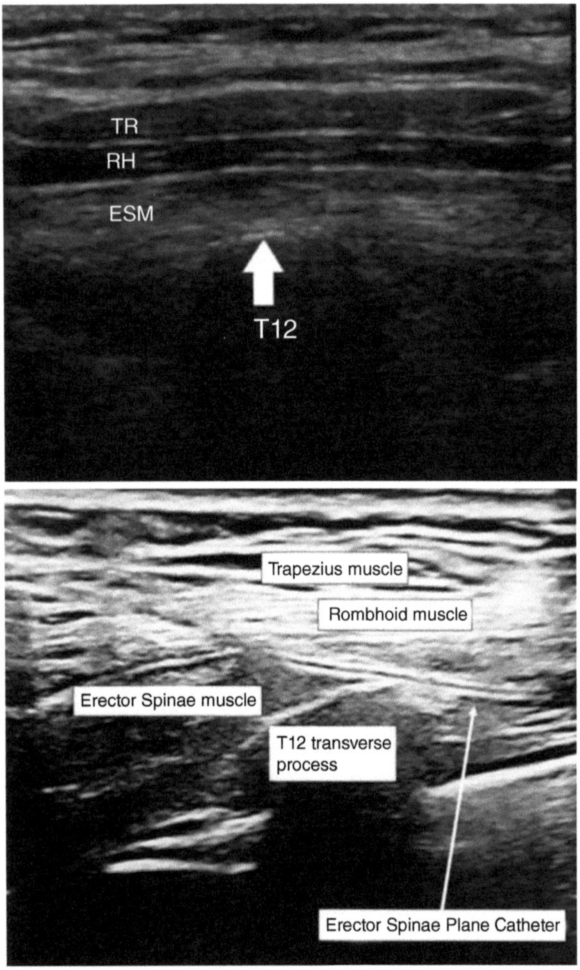

Fig. 13.6 (**a**) Sonoanatomy of the ESP block: trapezius (uppermost), rhomboid (middle), and erector spinae (lowermost) are identified. The hyperechoic T12 transverse process is individuated inferior to the erector spinae muscle. (**b**) Continuous ESP block. View of the catheter positioned under the erector spinae muscle. *TR* trapezius muscle, *RH* rhomboid muscle, *ESM* erector spinae muscle, *T4* transverse process

Table 13.4 Dosage and volumes for erector spinae plane (ESP) block

Dosages and volumes of local anesthetic (LA) for ESP block		
Volume of LA	Mixture of LA	Dosage
20–30 ml for side	Ropivacaine 0.375%–0.5% or levobupivacaine 0.25%–0.375%	Ropivacaine 3 mg/kg, levobupivacaine 2.5 mg/kg

By the placement of a peripheral nerve catheter in the interfascial plane, a continuous block can be performed (Fig. 13.6b).

Between 20 and 30 ml of 0.25% levobupivacaine or 0.375%, ropivacaine should be used. After injecting 10–20 ml of the local anesthetic solution, the catheter can thread easily into that space. It is prudent to thread 5–7 cm of the catheter into the space to avoid inadvertent dislodgement of the catheter.

Infection at the site of injection in the paraspinal region and patient refusal are absolute contraindications for performing an ESP block.

Complications are very rare because the site of injection is far from the pleura, major blood vessels, and the spinal cord. Infection at the needle insertion site, local anesthetic toxicity/allergy, vascular puncture, pleural puncture, pneumothorax, and failed block are the primary complications. Because of the few published data, more investigations (e.g., randomized controlled trials, RCTs) are needed to verify the safety, complication rates, and efficacy of this strategy. A recent evidence-based study, indeed, identified only four RCTs, and their endpoints were heterogeneous [56].

Table 13.4 shows the dosages and volumes of LA used for QLB in the adult patient.

References

1. Savoia G, Alampi D, Amantea B, Ambrosio F, Arcioni R, Berti M, Bettelli G, Bertini L, Bosco M, Casati A, Castelletti I, Carassiti M, Coluzzi F, Costantini A, Danelli G, Evangelista M, Finco G, Gatti A, Gravino E, Launo C, Loreto M, Mediati R, Mokini Z, Mondello E, Palermo S, Paoletti F, Paolicchi A, Petrini F, Piacevoli Q, Rizza A, Sabato AF, Santangelo E, Troglio E, Mattia C, SIAARTI Study Group. Postoperative pain treatment SIAARTI recommendations 2010. Short version. Minerva Anestesiol. 2010;76(8):657–67.
2. Osterbrink J, Evers GC. Der Einfluss pflegerischer Massnahmen auf Inzisionsschmerz und Opioidverbrauch in der postoperativen Phase [The influence of nursing measures on incision pain and the use of opioids in the postoperative period]. Pflege. 2000;13(5):306–14. German. https://doi.org/10.1024/1012-5302.13.5.306.
3. Wellenbrock S, Aitzetmüller MM, Klietz ML, Wiebringhaus P, Djedovic G, Hirsch T, Rieger UM. Measurement of postoperative quality of pain in abdominoplasty patients-an outcome oriented prospective study. J Clin Med. 2023;12(5):1745. https://doi.org/10.3390/jcm12051745. PMID: 36902531; PMCID: PMC10002866.
4. Meissner W, Komann M, Erlenwein J, Stamer U, Scherag A. The quality of postoperative pain therapy in German hospitals. Dtsch Arztebl Int. 2017;114:161–7. https://doi.org/10.3238/arztebl.2017.0161.
5. White PF, Kehlet H, Neal JM, Schricker T, Carr DB, Carli F, Fast-Track Surgery Study Group. The role of the anesthesiologist in fast-track surgery: from multimodal analgesia to

perioperative medical care. Anesth Analg. 2007;104(6):1380–96, table of contents. https://doi.org/10.1213/01.ane.0000263034.96885.e1. PMID: 17513630.
6. Oodit R, Biccard BM, Panieri E, Alvarez AO, Sioson MRS, Maswime S, Thomas V, Kluyts HL, Peden CJ, de Boer HD, Brindle M, Francis NK, Nelson G, Gustafsson UO, Ljungqvist O. Guidelines for perioperative care in elective abdominal and pelvic surgery at primary and secondary hospitals in Low-Middle-Income Countries (LMIC's): Enhanced Recovery After Surgery (ERAS) Society recommendation. World J Surg. 2022;46(8):1826–43. https://doi.org/10.1007/s00268-022-06587-w. Epub 2022 May 31. PMID: 35641574; PMCID: PMC9154207.
7. Hughes M, Ventham N, McNally S, et al. Analgesia after open abdominal surgery in the setting of enhanced recovery surgery. JAMA Surg. 2014;149(12):1224.
8. Block B, Liu S, Rowlingson A, et al. Efficacy of postoperative epidural analgesia. JAMA. 2003;290(18):2455.
9. Werawatganon T, Charuluxananan S. WITHDRAWN: patient controlled intravenous opioid analgesia versus continuous epidural analgesia for pain after intra-abdominal surgery. Cochrane Database Syst Rev. 2013;2013(3):CD004088. https://doi.org/10.1002/14651858.CD004088.pub3.
10. Pöpping D, Elia N, Van Aken H, et al. Impact of epidural analgesia on mortality and morbidity after surgery. Ann Surg. 2014;259(6):1056–67.
11. Baker H, Yates V, Addison D, et al. The effect of anaesthetist grade and frequency of insertion on epidural failure: a service evaluation in a United Kingdom teaching hospital. BMC Anesthesiol. 2015;15(1):5. https://doi.org/10.1186/1471-2253-15-5.
12. Bos EME, Haumann J, de Quelerij M, Vandertop WP, Kalkman CJ, Hollmann MW, Lirk P. Haematoma and abscess after neuraxial anaesthesia: a review of 647 cases. Br J Anaesth. 2018;120(4):693–704. https://doi.org/10.1016/j.bja.2017.11.105. Epub 2018 Feb 15. PMID: 29576110.
13. Horlocker TT, Vandermeuelen E, Kopp SL, Gogarten W, Leffert LR, Benzon HT. Regional anesthesia in the patient receiving antithrombotic or thrombolytic therapy: American Society of Regional Anesthesia and Pain Medicine evidence-based guidelines (fourth edition). Reg Anesth Pain Med. 2018;43(3):263–309. https://doi.org/10.1097/AAP.0000000000000763. Erratum in: Reg Anesth Pain Med. 2018;43(5):566. Vandermeuelen, Erik [corrected to Vandermeulen, Erik]. PMID: 29561531.
14. Toscano A, Capuano P, Galatà M, Tazzi I, Rinaldi M, Brazzi L. Safety of ultrasound-guided serratus anterior and erector spinae fascial plane blocks: a retrospective analysis in patients undergoing cardiac surgery while receiving anticoagulant and antiplatelet drugs. J Cardiothorac Vasc Anesth. 2022;36(2):483–8. https://doi.org/10.1053/j.jvca.2021.05.037. Epub 2021 May 24. PMID: 34148801.
15. Chin KJ, McDonnell JG, Carvalho B, Sharkey A, Pawa A, Gadsden J. Essentials of our current understanding: abdominal wall blocks. Reg Anesth Pain Med. 2017;42(2):133–83. https://doi.org/10.1097/AAP.0000000000000545.
16. Tsai HC, Yoshida T, Chuang TY, Yang SF, Chang CC, Yao HY, Tai YT, Lin JA, Chen KY. Transversus abdominis plane block: an updated review of anatomy and techniques. Biomed Res Int. 2017;2017:8284363. https://doi.org/10.1155/2017/8284363. Epub 2017 Oct 31. PMID: 29226150; PMCID: PMC5684553.
17. Carney J, Finnerty O, Rauf J, Bergin D, Laffey JG, Mc Donnell JG. Studies on the spread of local anaesthetic solution in transversus abdominis plane blocks. Anaesthesia. 2011;66(11):1023–30. https://doi.org/10.1111/j.1365-2044.2011.06855.x. Epub 2011 Aug 18. PMID: 21851346.
18. Rafi AN. Abdominal field block via the lumbar triangle revisited. Anaesthesia. 2012;67(12):1399–401. https://doi.org/10.1111/anae.12077. PMID: 23130727.
19. Hebbard P, Fujiwara Y, Shibata Y, Royse C. Ultrasound-guided transversus abdominis plane (TAP) block. Anaesth Intensive Care. 2007;35(4):616–7. PMID: 18020088.

20. Milan Z, Tabor D, McConnell P, Pickering J, Kocarev M, du Feu F, Barton S. Three different approaches to transversus abdominis plane block: a cadaveric study. Med Glas (Zenica). 2011;8:181–4.
21. Lee THW, Barrington MJ, Tran TMN, Wong D, Hebbard PD. Comparison of sensory blockade following posterior and subcostal approaches to ultrasound-guided transversus abdominis plane block. Anaesth Intensive Care. 2010;38:452–60.
22. Abdallah FW, Laffey JG, Halpern SH, Brull R. Duration of analgesic effectiveness after the posterior and lateral transversus abdominis plane block techniques for transverse lower abdominal incisions: a meta-analysis. Br J Anaesth. 2013;111:721–35.
23. Børglum J, Maschmann C, Belhage B, Jensen K. Ultrasound-guided bilateral dual transversus abdominis plane block: a new four-point approach. Acta Anaesthesiol Scand. 2011;55(6):658–63. https://doi.org/10.1111/j.1399-6576.2011.02430.x. Epub 2011 Apr 4. PMID: 21463262.
24. Toscano A, Cuccomarino S, Capuano P, Bonomo LD, Forcella KMR, Aprà F, Jannaci A, Brazzi L. Effectiveness of Subcostal Transversus Abdominis Plane Block in Subcutaneous Onlay Laparoscopic Approach (SCOLA) surgery: a retrospective observational study. Surg Laparosc Endosc Percutan Tech. 2021;31(6):760–4. https://doi.org/10.1097/SLE.0000000000000988. PMID: 34369482.
25. Alexander JC, Sunna M, Goldenmerry Y, Mootz A, O'Connor C, Ringqvist J, Bunker M, Joshi GP, Gasanova I. Comparison of transversus abdominis plane blocks with liposomal bupivacaine versus ropivacaine in open total abdominal hysterectomy. Proc (Bayl Univ Med Cent). 2022;35(6):746–50. https://doi.org/10.1080/08998280.2022.2090798. PMID: 36304627; PMCID: PMC9586627.
26. Tran DQ, Bravo D, Leurcharusmee P, Neal JM. Transversus abdominis plane block: a narrative review. Anesthesiology. 2019;131(5):1166–90. https://doi.org/10.1097/ALN.0000000000002842. PMID: 31283738.
27. Lancaster P, Chadwick M. Liver trauma secondary to ultrasound-guided transversus abdominis plane block. Br J Anaesth. 2010;104(4):509–10. https://doi.org/10.1093/bja/aeq046. PMID: 20228188.
28. Walker G. Transversus abdominis plane block: a note of caution! Br J Anaesth. 2010;104:265.
29. Dolan J, Lucie P, Geary T, et al. The rectus sheath block: accuracy of local anesthetic placement by trainee anesthesiologists using loss of resistance or ultrasound guidance. Reg Anesth Pain Med. 2009;34(3):247–50. https://doi.org/10.1097/AAP.0b013e31819a3f67.
30. Dolan J, Smith M. Visualization of bowel adherent to the peritoneum before rectus sheath block: another indication for use of ultrasound in regional anesthesia. Reg Anesth Pain Med. 2009;34(3):280–1. https://doi.org/10.1097/AAP.0b013e31819a4f84.
31. Chakraborty A, Khemka R, Datta T. Ultrasound-guided truncal blocks: a new frontier in regional anaesthesia. Indian J Anaesth. 2016;60(10):703–11. https://doi.org/10.4103/0019-5049.191665. PMID: 27761032; PMCID: PMC5064693.
32. Purdy M, Kinnunen M, Kokki M, Anttila M, Eskelinen M, Hautajärvi H, Lehtonen M, Kokki H. A prospective, randomized, open label, controlled study investigating the efficiency and safety of 3 different methods of rectus sheath block analgesia following midline laparotomy. Medicine (Baltimore). 2018;97(7):e9968. https://doi.org/10.1097/MD.0000000000009968. PMID: 29443788; PMCID: PMC5839819.
33. Bashandy GM, Elkholy AH. Reducing postoperative opioid consumption by adding an ultrasound-guided rectus sheath block to multimodal analgesia for abdominal cancer surgery with midline incision. Anesth Pain Med. 2014;4(3):e18263. https://doi.org/10.5812/aapm.18263. PMID: 25289373; PMCID: PMC4183078.
34. Smith BE, Suchak M, Siggins D, Challands J. Rectus sheath block for diagnostic laparoscopy. Anaesthesia. 1988;43(11):947–8. https://doi.org/10.1111/j.1365-2044.1988.tb05658.x. PMID: 2975148.

35. Allene MD. Assessment of the analgesic effectiveness of bilateral rectus sheath block as postoperative analgesia for midline laparotomy: prospective observational cohort study. Int J Surg Open. 2020;24:166–9.
36. Kwon HJ, Kim YJ, Kim Y, Kim S, Cho H, Lee JH, Kim DH, Jeong SM. Complications and technical consideration of ultrasound-guided rectus sheath blocks: a retrospective analysis of 4033 patients. Anesth Analg. 2023;136(2):365–72. https://doi.org/10.1213/ANE.0000000000006282. Epub 2022 Nov 29. PMID: 36638514.
37. Ueshima H, Otake H, Lin JA. Ultrasound-guided quadratus lumborum block: an updated review of anatomy and techniques. Biomed Res Int. 2017;2017:2752876. https://doi.org/10.1155/2017/2752876. Epub 2017 Jan 3. PMID: 28154824; PMCID: PMC5244003.
38. Tesarz J, Hoheisel U, Wiedenhöfer B, Mense S. Sensory innervation of the thoracolumbar fascia in rats and humans. Neuroscience. 2011;194:302–8. https://doi.org/10.1016/j.neuroscience.2011.07.066. Epub 2011 Aug 2. PMID: 21839150.
39. El-Boghdadly K, Elsharkawy H, Short A, Chin KJ. Quadratus lumborum block nomenclature and anatomical considerations. Reg Anesth Pain Med. 2016;41(4):548–9. https://doi.org/10.1097/AAP.0000000000000411. PMID: 27315184.
40. Elsharkawy H, El-Boghdadly K, Barrington M. Quadratus lumborum block: anatomical concepts, mechanisms, and techniques. Anesthesiology. 2019;130(2):322–35. https://doi.org/10.1097/ALN.0000000000002524. PMID: 30688787.
41. Ueshima H, Hiroshi O. Incidence of lower-extremity muscle weakness after quadratus lumborum block. J Clin Anesth. 2018;44:104.
42. Wikner M. Unexpected motor weakness following quadratus lumborum block for gynaecological laparoscopy. Anaesthesia. 2017;72:230–2.
43. Sá M, Cardoso JM, Reis H, Esteves M, Sampaio J, Gouveia I, Carballada P, Pinheiro C, Machado D. [Quadratus lumborum block: are we aware of its side effects? A report of 2 cases]. [Article in Portuguese.]. Rev Bras Anestesiol. 2017;68:396–9.
44. Gitman M, Barrington MJ. Local anesthetic systemic toxicity: a review of recent case reports and registries. Reg Anesth Pain Med. 2018;43(2):124–30. https://doi.org/10.1097/AAP.0000000000000721. PMID: 29303925.
45. Murouchi T, Iwasaki S, Yamakage M. Chronological changes in ropivacaine concentration and analgesic effects between transversus abdominis plane block and rectus sheath Block. Reg Anesth Pain Med. 2015;40(5):568–71. https://doi.org/10.1097/AAP.0000000000000288. PMID: 26222347.
46. Forero M, Adhikary SD, Lopez H, Tsui C, Chin KJ. The erector spinae plane block: a novel analgesic technique in thoracic neuropathic pain. Reg Anesth Pain Med. 2016;41(5):621–7. https://doi.org/10.1097/AAP.0000000000000451.
47. Tedesco M, Capuano P, Toscano A, Sepolvere G. Combined erector spinae plane block and serratus anterior plane block for thoracic surgery: is two better than one? Minerva Anestesiol. 2023;89(9):842–4. https://doi.org/10.23736/S0375-9393.23.17348-2. Epub 2023 May 9. PMID: 37158632.
48. Capuano P, Burgio G, Martucci G, Scarlata M, Bonicolini E, Tancredi G, Toscano A, Bertani A, Arcadipane A. Enhanced recovery after minimally invasive esophagectomy: could bilateral erector spinae block be the answer? Minerva Anestesiol. 2023;89(6):597–8. https://doi.org/10.23736/S0375-9393.22.17035-5. Epub 2022 Nov 23. PMID: 36416246.
49. Toscano A, Cremascoli L, Balzano S, Capuano P, Salonia C, Patrono D, Romagnoli R, Balagna R. Continuous bilateral erector spinae plane block for open hepatectomy. Minerva Anestesiol. 2024;90(4):348–50. https://doi.org/10.23736/S0375-9393.23.17854-0. Epub ahead of print. PMID: 38289297.
50. Toscano A, Barbero C, Capuano P, Costamagna A, Pocar M, Trompeo A, Pasero D, Rinaldi M, Brazzi L. Chronic postsurgical pain and quality of life after right minithoracotomy mitral valve operations. J Card Surg. 2022;37(6):1585–90. https://doi.org/10.1111/jocs.16400. Epub 2022 Mar 11. PMID: 35274774.

51. Marija T, Aleksandar D. Erector spinae plane block in various abdominal surgeries: a case series. Saudi J Anaesth. 2020;14(4):528–30. https://doi.org/10.4103/sja.SJA_31_20. Epub 2020 Sep 24. PMID: 33447200; PMCID: PMC7796768.
52. Chin KJ, El-Boghdadly K. Mechanisms of action of the erector spinae plane (ESP) block: a narrative review. Mécanismes d'action du bloc du plan des muscles érecteurs du rachis (erector spinae, ESP): un compte rendu narratif. Can J Anaesth. 2021;68(3):387–408. https://doi.org/10.1007/s12630-59.
53. Adhikary SD, Bernard S, Lopez H, Chin KJ. Erector spinae plane block versus retrolaminar block: a magnetic resonance imaging and anatomical study. Reg Anesth Pain Med. 2018;43(7):756–62. https://doi.org/10.1097/AAP.0000000000000798.
54. Schwartzmann A, Peng P, Maciel MA, Alcarraz P, Gonzalez X, Forero M. A magnetic resonance imaging study of local anesthetic spread in patients receiving an erector spinae plane block. Étude d'imagerie par résonance magnétique de la diffusion d'un anesthésique local chez des patients recevant un bloc du plan des muscles érecteurs du rachis. Can J Anaesth. 2020;67(8):942–8. https://doi.org/10.1007/s12630-020-01613-8.
55. Gao Y, Liu L, Cui Y, Zhang J, Wu X. Postoperative analgesia efficacy of erector spinae plane block in adult abdominal surgery: a systematic review and meta-analysis of randomized trials. Front Med (Lausanne). 2022;9:934866. https://doi.org/10.3389/fmed.2022.934866. PMID: 36267624; PMCID: PMC9578553.
56. De Cassai A, Bonvicini D, Correale C, Sandei L, Tulgar S, Tonetti T. Erector spinae plane block: a systematic qualitative review. Minerva Anestesiol. 2019;85(3):308–19. https://doi.org/10.23736/S0375-9393.18.13341-4. Epub 2019 Jan 4. PMID: 30621377.

Chapter 14
Minimally Invasive Lipoabdominoplasty (MILA)

Guillermo Di Biasio and Ezequiel M. Palmisano

14.1 Introduction

Abdominoplasty is called the simultaneous performance of a dermolipectomy plus repair of defects in the abdominal wall, and dermolipectomy is the removal of a dermo-fat flap from the abdomen [1–7].

Starting in the 1980s, great changes occurred with the arrival of liposuction.

In 1982 Villa Rovira [8] published a lipoaspiration in a dermolipectomy with extensive detachment.

Since then, works related to liposuction combined with abdominal surgery have begun to be published as a proposal to reduce abdominal flap detachment with the aim of reducing local complications in abdominoplasties [7].

In relation to abdominoplasty techniques, it can be considered a gray area in its traditional classifications, and it is the evaluation of abdominal flaccidity, since with current terminology (mild/moderate/severe) it is very subjective and difficult to measure objectively [6–8].

Ultrasound-assisted liposuction began in the late 1980s. It has been perfected, and today its advantages compared to traditional liposuction are well recognized, such as less trauma, less pain, faster recovery, and better skin tightening. More fat can be extracted, the body contour can be better modeled, and unconventional areas such as the face and legs, among others, can be aspirated [9, 10].

Reunion (J Plasma) is a technology that uses helium gas together with monopolar radiofrequency; together they generate helium plasma that acts directly on the fibro-septal network, producing its retractions and remodeling of the collagen fibers [11].

G. Di Biasio (✉)
Plastic Surgery Center Dr. Guillermo Di Biasio, Rosario, Argentina

E. M. Palmisano
Italian University Institute of Rosario (IUNIR), Rosario, Argentina

S. Cuccomarino et al. (eds.), *New Concepts in Diastasi Recti Surgery*,
https://doi.org/10.1007/978-3-031-74947-6_14

14.2 Historical Background of the MILA Tactic

The VER (Vaser/Endoscopy/Renuvion) tactic [12], today known as the MILA (minimally invasive lipoabdominoplasty) tactic [13], was born from the need to improve the aesthetic and functional result of the abdomen without requiring the indications of a traditional abdominoplasty or minidermolipectomy, causing high scars, requiring repairs of diastasis and suffering of the wound due to closure with too much tension (Fig. 14.1).

Another motivation arises as patients increase refusal to large scars and wish to preserve their original navel against a neonavel (Fig. 14.2).

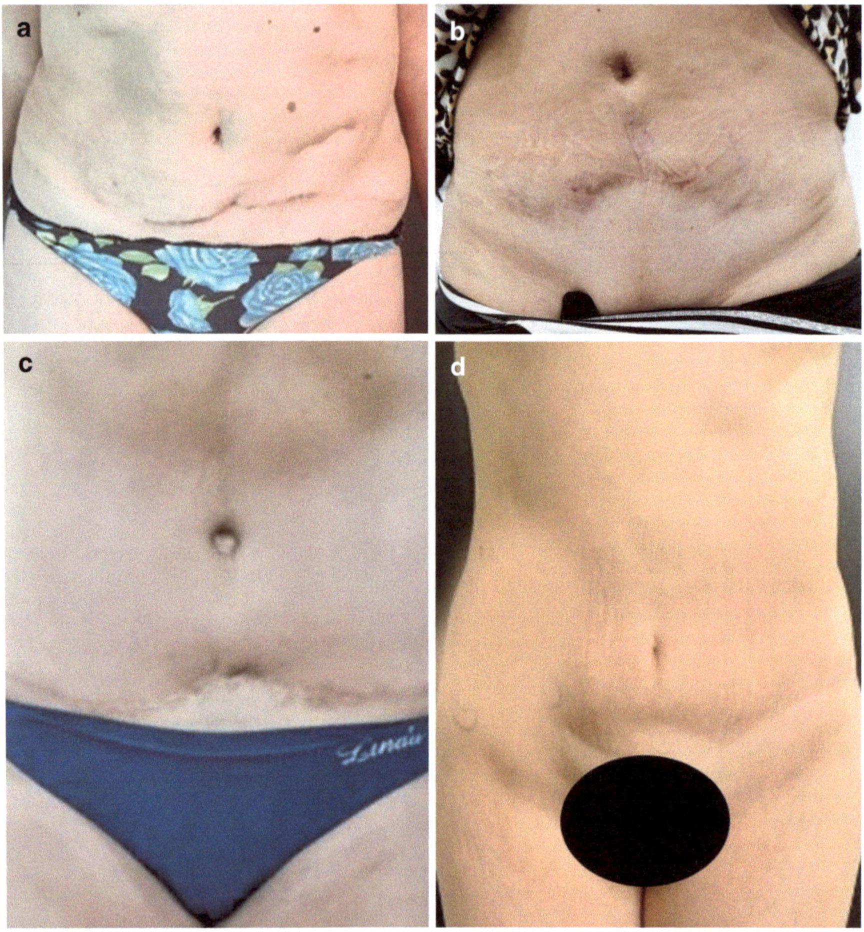

Fig. 14.1 (**a**, **b**, and **c**) High scars with stigmata of wound suffering due to tension closure. (**d**) Typical example of umbilical descent to leave a low scar when the supraumbilical flaccidity is not severe

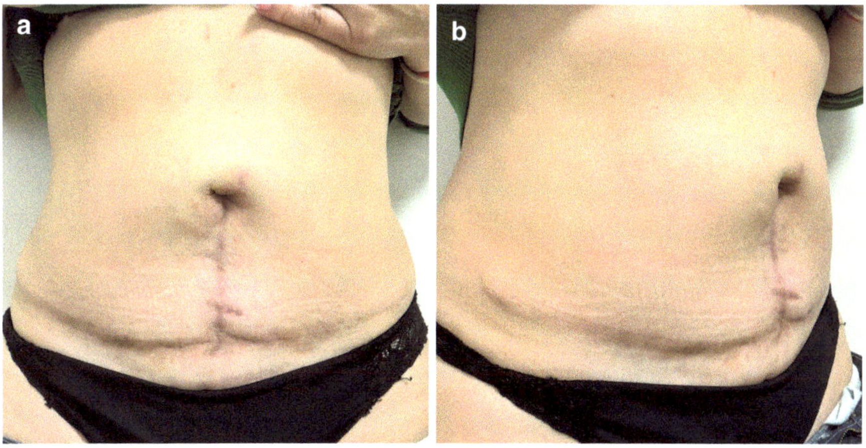

Fig. 14.2 Wide scar from abdominoplasty associated with neoumbilicus. (**a**) Front and (**b**) right anterior oblique

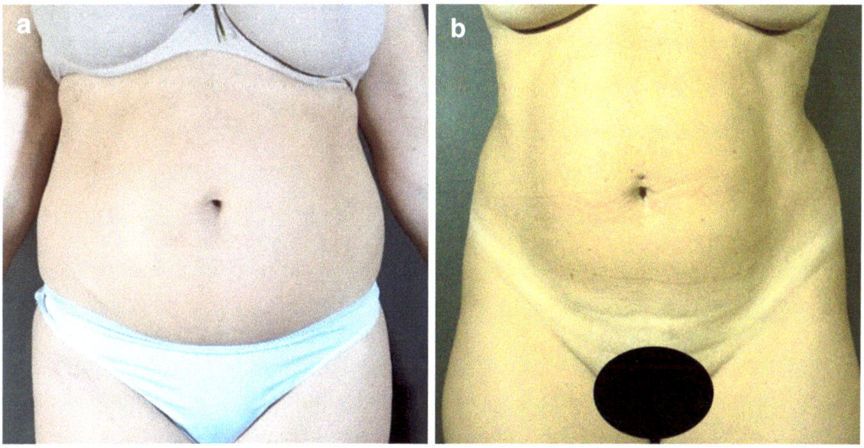

Fig. 14.3 (**a** and **b**) Both patients have a round navel, preserving its shape, ideal for the MILA technique

Mini-invasive techniques began to gain ground in the repair of abdominal diastasis; however, for a majority group of patients with abdominal sagging, the cosmetic component continued to result dissatisfied need for these procedures.

Multiple factors have led to the scenario of the development of this technique where the most important point is to evaluate the upper abdominal flaccidity and the shape of the navel (Fig. 14.3).

14.3 Indication

- Abdominal diastasis with or without midline defects (hernias) associated with mild moderate abdominal flaccidity (classification 2 and 3 by Matarazzo [14] and 2, 3, and 4 by Bazzola).
- Patient who refuse abdominoplasty/minidermolipectomy scar and a neonavel.
- Visceral fat percentage in healthy range.
- Family planning completed.
- Age has no limits as long as they meet the above requirements, and there is no formal contraindication for surgery.

14.4 Surgical Technique

It consists of three surgical stages: first stage, ultrasonic liposuction; second stage, REPA (endoscopic pre-aponeurotic repair); and third stage, final tightening, treatment of sagging.

14.4.1 First Stage: Vaser

After marking the patient (Fig. 14.4) and from two incisions (Fig. 14.5) 4 or 5 cm from the suprapubic midline (coinciding with operator ports of the second stage), we begin the infiltration of the subcutaneous fatty tissue with a combination of 1000 cm^3 of sterile physiological solution, 1 ampoule of 2% lidocaine, and 1 ampoule of 1% adrenaline. A final volume between 2 and 3 liters is used, depending on the surgeon's habit. The incisions are expanded to 5 mm by applying ultrasound (Vaser) for 1 min for every 100 cm^3 of infiltrated liquid, and then aspiration is carried out with cannulas "without pinch maneuver." It is recommended not to use "aggressive cannulas," such as a stripper, Basket, or any other that could damage the connective tissue.

14.4.2 Second Stage: Endoscopy/REPA

A 2 cm suprapubic incision is made (Fig. 14.6) (this size of incision allows us to satisfactorily conclude the reapproximation of the rectus muscles with an open technique). We made a cuticular pouch with polypropylene 1, whose purpose is to prevent peritrocar CO2 leakage, and we proceeded to place a 10 mm trocar, through which the 30° working optic was introduced (Fig. 14.7) and the work space was created with CO2 at 12 mmHg. We begin the dissection of the fibroseptal network

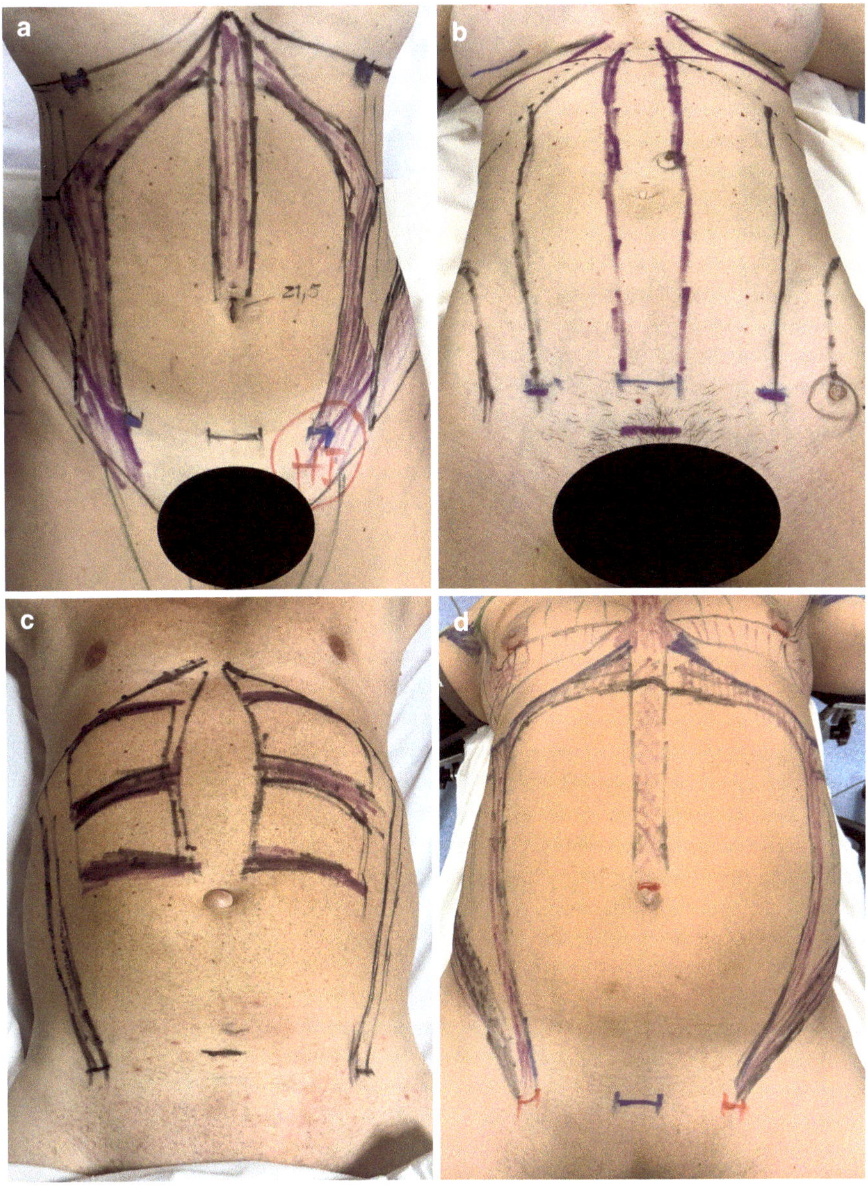

Fig. 14.4 Previous marking of the patient. (**a** and **b**) Women. (**c** and **d**) Men

(Fig. 14.8) with a monopolar hook or scissors, making an extended channel up to the xiphoid appendix limited to the size of the abdominal diastasis and ensuring sufficient space for the placement of the mesh with an overlap of at least 3 cm to its correct deployment (Fig. 14.9). The rectus muscles are reapproximated with symmetrical barbed suture of 0 gauge polydioxanone, with a 26 mm needle (CT2)

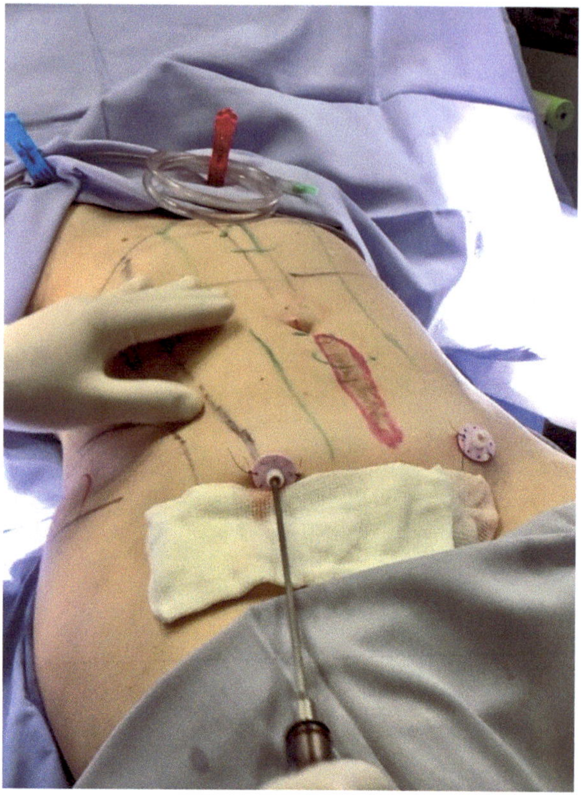

Fig. 14.5 Initial incisions for introduction of Vaser® ultrasonic liposuction cannulas

(Fig. 14.10), at which time the CO2 pressure is lowered to between 6 and 8 mmHg. A flat, macroporous polypropylene prosthesis of medium density (9 to 11 cm considering an abdominal diastasis of 3 to 5 cm) is placed and fixed with absorbable staples, adhesive, or continuous 2–0 polydioxanone suture (Fig. 14.11).

14.4.2.1 Volumization

Infiltration of the abdominal muscles (rectus, internal oblique, and transverse muscles) with fat tissue can be performed under direct vision if the case requires it. Control with ultrasound is suggested.

14.4.3 Third Stage: Renuvion

Once the instruments have been removed from the operator ports of the endoscopic access, the cannulas are introduced through the same incisions to conclude with the final tensioning using the Renuvion technique (Fig. 14.12).

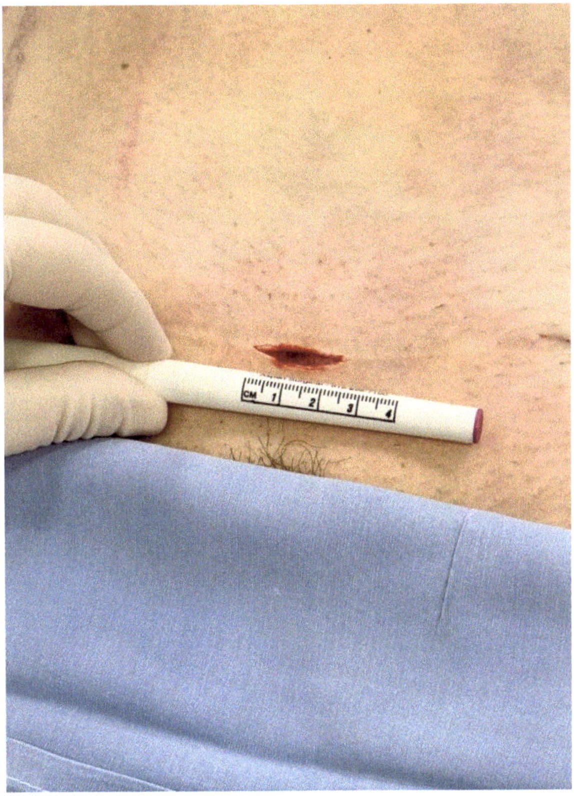

Fig. 14.6 2 cm suprapubic incision intended for placement of the optic port and final open suture route of the caudal diastasis

It is a technology that combines monopolar radiofrequency with helium gas [15–20]; in this combination, the gas is ionized and generates helium plasma fourth state of matter acting directly on the fibroseptal network in two ways:

First: direct contact with helium plasma.

Second: with the flow of our patented RF through the plasma to the tissue.

Collagen reacts predictably to the application of heat.

At higher temperatures, shorter treatment times can be used to achieve maximum shrinkage [5, 16–19].

At 65 °C collagen contracts 40% in ~2.5 min.

At 70 °C collagen contracts 40% in ~42 s.

With 85 °C collagen contracts 60% in 0.044 s and 50% more collagen contraction, ~3500 times faster, compared to a treatment temperature of 65 °C.

Currently we use APR 27 handpiece between 70 and 80 power and 2.5 to 3 liters of helium flow depending on the area to be treated. These new handpieces release plasma in 360 degrees making plasma distribution more uniform.

Stroke: It is the only application of energy. This is done anterogradely and retrogradely or retrogradely only. The speed with which it passes is 1 to 3 cm per second.

The separation between the strokes should be between 1.5 cm and 2 cm.

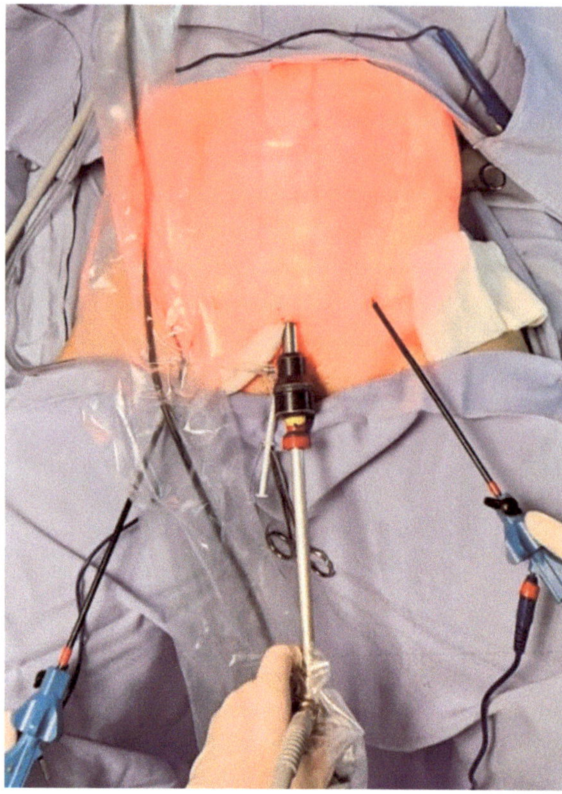

Fig. 14.7 Final layout of the endoscopic work ports

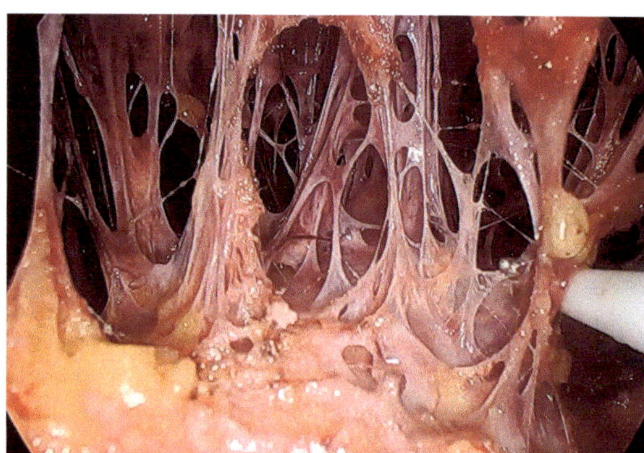

Fig. 14.8 Endoscopic visualization of the fibroseptal network

The number of strokes is variable; there are as many as necessary to cover the area to be treated.

Passes: it is the sum of several strokes, the amount varies according to the degree of flaccidity, and between four to six passes are made.

Speed: 1 to 3 cm per second, always try to do it slowly.

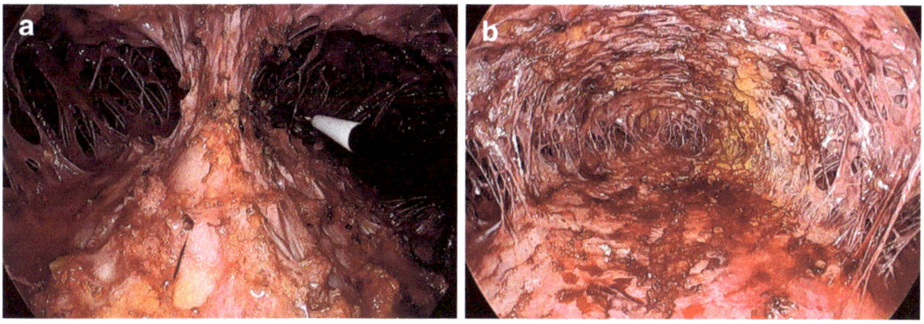

Fig. 14.9 (**a**) Endoscopic visualization of umbilical scar and (**b**) completely dissected supra-aponeurotic space

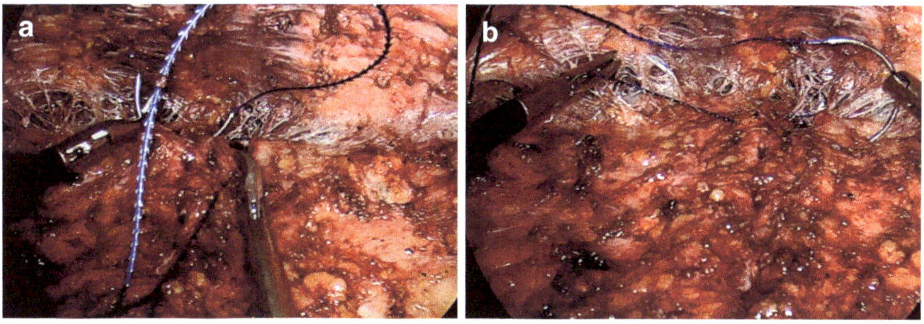

Fig. 14.10 (**a** and **b**) Reapproximation of rectus muscles with barbed suture surget

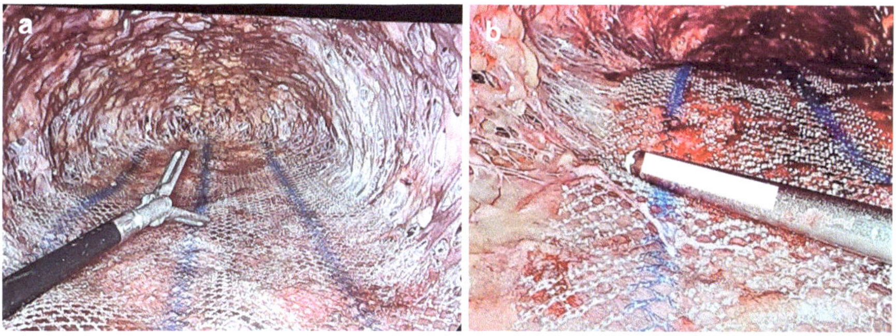

Fig. 14.11 (**a**) Placement of medium-density macropore polypropylene mesh and (**b**) fixation of the mesh with absorbable fasteners

The last step is the safety aspiration to remove residual helium.

Only 1% of the helium gas combines to form helium plasma; the rest of the gas serves for cooling and escapes through the incisions.

It is recommended to leave the wounds open or drain, the duration of the latter is variable, and it is at the discretion of the surgeon and the patient's evolution.

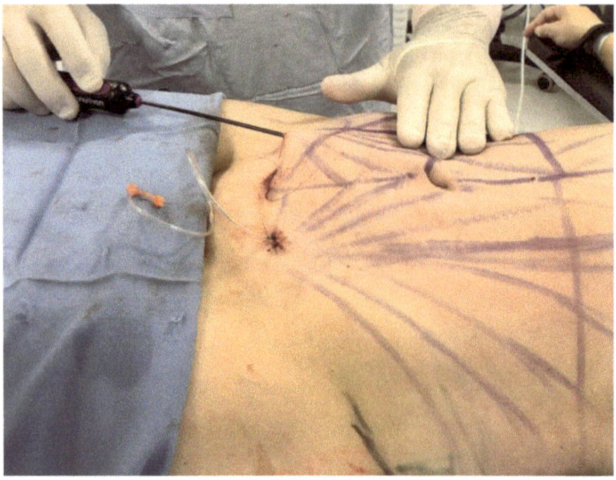

Fig. 14.12 Final tightening of the skin using the Renuvion® technique

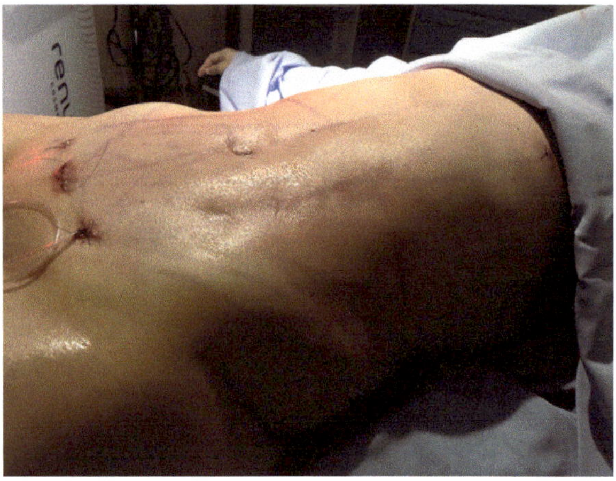

Fig. 14.13 Example of immediate result

At the end of the third stage, the incisions are closed with 3-0 intradermal nylon suture after placement of tubular or aspiration plane drainage (Fig. 14.13), which is removed according to the rate, generally between 7 and 10 days or when the rate is lower at 30cm^3 and its serous appearance.

Early mobilization after anesthesia recovery.

Low molecular weight heparin. One dose 12 h after the procedure.

Postoperative analgesia is indicated with 40 mg ketorolac every 8 h during the first 48 h; thereafter, 20 mg every 12 h with paracetamol rescue of 1 g every 12 h as needed associated with cefadroxil of 1 g every 12 h for 3–5 days (in those allergic to penicillin, we use ciprofloxacin 500 mg every 12 h during the same time).

Diet rich in fiber and intake of no less than 2 or 3 liters of fluids to compensate for losses.

Medium compression girdle with padding is indicated.

It is associated with the application of special elastic adhesive tapes on the area after the operation (taping) in order to reduce edema, ecchymosis, and fibrosis. When it is not feasible to apply it in the immediate postoperative period, its placement should not be delayed beyond 24 h.

It is indicated with manual lymphatic drainage from the first day of the operation.

The performance of hypopressive exercises is indicated according to kinesiology criterion depending on the clinical evolution. Clinical and ultrasound follow-up is carried out in the short, medium, and long term (Fig. 14.14).

a

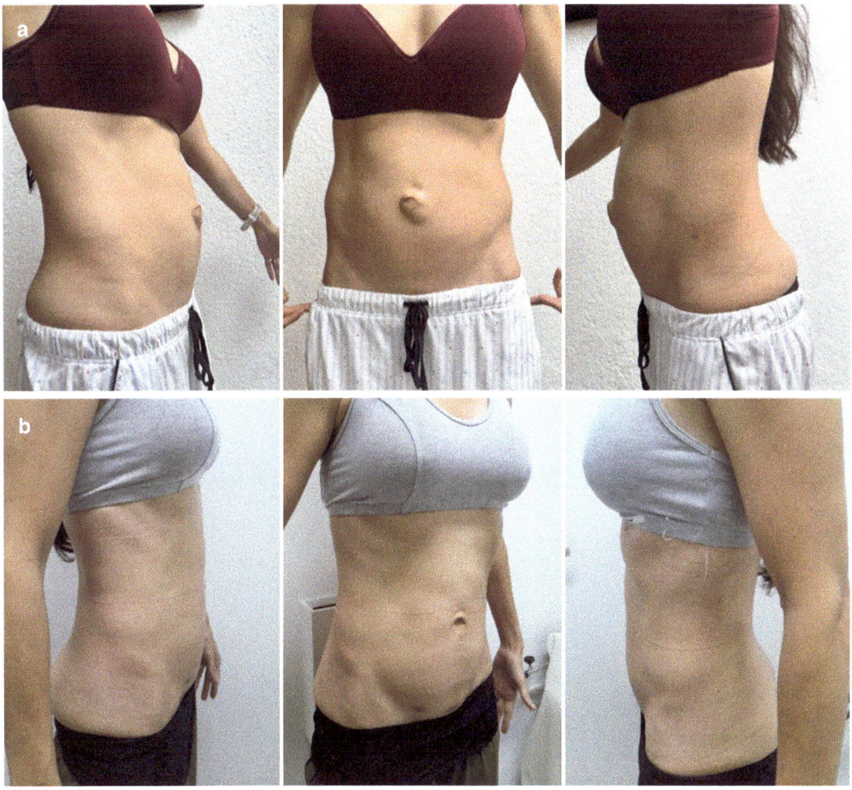

Fig. 14.14 (**a**, **b**, and **c**) Examples of long-term results

b

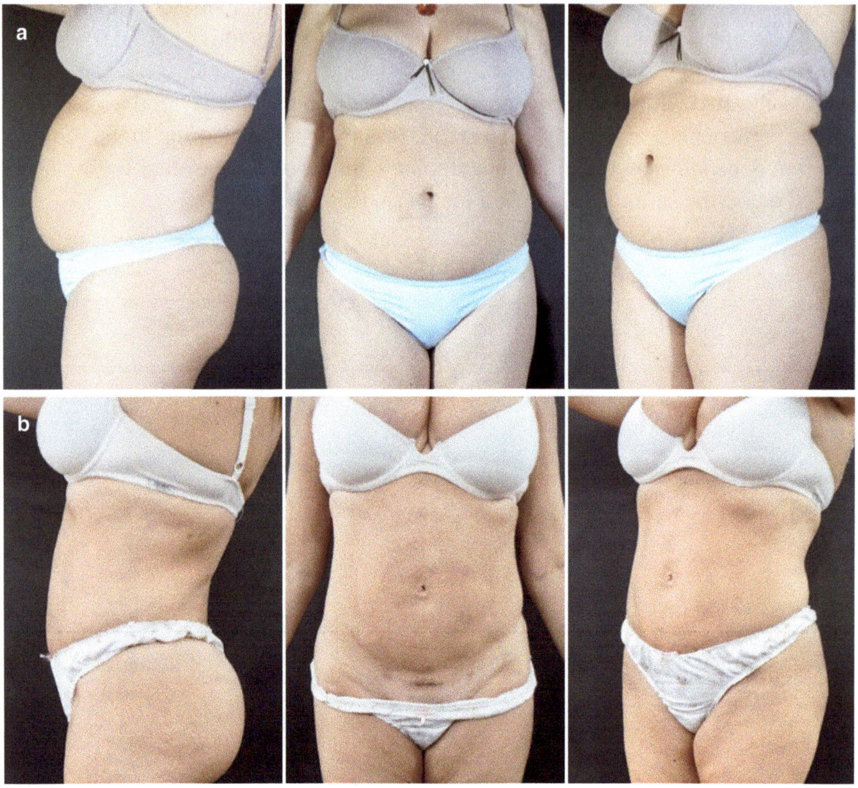

Fig. 14.14 (continued)

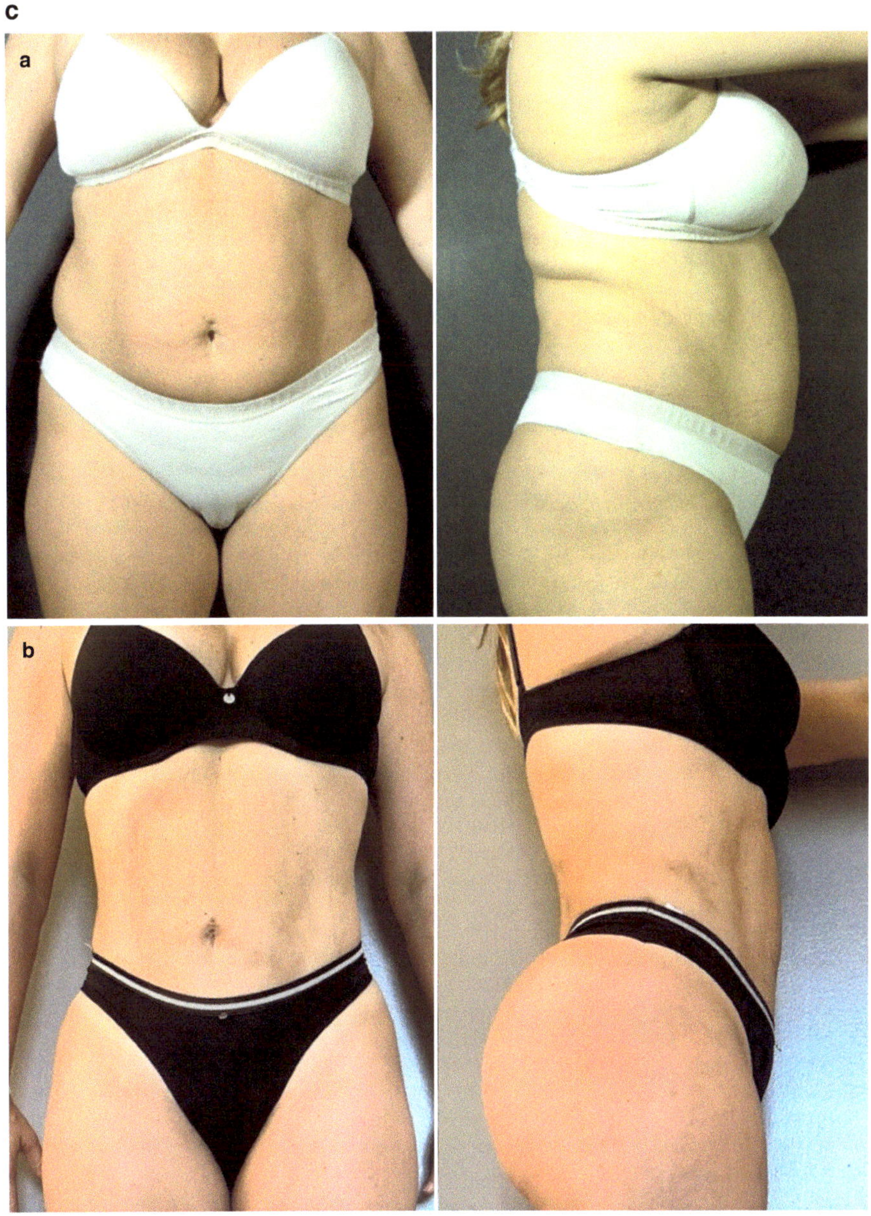

Fig. 14.14 (continued)

References

1. Kelly HA. Report of gynecological cases. Johns Hopkins Med. 1989;10:197.
2. Gaudet F, Morestin H. French congress of surgeons, vol. vol 82. Paris; 1905. p. 125.
3. Gonzalez-Ulloa M. Belt lipectomy. Br J Plast Surg. 1960;13:179–86. https://doi.org/10.1016/s0007-1226(60)80035-5.
4. Pitanguy I. Abdominoplastias [Abdominal plastic surgery]. Hospital (Rio J). 1967;71(6):1541–56. Portuguese
5. Rebello C, Franco T. Abdomioplastia through submamary incisión. In: Intern Cong- international Soc. of Aesthetic Plastic. Surg. Rio de Janeiro. Madrid: Ed. Publicaciones Controladas; 1972. p. 58.
6. Hakme F. Technical details in abdominoplasty associated with liposuction. Rev Bras Cir. 1985;75(5):331–7.
7. Saldanha OR. Lipoabdominoplasty without undermining. Aesth Surg J. 2001;21:518–26.
8. Villa RR. Liposuccion en cirugía plástica y estética. España: Ed Salvat; 1988. p. 81–5.
9. Zocchi M. Ultrasonic liposculpturing. Aesth Plast Surg. 2020;44(4):1218–29. https://doi.org/10.1007/s00266-020-01824-w. PMID: 32766910.
10. Adamo C, Mazzocchi M, Rossi A, Scuderi N. Ultrasonic liposculpturing: extrapolations from the analysis of in vivo sonicated adipose tissue. Plast Reconstr Surg. 1997;100(1):220–6. https://doi.org/10.1097/00006534-199707000-00033. PMID: 9207679.
11. Masghati S, Pedroso J, Gutierrez M, Stocwell E, Volker W, Howard DL. Comparative thermal effects of J-Plasma®, Monopolar, Argon, and Laser electrosurgery in a Porcine Tissue Model. Surg Technol Int. 2019;34:1–5.
12. Palmisano EM, Di Biasio G. Alternativa de manejo miniinvasivo para el tratamiento de pacientes con diástasis abdominal y colgajo dermograso mediante la táctica VER: Vaser® + endoscopia + Renuvion®. Rev Hispanoam Hernia. 2022;10(4):167–71.
13. Claus C, Palmisano EM. MILA (Minimally invasive lipoabdominoplasty) for diastasis recti. Are general surgeons and plastic surgeons fighting or playing together? Rev Argent Cir. 2023;115(4):393–5. Retrieved from https://revista.aac.org.ar/index.php/RevArgentCirug/article/view/637.
14. Matarasso A. Abdominoplasty: Q System of classification and treatment for combined abdominoplasty and suction assisted lipectomy. Aesthe Plas Surg. 1991;15:111.
15. Duncan DI, Roman S. Helium plasma subdermal tissue contraction method of action. Biomedic J Sci Tech Res. 2020;31(2):24063–8.
16. Feldman LS, Fuchshuber PR, Jones DB. The SAGES manual on the Fundamental Use of Surgical Energy (FUSE). New York: Springer; 2012. ISBN 978-1-4614-2073-6.
17. Chen SS, Wright NT, Humphrey JD. Heat- induced changes in the mechanics of a collagenous tissue: isothermal free shrinkage. J Biomech Eng. 1997;109:372–8.
18. MacDonald MB. Conductive keratoplasty: a radiofrequency-based technique for the correction of hyperopia. Trans Am Ophthalmol Soc. 2005;103:512–36.
19. Chen SS, Humprey JD. Heat-induced changes in the mechanics of de collagenous tissue: pseudoelastic behavior at 37° C. J Biomech. 1998;31:211–6.
20. Wright NT, Humprey JD. Denaturation of collagen during heating: an irreversible rate process. Annu Rev Biomed Eng. 2004;4:109–28.

Chapter 15
The Role of Physiotherapy

Marcel Caufriez and Fabrizio Botanica

15.1 Introduction

During the last decade, the treatment of diastasis recti has received more and more attention, and studies have reported positive results after surgical repair [1–3].

Although numerous reviews have been published, there is still no consensus on which is the best treatment due to contradictory results and insufficient follow-up times [4–6].

However, guidelines have been published about the treatment of diastasis [7, 8] and the recommendation of treatments of first line; it is training for the stability of the abdominal core [9, 10]; there is still much debate about the best method to use, and its duration and results vary between studies [9, 11–14].

If the core training fails, the guidelines propose surgical repair, also considering other parameters such us interrectal distance (IRD) and a maximum BMI limit [7, 8].

Evidences show that different surgical techniques reduce recurrencies and postpartum complications in the patients who have not shown improvement with a core training program [2, 3, 15].

Specifically, the role of physiotherapy is reviewed in the literature, specially in the case of conservative treatment of diastasis; most studies are performed in the pre- and postpartum period, correlating diastasis with pregnancy and physical activity performed after it (e.g., carrying babies in a baby carrier) [16–23].

M. Caufriez
Université Libre de Bruxelles, Brussels, Belgium

Laboratory for Experimental and Applied Human Ecophysiology, Palma, Spain

F. Botanica (✉)
Scientific Research Committee, ACHC (Abdominal Core Health Center), Cuneo-Torino, Italy
e-mail: fabriziobotanica@abdominalcorehealthcenter.com

S. Cuccomarino et al. (eds.), *New Concepts in Diastasi Recti Surgery*,
https://doi.org/10.1007/978-3-031-74947-6_15

In relation to surgery, it has recently been shown that it is useful to associate the operation, both before and after it, with physiotherapy and also with complementary therapy such as yoga, pilates, and acupuncture [24, 25] in a concept defined as TOR (training, operation, and rehabilitation) [26].

15.2 Abdominal Core Health Concept

Both surgical and conservative treatment of diastasis recti should be considered as the correction of a pathology that affects a sector that is part of a complex functional unit that is defined as abdominal core, composed of the thoracic diaphragm, pelvic floor, abdominal wall, and lumbar spine. The abdominal core allows the patient to run, jump, sit, stand, turn, work, do exercise, urinate, and defecate without effort [27].

This concept becomes even more fundamental if, in addition to the functional observation of the region, the symptoms associated with the presence of diastasis are taken into account, such as low back pain, muscle weakness, abdominal pain, incorrect posture, stress urinary incontinence, gastroesophageal reflux, etc. [28–33].

Diastasis recti occurs when abdominal pressure is greater than the tissue resistance of the abdominal wall. From here it can be deduced that the role of pre- and postoperative physiotherapy should be aimed at identifying and correcting these two parameters first, to improve the surgeon's work during surgery and, above all, accelerate postoperative recovery and reduce the risk of recurrences.

Taking these aspects into account, it is difficult to protocolize a preoperative and postoperative physiotherapy process, and the key to good patient management is, in our opinion, considering some fundamental aspects of diastasis recti and building a tailored path for the patient in order to achieve the best possible surgical result, accelerate postoperative recovery, and reduce postoperative complications.

Therefore, the intervention must be personalized on the basis of a precise physiotherapeutic evaluation, in which the data must be objective and well quantifiable, with certified instruments that allow the repeatability of the test.

The main components to take into account are a muscular balance of the different muscular components of the core (diaphragmatic, abdominal, and pelvic), the management of abdominal pressure (especially in the presence of other symptoms such as gastroesophageal reflux, hernias, stress urinary incontinence, or prolapse), the stimulation of collagen turnover at the level of the linea alba, and the decrease in inflammatory levels.

Therefore, if the work is well structured, the multidisciplinary team should be able to recognize the best moment to do the surgical intervention.

15.3 Physiotherapy Evaluation

In light of what has been explained, the physiotherapeutic evaluation in the approach to diastasis must take into account all the aspects that could have favored its appearance: increase in abdominal pressure, alteration of the collagen component, deficit in muscle proprioception, as well as the co-presence of perineal (incontinence, prolapse), respiratory, abdominal (hernias, gastroesophageal reflux), or spinal symptoms.

15.3.1 Medical History

The patient's anamnestic examination should include the different specific rating scales related to the quantification of pain and quality of life. In our opinion, it should also include an in-depth exploration of overall musculoskeletal, respiratory, gastrointestinal, and urogenital functionality.

15.3.2 Objective Exam

The objective examination of the patient must specifically evaluate the abdominal wall, the pelvic muscles, and, more generally, the overall postural attitude.

Therefore, it will be necessary to examine the abdominal skin reflexes, the resistance of the rectus muscles to manual separation, the presence of previous scars, and possible asymmetries of the linea alba and the muscles.

At the perineal level, it is good to observe the presence of the different reflexes, performing a careful muscular examination, as well as the presence of a possible descent of the internal organs and the behavior of their support component, such as the intra-abdominal, when the pressure varies; the last is an important element to more precisely define the current physiology of the core.

15.3.3 Instrumental Tests

The instrumental tests to be used in the field of physiotherapy evaluation should include functional evaluation by ultrasound, electromyography, biofeedback, spirometry, and perineal tonimetry.

Ultrasound evaluation should be aimed at establishing correct respiratory synergy between the thoracic diaphragm, oblique muscles, and abdominal recti.

In our opinion, the important information to obtain are the dimensions of the muscle bellies (in comparison with the lateral controls and the other muscles examined) and possible structural alterations (such as the alteration of the semilunar line); the values must be obtained at rest and with an active maneuver that causes an increase in abdominal pressure.

Electromyography allows us to exclude lesions and/or physiological alterations (mono or bilateral) of the peripheral nervous component, while the use of biofeedback can give a useful indication to establish to what extent the patient's proprioception in the same muscles is altered (and to what extent it will be recoverable).

The spirometric evaluation should provide useful data to evaluate the entity of the diaphragmatic thrust on the abdominal core at rest and under stress, studying the presence of possible respiratory restrictions and dysnecias of the inspiratory muscles.

On the other hand, perineal tonimetry provides an objective parameter of the quality of the tonic and phasic muscle components and unlike the "test" normally used (force evaluation with the operator's fingers giving a value from 0 to 4) provides objective numerical data that cannot be influenced by the therapist.

Profilometer: the use of the profilometer makes it possible to evaluate the modification of the linea alba during a calibrated expiratory effort. It is a test that requires good execution experience to reduce the influence of operator error but that, in our experience, can provide important information about the failure of the abdominal wall under stress (increased pressure).

15.4 What Exercise of Physiotherapy?

Exercises used in the diastasis recti treatment protocol must take into account some fundamental factors such as the synergistic activation of the abdominal wall and pelvic muscles and the role of the core as a shock absorber and container of abdominal pressure; it should not allow a greater widening of the straight lines at the time of its execution.

The synergistic activation of the pelvic and abdominal muscles is well highlighted in the literature; several studies have shown that voluntary contraction of the abdominal muscles leads to a reverse co-contraction of the perineal muscles [9, 34–38]. Therefore it seems that the contraction of the perineum can be used to train the abdominal fascia and reduce diastasis [39, 40]. There are numerous studies that demonstrate how the activation of one region reflexively triggers the activation of the other [41–49].

Hypopressive exercises are widely studied in the literature both as a method of rehabilitation of pelvic dysfunctions and in the treatment of diastasis, and the results validate their effectiveness [50–53] especially due to the effects not only on the abdominal muscles but also on the respiratory thoracic and perineal muscles [53].

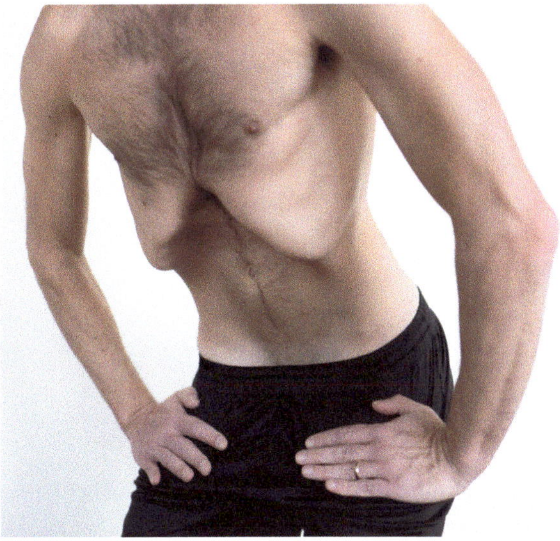

Fig. 15.1 Propaedeutic hypopressive exercise

Various studies have compared hypopressive gymnastics with the execution of exercises to strengthen the pelvic floor; some showed no differences between the study groups [54–56]; others, however, showed better results if both works were carried out at the same time [55–57].

Physical activity also plays a fundamental role in modulating inflammation; therefore, it is important to regulate the specific muscle training of the abdominal core at a specific intensity that varies depending on the patient's training [58–62].

Given this, hypopressive gymnastics seems to be the first option in the management of diastasis, especially if it is considered that the latter is part of a complex functional unit such as the core (Fig. 15.1).

15.5 Biofeedback and RUSI

The use of biofeedback is widely documented and is of fundamental importance to repropiocept the correct neurophysiology of the abdominal core.

Different modalities of biofeedback are described in the literature; however, the most used are ultrasound, pressure, and electromyography [63].

Several studies have verified the use of different methods without being able to show differences [64–67].

Ultrasound biofeedback and its use in rehabilitation (RUSI) are quick, easy, risk-free, non-invasive, and economical; it is generally used to evaluate muscle morphology (thickness, cross-sectional area, and volume), quality (echogenicity, adipose infiltration), and function [68–75].

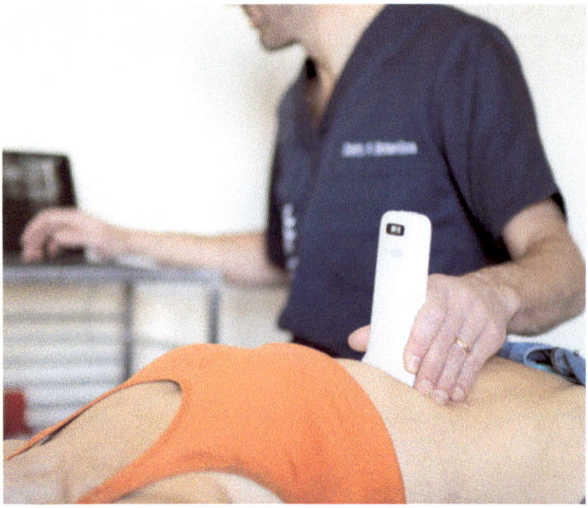

Fig. 15.2 RUSI—functional evaluation of abdominal muscles

We consider it a fundamental part in the management of the abdominal core since it allows us to:

- Measure muscle sections and assess any dominant laterality
- Have a simultaneous view of muscle activations at different depths (this is important to evaluate, for example, in a respiratory action, the coordination between the oblique and transverse abdominal muscles)
- Have a global vision of the muscular functioning of the entire behavior of the associated joint component
- Have real visual feedback and not numerical or audible feedback, which may be more motivating for some patients [68]

Pressure biofeedback is generally used in the perineal area to obtain values regarding intravaginal and anorectal pressures in response to correct or incorrect activation of the abdominal and respiratory muscles [76, 77].

Electromyography is well studied, especially in the perineal area [78–83]; it certainly provides more objective and repeatable data, but it is more invasive and annoying for the patient, with the consequent risk of loss of effectiveness of the intervention. Alternatively, surface electromyography is not invasive but does not allow analysis of deep muscles [84–86] (Fig. 15.2).

15.6 Increased Intra-abdominal Pressure and the Role of the Diaphragm

Intra-abdominal pressure is defined as the stationary pressure present within the abdominal cavity and resulting from the interaction between the abdominal wall and the visceras [87–93].

As mentioned above, diastasis occurs when abdominal pressure is greater than the tissue resistance of the linea alba.

Furthermore, if we consider the abdominal cavity and abdominal muscles as a complex functional unit, two physical laws that participate in the upkeep of physiology can be taken into account: Laplace's law, according to which the tension in the anterior wall is directly proportional to its thickness; and Pascal's principle, according to which the pressure exerted on the abdominal core is transmitted equally and unchanged to all parts of the muscles [27].

It has been shown that intra-abdominal pressure is strongly correlated with abdominal wall tension monitored over the inguinal ligament and in the upper lumbar trigone area and can be measured from this. The same study showed comparable results between anorectal manometry and indirect abdominal wall manometry [94, 95].

The risk factors most commonly considered in the case of diastasis are obesity, a previous pregnancy, and an alteration in the quality of the tissues (especially collagen); the first two are strictly related to an increase in abdominal pressure; on the other hand, the tissue alteration is related to age and/or to a hormonally based histological alteration, which may be linked to pregnancy, age, genetic factors, or complications of unhealthy conditions in the endocrinological field.

The diaphragm is made up of 60% type I muscle fibers, which gives it a predominant tonic-postural meaning; from them it is deduced that global postural analysis should be an integral part of the evaluation of the abdominal core.

In addition, it has been shown that intra-abdominal pressure oscillates according to the respiratory phases and the resistance of the abdominal wall [87–93].

We are convinced that a condition of hypertonicity of the diaphragm muscle can be a cause of increased abdominal pressure: if diaphragmatic hypertonicity is associated with acute effort (coughing) or prolonged effort (weight lifting), this risk increases.

Few studies have addressed the topic, and none of them have established a clear correlation between diaphragmatic hypertonicity and increased intra-abdominal pressure. This is probably due to the adaptability of all the structures that make up the abdominal core.

Furthermore, increased diaphragmatic tone can be a cause of gastroesophageal reflux [96, 97], which is very common in patients with diastasis and which improves or disappears in a very high percentage of cases after surgery, so the co-presence of this pathology could be evaluated to consider abdominal hyperpressure as a cause of diastasis.

Some studies have shown that the use of equipment that trains respiratory muscles in situations of isocapnic hyperpnea has positive results on tissue oxygenation [98, 99] and abdomino-thoracic coordination [98] without increasing maximum inspiratory pressure [100] (Fig. 15.3).

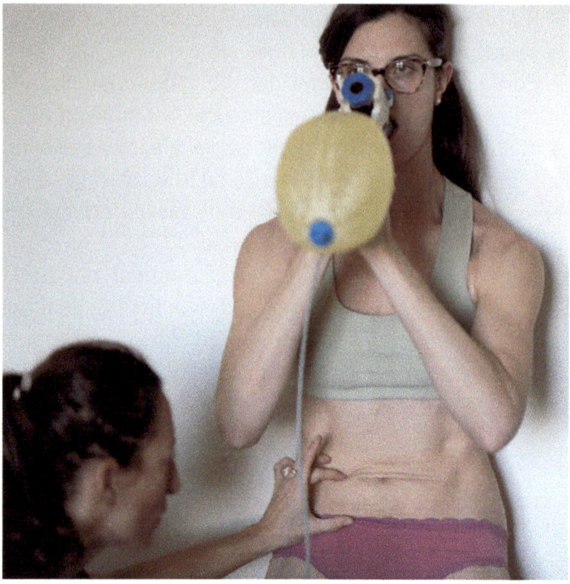

Fig. 15.3 Diaphragmatic neuromuscular rehabilitation in condition of isocapnic hyperpnea

15.7 The Role of Collagen

The rectus abdominal muscles are essentially tonic muscles (such as the obliques and transversus) and have 70% type I muscle fibers; its functions are, among others, to maintain and protect the abdominal viscera and stabilize posture in general, the pelvic region, and the lumbar spine [99–104].

It is currently demonstrated that the tone of the abdominal fascia is related in women to the tone of the perineum and that parietal abdominal hypotonia can be associated with the presence of stress urinary incontinence or descent of the pelvic organs [103–106].

These functions are possible if the muscle insertions are functional: each rectus abdominis muscle inserts laterally into the internal oblique (in 90% of cases) and contralaterally into the other rectus muscle through the linea alba [30, 107, 108].

The histological constitution of the linea alba includes collagen fibers of type I and type III [109, 110].

The resistance of the linea alba during physical effort depends on the increase in abdominal pressure, the amount of collagen, and the orientation of the fibers (collagen has anisotropic properties, and the best orientation of the fibers seems to be oblique) [111–113].

In women, diastasis has a high incidence after pregnancy; most of them do not recover their pre-pregnancy condition (reference time at 3 years) and persist over time, worsening with physical effort (sports, weight lifting) and with age [114–120].

Currently we do not know the prevalence of dysfunctions or pathologies related to diastasis recti in women, many of them ask for a specialist consultation 3 months after giving birth, and the aesthetic reason seems to be the most frequent [105, 119].

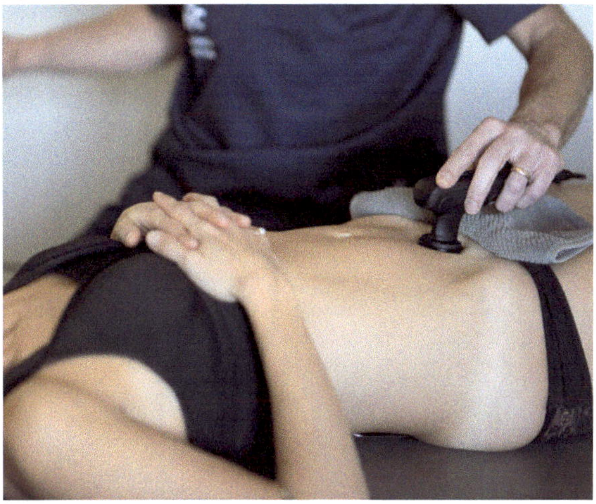

Fig. 15.4 Collagenic turnover stimulation using capacitive radiofrequency (hyperthermia)

We think that in a state of diastasis associated with hypotonia of the abdominal wall, it could give rise to functional low back pain (without traumatic origin) and be the cause of perineal symptoms.

In fact, some studies associate the presence of diastasis recti with a decrease in stability of the lumbar spine and the presence of pelvic dysfunctions such as prolapses and incontinence [99–104].

According to one of our studies, the use of capacitive radiofrequency (hyperthermia) has positive effects on the reduction of diastasis, as well as on the muscle structure of both the rectus and transverse muscles.

Furthermore, this work carried out before the operation allows for better integration of the mesh precisely thanks to the stimulation of collagen renewal (Fig. 15.4).

15.8 Stimulation of Microcirculation and Lymphatic Drainage

During the preparation phase for the surgical procedure and in the postoperative period, the role of physiotherapy should also be aimed at obtaining the best physiology of the microcirculation of the abdominal wall, increasing lymphatic drainage and vascularization.

For this purpose, both manual lymphatic drainage [56, 121, 122] and the application of neuromuscular tape are useful [123, 124]; analyzing the published studies, the choice to do both seems better, since the application of the tape could amplify and prolong the effect of manual work over time [121–124].

In addition, capacitive and/or resistive radiofrequency work has proven to be useful to improve drainage at the level of the superficial fascia [122] and increase superficial microcirculation [125–127] as well as the viscoelasticity of muscle tissue [128].

The significant increase in superficial microcirculation appears to last at least 24–48 h [129, 130]. Combining radiofrequency with manual therapy increases the effectiveness of the work [125–128].

References

1. Emanuelsson P, Gunnarsson U, Strigård K, Stark B. Early complications, pain, and quality of life after reconstructive surgery for abdominal rectus muscle diastasis: a 3-month follow-up. J Plast Reconstr Aesthet Surg. 2014;67(8):1082–8.
2. Emanuelsson P, Gunnarsson U, Dahlstrand U, Strigård K, Stark B. Operative correction of abdominal rectus diastasis (ARD) reduces pain and improves abdominal wall muscle strength: a randomized, prospective trial comparing retromuscular mesh repair to double-row, self-retaining sutures. Surgery. 2016;160(5):1367–75.
3. Olsson A, Kiwanuka O, Wilhelmsson S, Sandblom G, Stackelberg O. Cohort study of the effect of surgical repair of symptomatic diastasis recti abdominis on abdominal trunk function and quality of life. BJS Open. 2019;3(6):750–8.
4. Akram J, Matzen SH. Rectus abdominis diastasis. J Plast Surg Hand Surg. 2014;48(3):163–9.
5. Mommers EHH, Ponten JEH, Al Omar AK, de Vries Reilingh TS, Bouvy ND, Nienhuijs SW. The general surgeon's perspective of rectus diastasis. A systematic review of treatment options. Surg Endosc. 2017;31(12):4934–49.
6. Michalska A, Rokita W, Wolder D, Pogorzelska J, Kaczmarczyk K. Diastasis recti abdominis—a review of treatment methods. Ginekol Pol. 2018;89(2):97–101.
7. Carlstedt A, Bringman S, Egberth M, Emanuelsson P, Olsson A, Petersson U, Pålstedt J, Sandblom G, Sjödahl R, Stark B, Strigård K, Tall J, Theodorsson E. Management of diastasis of the rectus abdominis muscles: recommendations for Swedish national guidelines. Scand J Surg. 2021;110(3):452–9.
8. Reinpold W, Köckerling F, Bittner R, Conze J, Fortelny R, Koch A, Kukleta J, Kuthe A, Lorenz R, Stechemesser B. Classification of rectus diastasis-a proposal by the German Hernia Society (DHG) and the International Endohernia Society (IEHS). Front Surg. 2019;6:1.
9. Lee D, Hodges PW. Behavior of the linea alba during a curl-up task in diastasis rectus abdominis: an observational study. J Orthop Sports Phys Ther. 2016;46(7):580–9.
10. Thabet AA, Alshehri MA. Efficacy of deep core stability exercise program in postpartum women with diastasis recti abdominis: a randomised controlled trial. J Musculoskelet Neuronal Interact. 2019;19(1):62–8.
11. Cavalli M, Aiolfi A, Bruni PG, Manfredini L, Lombardo F, Bonfanti MT, Bona D, Campanelli G. Prevalence and risk factors for diastasis recti abdominis: a review and proposal of a new anatomical variation. Hernia. 2021;25(4):883–90.
12. Benjamin DR, van de Water AT, Peiris CL. Effects of exercise on diastasis of the rectus abdominis muscle in the antenatal and postnatal periods: a systematic review. Physiotherapy. 2014;100(1):1–8.
13. Gallus KM, Golberg KF, Field R. Functional improvement following diastasis rectus abdominus repair in an active duty navy female. Mil Med. 2016;181(8):e952–4.
14. Gluppe SL, Hilde G, Tennfjord MK, Engh ME, Bø K. Effect of a postpartum training program on the prevalence of diastasis recti abdominis in postpartum primiparous women: a randomized controlled trial. Phys Ther. 2018;98(4):260–8.
15. Rodrigues MA, Nahas FX, Reis RP, Ferreira LM. Does diastasis width influence the variation of the intra-abdominal pressure after correction of rectus diastasis? Aesthet Surg J. 2015;35(5):583–8.

16. Keshwani N, Mathur S, McLean L. The impact of exercise therapy and abdominal binding in the management of diastasis recti abdominis in the early post-partum period: a pilot randomized controlled trial. Physiother Theory Pract. 2021;37(9):1018–33.
17. Bixo L, Sandblom G, Österberg J, Stackelberg O, Bewö K, Olsson A. Association between inter-recti distance and impaired abdominal core function in post-partum women with diastasis recti abdominis. J Abdom Wall Surg. 2022;1:10909.
18. Boissonnault JS, Blaschak MJ. Incidence of diastasis recti abdominis during the childbearing year. Phys Ther. 1988;68(7):1082–6.
19. Hu J, Gu J, Yu Z, Yang X, Fan J, You L, Hua Q, Zhao Y, Yan Y, Bai W, Xu Z, You L, Chen C. Efficacy of standardized rehabilitation in the treatment of diastasis rectus abdominis in postpartum women. Int J Gen Med. 2021;14:10373–83.
20. Gluppe S, Engh ME, Bø K. What is the evidence for abdominal and pelvic floor muscle training to treat diastasis recti abdominis postpartum? A systematic review with meta-analysis. Braz J Phys Ther. 2021;25(6):664–75.
21. Ghandali NY, Iravani M, Habibi A, Cheraghian B. The effectiveness of a pilates exercise program during pregnancy on childbirth outcomes: a randomised controlled clinical trial. BMC Pregnancy Childbirth. 2021;21(1):480.
22. Fukano M, Tsukahara Y, Takei S, Nose-Ogura S, Fujii T, Torii S. Recovery of abdominal muscle thickness and contractile function in women after childbirth. Int J Environ Res Public Health. 2021;18(4):2130.
23. Gluppe SB, Engh ME, Bø K. Immediate effect of abdominal and pelvic floor muscle exercises on interrecti distance in women with diastasis recti abdominis who were parous. Phys Ther. 2020;100(8):1372–83.
24. Poulose BK, Adrales GL, Janis JE. Abdominal core health-a needed field in surgery. JAMA Surg. 2020;155(3):185–6.
25. Lee N, Bae YH, Fong SSM, Lee WH. Effects of pilates on inter-recti distance, thickness of rectus abdominis, waist circumference and abdominal muscle endurance in primiparous women. BMC Womens Health. 2023;23(1):626.
26. Olsson A, Woxnerud K, Kiwanuka O, Sandblom G, Stackelberg O. The TOR concept (training, operation, and rehabilitation) applied to a cohort of postpartum women with training-resistant symptomatic rectus diastasis: evaluation 1 year after surgery. BJS Open. 2023;7(1):zrac162.
27. Poulose BK. Abdominal core health: what is it? Surg Clin North Am. 2023;103(5):827–34.
28. Hills NF, Graham RB, McLean L. Comparison of trunk muscle function between women with and without diastasis recti abdominis at 1 year postpartum. Phys Ther. 2018;98(10):891–901.
29. Benjamin DR, Frawley HC, Shields N, van de Water ATM, Taylor NF. Relationship between diastasis of the rectus abdominis muscle (DRAM) and musculoskeletal dysfunctions, pain and quality of life: a systematic review. Physiotherapy. 2019;105(1):24–34.
30. Keshwani N, Mathur S, McLean L. Relationship between interrectus distance and symptom severity in women with diastasis recti abdominis in the early postpartum period. Phys Ther. 2018;98(3):182–90.
31. Parker MM, Dugan S. Diastasis rectus abdominis and lumbo-pelvic pain and dysfunction–are they related? J Women's Health Phys Ther. 2009;33(2):15–22.
32. Doubkova L, Andel R, Palascakova-Springrova I, Kolar P, Kriz J, Kobesova A. Diastasis of rectus abdominis muscles in low back pain patients. J Back Musculoskelet Rehabil. 2018;31(1):107–12.
33. Liaw LJ, Hsu MJ, Liao CF, Liu MF, Hsu AT. The relationships between inter-recti distance measured by ultrasound imaging and abdominal muscle function in postpartum women: a 6-month follow-up study. J Orthop Sports Phys Ther. 2011;41(6):435–43.
34. Zachovajeviene B, Siupsinskas L, Zachovajevas P, Venclovas Z, Milonas D. Effect of diaphragm and abdominal muscle training on pelvic floor strength and endurance: results of a prospective randomized trial. Sci Rep. 2019;9(1):19192.

35. Benjamin DR, Frawley HC, Shields N, Peiris CL, van de Water ATM, Bruder AM, Taylor NF. Conservative interventions may have little effect on reducing diastasis of the rectus abdominis in postnatal women—a systematic review and meta-analysis. Physiotherapy. 2023;119:54–71.
36. Brown SH, McGill SM. A comparison of ultrasound and electromyography measures of force and activation to examine the mechanics of abdominal wall contraction. Clin Biomech (Bristol, Avon). 2010;25(2):115–23.
37. Ishida H, Watanabe S. Changes in lateral abdominal muscles' thickness immediately after the abdominal drawing-in maneuver and maximum expiration. J Bodyw Mov Ther. 2013;17(2):254–8.
38. Vasseljen O, Fladmark AM. Abdominal muscle contraction thickness and function after specific and general exercises: a randomized controlled trial in chronic low back pain patients. Man Ther. 2010;15(5):482–9.
39. Neumann P, Gill V. Pelvic floor and abdominal muscle interaction: EMG activity and intra-abdominal pressure. Int Urogynecol J Pelvic Floor Dysfunct. 2002;13(2):125–32.
40. Madill SJ, McLean L. Quantification of abdominal and pelvic floor muscle synergies in response to voluntary pelvic floor muscle contractions. J Electromyogr Kinesiol. 2008;18(6):955–64.
41. Hodges PW, Richardson CA. Contraction of the abdominal muscles associated with movement of the lower limb. Phys Ther. 1997;77(2):132–42; discussion 142-4.
42. Robledo-Resina IDM, Romero-Morales C, Martín-Casas P, Villafañe JH, Abuín-Porras V. Relationship between female sexual dysfunction and trunk stability post-stroke: a cross-sectional study. Medicina (Kaunas). 2024;60(2):324.
43. Carriere B. Fitness for the pelvic floor. Stuttgart: Thieme; 2002. p. 14–37.
44. Tajiri K, Huo M, Akiyama S, Fujisawa S, Maruyama H. Measurement reliability and kinetic chain of the thickness of the transverse abdominal muscle and action potential of the levator ani muscle. J Phys Ther Sci. 2010;22:451–4.
45. Critchley D. Instructing pelvic floor contraction facilitates transversus abdominis thickness increase during low-abdominal hollowing. Physiother Res Int. 2002;7(2):65–75.
46. Madill SJ, McLean L. Relationship between abdominal and pelvic floor muscle activation and intravaginal pressure during pelvic floor muscle contractions in healthy continent women. Neurourol Urodyn. 2006;25(7):722–30.
47. Rzymski P, Burzyński B, Knapik M, Kociszewski J, Wilczak M. How to balance the treatment of stress urinary incontinence among female athletes? Arch Med Sci. 2020;17(2):314–22.
48. Sapsford RR, Hodges PW, Richardson CA, Cooper DH, Markwell SJ, Jull GA. Co-activation of the abdominal and pelvic floor muscles during voluntary exercises. Neurourol Urodyn. 2001;20(1):31–42.
49. Bø K, Stien R. Needle EMG registration of striated urethral wall and pelvic floor muscle activity patterns during cough, Valsalva, abdominal, hip adductor, and gluteal muscle contractions in nulliparous healthy females. Neurourol Urodyn. 1994;13(1):35–41.
50. Arranz-Martín B, Navarro-Brazález B, Sánchez-Sánchez B, McLean L, Carazo-Díaz C, Torres-Lacomba M. The impact of hypopressive abdominal exercise on linea alba morphology in women who are postpartum: a short-term cross-sectional study. Phys Ther. 2022;102(8):pzac086.
51. Molina-Torres G, Moreno-Muñoz M, Rebullido TR, Castellote-Caballero Y, Bergamin M, Gobbo S, Hita-Contreras F, Cruz-Diaz D. The effects of an 8-week hypopressive exercise training program on urinary incontinence and pelvic floor muscle activation: a randomized controlled trial. Neurourol Urodyn. 2023;42(2):500–9.
52. Da Cuña-Carrera I, Alonso-Calvete A, Soto-González M, Lantarón-Caeiro EM. How do the abdominal muscles change during hypopressive exercise? Medicina (Kaunas). 2021;57(7):702.
53. Ramírez-Jiménez M, Alburquerque-Sendín F, Garrido-Castro JL, Rodrigues-de-Souza D. Effects of hypopressive exercises on post-partum abdominal diastasis, trunk circumfer-

ence, and mechanical properties of abdominopelvic tissues: a case series. Physiother Theory Pract. 2023;39(1):49–60.
54. Bernardes BT, Resende AP, Stüpp L, Oliveira E, Castro RA, Bella ZI, Girão MJ, Sartori MG. Efficacy of pelvic floor muscle training and hypopressive exercises for treating pelvic organ prolapse in women: randomized controlled trial. Sao Paulo Med J. 2012;130(1):5–9.
55. Navarro-Brazález B, Prieto-Gómez V, Prieto-Merino D, Sánchez-Sánchez B, McLean L, Torres-Lacomba M. Effectiveness of hypopressive exercises in women with pelvic floor dysfunction: a randomised controlled trial. J Clin Med. 2020;9(4):1149.
56. Sperstad JB, Tennfjord MK, Hilde G, Ellström-Engh M, Bø K. Diastasis recti abdominis during pregnancy and 12 months after childbirth: prevalence, risk factors and report of lumbopelvic pain. Br J Sports Med. 2016;50(17):1092–6.
57. Katz CMS, Barbosa CP. Effects of hypopressive exercises on pelvic floor and abdominal muscles in adult women: a systematic review of randomized clinical trials. J Bodyw Mov Ther. 2024;37:38–45.
58. Della Guardia L, Codella R. Exercise tolls the bell for key mediators of low-grade inflammation in dysmetabolic conditions. Cytokine Growth Factor Rev. 2021;62:83–93.
59. Faraldi M, Gomarasca M, Sansoni V, Perego S, Banfi G, Lombardi G. Normalization strategies differently affect circulating miRNA profile associated with the training status. Sci Rep. 2019;9(1):1584.
60. Veronese N, Soysal P, Demurtas J, Solmi M, Bruyère O, Christodoulou N, Ramalho R, Fusar-Poli P, Lappas AS, Pinto D, Frederiksen KS, Corbi GM, Karpenko O, Georges J, Durães J, Schlögl M, Yilmaz O, Sieber C, Shenkin SD, Smith L, Reginster JY, Maggi S, Limongi F, Ars J, Barbagallo M, Cherubini A, Quinn T, Alzheimer Europe; European College of Neuropsychopharmacology; European Geriatric Medicine Society (Lead Society); European Interdisciplinary Council on Ageing; European Society of Clinical and Economic Aspects of Osteoporosis and Osteoarthritis; International Association of Gerontology and Geriatrics-European Region; Scottish Brain Health ARC; World Psychiatry Association-Preventive Psychiatry Section; endorsed by the European Academy of Neurology. Physical activity and exercise for the prevention and management of mild cognitive impairment and dementia: a collaborative international guideline. Eur Geriatr Med. 2023;14(5):925–52.
61. Lin W, Song H, Shen J, Wang J, Yang Y, Yang Y, Cao J, Xue L, Zhao F, Xiao T, Lin R. Functional role of skeletal muscle-derived interleukin-6 and its effects on lipid metabolism. Front Physiol. 2023;14:1110926.
62. Jin L, Diaz-Canestro C, Wang Y, Tse MA, Xu A. Exerkines and cardiometabolic benefits of exercise: from bench to clinic. EMBO Mol Med. 2024;16(3):432–44.
63. Costa LO, Maher CG, Latimer J, Smeets RJ. Reproducibility of rehabilitative ultrasound imaging for the measurement of abdominal muscle activity: a systematic review. Phys Ther. 2009;89(8):756–69.
64. Kiesel KB, Underwood FB, Mattacola CG, Nitz AJ, Malone TR. A comparison of select trunk muscle thickness change between subjects with low back pain classified in the treatment-based classification system and asymptomatic controls. J Orthop Sports Phys Ther. 2007;37(10):596–607.
65. Teyhen DS, Rieger JL, Westrick RB, Miller AC, Molloy JM, Childs JD. Changes in deep abdominal muscle thickness during common trunk-strengthening exercises using ultrasound imaging. J Orthop Sports Phys Ther. 2008;38(10):596–605.
66. Tsao H, Hodges PW. Persistence of improvements in postural strategies following motor control training in people with recurrent low back pain. J Electromyogr Kinesiol. 2008;18(4):559–67.
67. Daigle F, Léonard G, Émond M, Benoit-Piau J, Gaudreault N. Comparison of the pressure biofeedback unit and real-time ultrasound imaging as feedback tools to contract the transversus abdominis muscle: a randomized controlled trial in healthy older adults. J Geriatr Phys Ther. 2022;45(1):25–33.

68. Whittaker JL, Teyhen DS, Elliott JM, Cook K, Langevin HM, Dahl HH, Stokes M. Rehabilitative ultrasound imaging: understanding the technology and its applications. J Orthop Sports Phys Ther. 2007;37(8):434–49.
69. Manzaneda Cipriani RM, Viaro M, Adrianzen G, Flores E, Duran Vega H, Babaitis R, Dal Ponte Zatt JV, Salonia Goldmann I, Kornalewski de Oliveira R, de Souza BL. Ultrasonography as a tool to improve preoperative marking in body contour surgery. Plast Reconstr Surg Glob Open. 2023;11(11):e5431.
70. Wijntjes J, van Alfen N. Muscle ultrasound: present state and future opportunities. Muscle Nerve. 2021;63(4):455–66.
71. Rahmani N, Mohseni-Bandpei MA, Vameghi R, Salavati M, Abdollahi I. Application of ultrasonography in the assessment of skeletal muscles in children with and without neuromuscular disorders: a systematic review. Ultrasound Med Biol. 2015;41(9):2275–83.
72. Mah JK, van Alfen N. Neuromuscular ultrasound: clinical applications and diagnostic values. Can J Neurol Sci. 2018;45(6):605–19.
73. van Alfen N, Gijsbertse K, de Korte CL. How useful is muscle ultrasound in the diagnostic workup of neuromuscular diseases? Curr Opin Neurol. 2018;31(5):568–74.
74. Pillen S, Arts IM, Zwarts MJ. Muscle ultrasound in neuromuscular disorders. Muscle Nerve. 2008;37(6):679–93.
75. Simon NG. Dynamic muscle ultrasound—another extension of the clinical examination. Clin Neurophysiol. 2015;126(8):1466–7.
76. Kim BI, Hwang-Bo G, Kim HR. Comparison of abdominal muscle thickness with vaginal pressure changes in healthy women. J Phys Ther Sci. 2014;26(3):427–30.
77. Bharucha AE, Basilisco G, Malcolm A, Lee TH, Hoy MB, Scott SM, Rao SSC. Review of the indications, methods, and clinical utility of anorectal manometry and the rectal balloon expulsion test. Neurogastroenterol Motil. 2022;34(9):e14335.
78. Liang P, Liang M, Shi S, Liu Y, Xiong R. Rehabilitation programme including EMG-biofeedback- assisted pelvic floor muscle training for rectus diastasis after childbirth: a randomised controlled trial. Physiotherapy. 2022;117:16–21.
79. Chmielewska D, Stania M, Kucab-Klich K, Błaszczak E, Kwaśna K, Smykla A, Hudziak D, Dolibog P. Electromyographic characteristics of pelvic floor muscles in women with stress urinary incontinence following sEMG-assisted biofeedback training and Pilates exercises. PLoS One. 2019;14(12):e0225647.
80. Haslam J. "Biofeedback" in therapeutic management of incontinence and pelvic pain: pelvicorgan disorders. 2nd ed. Springer-Verlag Ltd; 2008. p. 105–10.
81. Grape HH, Dedering A, Jonasson AF. Retest reliability of surface electromyography on the pelvic floor muscles. Neurourol Urodyn. 2009;28(5):395–9.
82. Dannecker C, Wolf V, Raab R, Hepp H, Anthuber C. EMG-biofeedback assisted pelvic floor muscle training is an effective therapy of stress urinary or mixed incontinence: a 7-year experience with 390 patients. Arch Gynecol Obstet. 2005;273(2):93–7.
83. Bertotto A, Schvartzman R, Uchôa S, Wender MCO. Effect of electromyographic biofeedback as an add-on to pelvic floor muscle exercises on neuromuscular outcomes and quality of life in postmenopausal women with stress urinary incontinence: a randomized controlled trial. Neurourol Urodyn. 2017;36(8):2142–7.
84. May S, Littlewood C, Bishop A. Reliability of procedures used in the physical examination of non-specific low back pain: a systematic review. Aust J Physiother. 2006;52(2):91–102.
85. Terwee CB, Bot SD, de Boer MR, van der Windt DA, Knol DL, Dekker J, Bouter LM, de Vet HC. Quality criteria were proposed for measurement properties of health status questionnaires. J Clin Epidemiol. 2007;60(1):34–42.
86. de Vet HC, Terwee CB, Knol DL, Bouter LM. When to use agreement versus reliability measures. J Clin Epidemiol. 2006;59(10):1033–9.
87. Viana RA. Enfermagem em terapia intensiva: práticas baseadas em evidências. São Paulo: Atheneu; 2011. p. 560.

88. Viana RA, Whitaker IY. Enfermagem em terapia intensiva: práticas e vivências. Porto Alegre: Artmed; 2011. p. 546.
89. Knobel E. Terapia intensiva: enfermagem. São Paulo: Atheneu; 2006. p. 656.
90. Baird MS, Bethel S. Manual de enfermagem no cuidado crítico: intervenções de enfermagem e condutas colaborativas. 6a ed. Rio de Janeiro: Elsevier; 2012. p. 1016.
91. Bersani AL, Gomes JO, Braga IL, Guimarães HP, Lopes RD. Síndrome compartimental abdominal. Rev Bras Clin Med. 2009;7:313–21.
92. Jeronimo RA, Cheregatti A. Técnicas de UTI. São Paulo: Rideel; 2010. p. 344.
93. Kirkpatrick AW, Roberts DJ, De Waele J, Jaeschke R, Malbrain ML, De Keulenaer B, Duchesne J, Bjorck M, Leppaniemi A, Ejike JC, Sugrue M, Cheatham M, Ivatury R, Ball CG, Reintam Blaser A, Regli A, Balogh ZJ, D'Amours S, Debergh D, Kaplan M, Kimball E, Olvera C. Pediatric guidelines Sub-Committee for the World Society of the Abdominal Compartment Syndrome. Intra-abdominal hypertension and the abdominal compartment syndrome: updated consensus definitions and clinical practice guidelines from the World Society of the Abdominal Compartment Syndrome. Intensive Care Med. 2013;39(7):1190–206.
94. Olsson A, Kiwanuka O, Wilhelmsson S, Sandblom G, Stackelberg O. Surgical repair of diastasis recti abdominis provides long-term improvement of abdominal core function and quality of life: a 3-year follow-up. BJS Open. 2021;5(5):zrab085.
95. Novak J, Jacisko J, Busch A, Cerny P, Stribrny M, Kovari M, Podskalska P, Kolar P, Kobesova A. Intra-abdominal pressure correlates with abdominal wall tension during clinical evaluation tests. Clin Biomech (Bristol, Avon). 2021;88:105426.
96. Lee YY, McColl KE. Disruption of the gastroesophageal junction by central obesity and waist belt: role of raised intra-abdominal pressure. Dis Esophagus. 2015;28(4):318–25.
97. Mitchell DR, Derakhshan MH, Wirz AA, Ballantyne SA, McColl KEL. Abdominal compression by waist belt aggravates gastroesophageal reflux, primarily by impairing esophageal clearance. Gastroenterology. 2017;152(8):1881–8.
98. Bernardi E, Pomidori L, Bassal F, Contoli M, Cogo A. Respiratory muscle training with normocapnic hyperpnea improves ventilatory pattern and thoracoabdominal coordination, and reduces oxygen desaturation during endurance exercise testing in COPD patients. Int J Chron Obstruct Pulmon Dis. 2015;10:1899–906.
99. Oueslati F, Saey D, Vézina FA, Nadreau É, Martin M, Maltais F. Acute cardiopulmonary and muscle oxygenation responses to normocapnic hyperpnea exercise in COPD. Med Sci Sports Exerc. 2022;54(1):47–56.
100. Walker DJ, Ertl T, Walterspacher S, Schlager D, Roecker K, Windisch W, Kabitz HJ. Respiratory muscle function during a six-week period of normocapnic hyperpnoea training. Respir Physiol Neurobiol. 2013;188(2):208–13.
101. Ainscough-Potts AM, Morrissey MC, Critchley D. The response of the transverse abdominis and internal oblique muscles to different postures. Man Ther. 2006;11(1):54–60.
102. Beillas P, Lafon Y, Smith FW. The effects of posture and subject-to-subject variations on the position, shape and volume of abdominal and thoracic organs. Stapp Car Crash J. 2009;53:127–54.
103. Bjerkefors A, Ekblom MM, Josefsson K, Thorstensson A. Deep and superficial abdominal muscle activation during trunk stabilization exercises with and without instruction to hollow. Man Ther. 2010;15(5):502–7.
104. Botanlioglu H, Kantarci F, Kaynak G, Unal Y, Ertan S, Aydingoz O, Erginer R, Unlu MC, Mihmanli I, Babacan M. Shear wave elastography properties of vastus lateralis and vastus medialis obliquus muscles in normal subjects and female patients with patellofemoral pain syndrome. Skeletal Radiol. 2013;42(5):659–66.
105. Critchley DJ, Coutts FJ. Abdominal muscle function in chronic low back pain patients—measurement with real-time ultrasound scanning. Physiotherapy. 2002;88(6):322–32.
106. Spitznagle TM, Leong FC, Van Dillen LR. Prevalence of diastasis recti abdominis in a urogynecological patient population. Int Urogynecol J Pelvic Floor Dysfunct. 2007;18(3):321–8.

107. Arab AM, Chehrehrazi M. Ultrasound measurement of abdominal muscles activity during abdominal hollowing and bracing in women with and without stress urinary incontinence. Man Ther. 2011;16(6):596–601.
108. Parson SH. Clinically oriented anatomy. (6th ed.). J Anat. 2009;215(4):474.
109. Caufriez MLP. Syllabus de Neuromyostatique Viscérale. Bruxelles: M.C. Editions; 2018.
110. Askar OM. Surgical anatomy of the aponeurotic expansions of the anterior abdominal wall. Ann R Coll Surg Engl. 1977;59(4):313–21.
111. Brown SH, Carr JA, Ward SR, Lieber RL. Passive mechanical properties of rat abdominal wall muscles suggest an important role of the extracellular connective tissue matrix. J Orthop Res. 2012;30(8):1321–6.
112. Förstemann T, Trzewik J, Holste J, Batke B, Konerding MA, Wolloscheck T, Hartung C. Forces and deformations of the abdominal wall-a mechanical and geometrical approach to the linea alba. J Biomech. 2011;44(4):600–6.
113. Grässel D, Prescher A, Fitzek S, Keyserlingk DG, Axer H. Anisotropy of human linea alba: a biomechanical study. J Surg Res. 2005;124(1):118–25.
114. Hadjikov L, Kirilova M, Stoytchev S, Pashkouleva D. Visco-elastic mechanical behaviour of human abdominal fascia. Biomechanics. 2007;1:39–46.
115. Hernández B, Peña E, Pascual G, Rodríguez M, Calvo B, Doblaré M, Bellón JM. Mechanical and histological characterization of the abdominal muscle. A previous step to modelling hernia surgery. J Mech Behav Biomed Mater. 2011;4(3):392–404.
116. Nahabedian MY. Management strategies for diastasis recti. Semin Plast Surg. 2018;32(3):147–54.
117. Ha W, Song SY, Yoon CS, Kim KN. Severe irreversible diastasis recti abdominis and abdominal hernia in postpartum women: rare case report. Int Surg. 2016. https://doi.org/10.9738/intsurg-d-15-00204.1.
118. Fan C, Guidolin D, Ragazzo S, Fede C, Pirri C, Gaudreault N, Porzionato A, Macchi V, De Caro R, Stecco C. Effects of cesarean section and vaginal delivery on abdominal muscles and fasciae. Medicina (Kaunas). 2020;56(6):260.
119. Theodorsen NM, Strand LI, Bø K. Effect of pelvic floor and transversus abdominis muscle contraction on inter-rectus distance in postpartum women: a cross-sectional experimental study. Physiotherapy. 2019;105(3):315–20.
120. Coldron Y, Stokes MJ, Newham DJ, Cook K. Postpartum characteristics of rectus abdominis on ultrasound imaging. Man Ther. 2008;13(2):112–21.
121. Bassalobre M, Liebano RE, da Silva MP, Castiglioni MLV, Sadala AY, Ferreira LM, Nahas FX. Changes in the pattern of superficial lymphatic drainage of the abdomen after abdominoplasty. Plast Reconstr Surg. 2022;149(6):1106e–13e.
122. Albertin G, Astolfi L, Fede C, Simoni E, Contran M, Petrelli L, Tiengo C, Guidolin D, De Caro R, Stecco C. Detection of lymphatic vessels in the superficial fascia of the abdomen. Life (Basel). 2023;13(3):836.
123. Guney-Deniz H, Kinikli GI, Aykar S, Sevinc C, Caglar O, Atilla B, Yuksel I. Manual lymphatic drainage and Kinesio taping applications reduce early-stage lower extremity edema and pain following total knee arthroplasty. Physiother Theory Pract. 2023;39(8):1582–90.
124. Tsai HJ, Hung HC, Yang JL, Huang CS, Tsauo JY. Could Kinesio tape replace the bandage in decongestive lymphatic therapy for breast-cancer-related lymphedema? A pilot study. Support Care Cancer. 2009;17(11):1353–60.
125. Kasimis K, Iakovidis P, Lytras D, Koutras G, Chatziprodromidou IP, Fetlis A, Ntinou SR, Keklikoglou NM, Samiotaki A, Chasapis G, Tarfali G, Apostolou T. Short-term effects of manual therapy plus capacitive and resistive electric transfer therapy in individuals with chronic non-specific low back pain: a randomized clinical trial study. Medicina (Kaunas). 2023;59(7):1275.
126. Barassi G, Mariani C, Supplizi M, Prosperi L, Di Simone E, Marinucci C, Pellegrino R, Guglielmi V, Younes A, Di Iorio A. Capacitive and resistive electric transfer therapy: a com-

parison of operating methods in non-specific chronic low back pain. Adv Exp Med Biol. 2022;1375:39–46.
127. Tashiro Y, Suzuki Y, Nakayama Y, Sonoda T, Yokota Y, Kawagoe M, Tsuboyama T, Aoyama T. The effect of capacitive and resistive electric transfer on non-specific chronic low back pain. Electromagn Biol Med. 2020;39(4):437–44.
128. Szabo DA, Neagu N, Teodorescu S, Predescu C, Sopa IS, Panait L. TECAR therapy associated with High-Intensity Laser Therapy (HILT) and manual therapy in the treatment of muscle disorders: a literature review on the theorised effects supporting their use. J Clin Med. 2022;11(20):6149.
129. Siereńska J, Sotomska Z, Madej-Łukasiak D, Wąż P, Grzybowska ME. The use of capacitive and resistive energy transfer in postpartum pain management in women after perineal trauma. J Clin Med. 2023;12(18):6077.
130. Bretelle F, Fabre C, Golka M, Pauly V, Roth B, Bechadergue V, Blanc J. Capacitive-resistive radiofrequency therapy to treat postpartum perineal pain: a randomized study. PLoS One. 2020;15(4):e0231869.

Chapter 16
Long-Term Outcomes and Prevention of Postoperative Complications in Diastasis Recti Surgery

Derlin M. Juárez Muas

Diastasis of the rectus abdominis (DRA) is a dysfunction of the linea alba (LA), resulting from an abnormal separation of the two rectus muscles. Present in a third of women after giving birth, it is characterized by an enlarged and weakened linea alba due to mechanical changes in the abdomen and hormonal changes during pregnancy. It can manifest as a bulging or sagging of the abdominal midline and is associated with midline hernias in between 92 and 96% [1–3]. DRA is a sequelae of pregnancy and the puerperium; it causes dysfunctions of the abdominal core such as back pain, incorrect posture, weakness of the abdominal wall muscles, predisposing to constipation due to a decrease in the function of the abdominal press, and alteration of the pelvic floor which predispose to the pathology urogenital [1, 3–9].

Surgical treatment of DRA by general surgeons has gained interest over the past decade with the advent of the minimally invasive endoscopic approach [10, 11], and numerous scientific studies have reported satisfactory short- and long-term results of surgical repair of DRA [3, 12–16].

A work published by Olsson et al. in 2021 [1] reports that, 1 year after surgery, surgical repair performed by plication of the linea alba using absorbable material resulted in significant improvements in central abdominal function, regardless of preoperative interrectal distance, as well as a decrease in urinary incontinence and improved quality of life, which implies that surgical repair of the DRA restores the anatomy and recovers the function of the abdominal core [1, 16]. The initial management of DRA, as well as the preparation of the abdominal wall in surgical

D. M. Juárez Muas (✉)
Argentine Hernia Association of Surgery, Salta, Argentina

Argentine Hernia Association, Salta, Argentina

Hispano-American Hernia Society, Salta, Argentina

Public Maternal-Child Hospital, Salta, Argentina

National University of Tucumán, Tucumán, Argentine

S. Cuccomarino et al. (eds.), *New Concepts in Diastasi Recti Surgery*,
https://doi.org/10.1007/978-3-031-74947-6_16

prehabilitation, is entrusted to the physiotherapist [15, 17–19]. If physical therapy fails, guidelines propose surgical repair under certain circumstances, such as a specific minimum interrectal distance (IRD) and a specific maximum BMI [1, 20, 21].

According to the "Classification of Rectus Diastasis—A Proposal" of the German Hernia Society (DHG) and the International Endohernia Society (IEHS) [21], interrectal separation greater than 5 cm is defined as severe DR, using the classification proposed by Ranney in 1990 [22], without discriminating against DRA with a transverse diameter greater than 8 cm, as we mentioned in the previous chapters and in the work Adjuvant Botulinum Toxin for Endoscopic Management (Preaponeurotic Endoscopic Repair) of Severe Diastasis Recti by Muas DM, Palmisano EM, Santonja GP, and Paz OR. in 2021 [23], in which we propose to divide the group into DRA W3, into DRA W3 A (from 5 to 8 cm), a situation in which there are usually not many inconveniences to perform the plication of the rectus, and DRA W3 B in diastasis del straight ones larger than 8 cm. In these cases, closure of the midline without tension is practically impossible. The support of neoadjuvant techniques such as TBA or the release of the external oblique muscle (uni- or bilateral) is necessary to be able to perform a suture with less tension. With the support of these techniques, the surgical conduct used, the surgical gestures necessary to obtain tension-free midline closure, and the probability of different preoperative and postoperative morbidities are the same in both groups.

The aim of this chapter is to show the long-term results and main morbidities of endoscopic management of DRA, emphasizing its preventive measures. A work on this specific topic was published by Juárez Muas et al. in 2023 [3] on 502 patients with average follow-up of 52 months (range, 25–96 months). The mean age was 41.46 ± 8.24 years. 92.8% were women with a mean body mass index (BMI) of 25.99 ± 2.98 kg/cm2. The anesthetic risk was ASA I and II in 100%. The mean transverse distance of the DRA was 46.93 ± 16.27 mm. DRA was associated with midline hernias in 98% of patients: umbilical hernia (74.5%), followed by epigastric hernia (10.6%) and umbilical hernia + epigastric hernia (8.2%). Reconstruction of the linea alba was performed using 0 gauge barbed suture in 80% of cases, 1 gauge (10.2%), or 2–0 gauge (9.4%). To reinforce the plication, a macroporous polypropylene mesh was used in 100% of cases: low weight (62%), medium weight (35.7%), high weight (1.2%), and ultralight (1.2%). The prosthesis was fixed with staples in 60% of cases (absorbable, 88%), adhesives in 24% (n-butyl cyanoacrylate), and polyglactin 910 sutures in 16%. The mean surgical time was 96 ± 35 min. The suction drains were left in 100% of cases: single in 26% and double in 74% [3]. The complications and their management were as follows:

16.1 Intraoperative Complications

Adverse events during surgery occurred in 3.4% of cases (Fig. 16.1). Intraoperative bleeding occurred in 1% of cases. It can be due to different situations: bleeding from periumbilical perforating vessels (0.2%), bleeding during plication with barbed suture or from trauma due to the needle (0.4%), and bleeding from tacks during

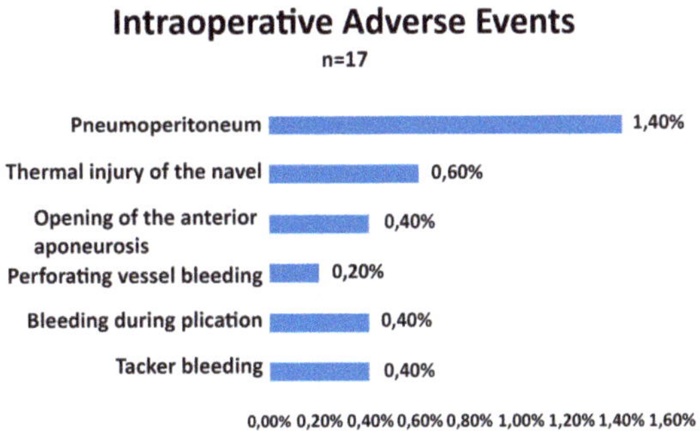

Fig. 16.1 Intraoperative adverse events

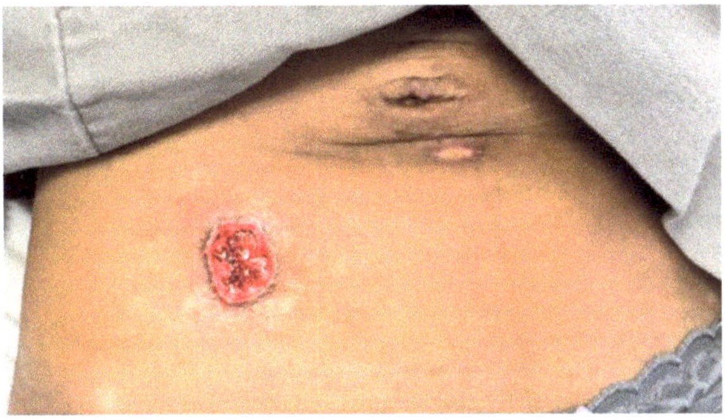

Fig. 16.2 Thermal skin injury

mesh fixation (0.4%) [3]. It is advisable to wash the neocavity before positioning and fixing the prosthesis to have clear anatomical landmarks. Additionally, you may choose to use adhesives to prevent bleeding through invasive means of fixation.

The premise to avoid these situations is to perform an accurate dissection with exhaustive hemostasis to have a correct vision of the small vessels, perforating vessels, and anterior aponeurosis, thus avoiding bleeding which may make dissection on the correct plane difficult, to reduce the risk of opening of the hernia sac at the umbilical level and entry into the retrorectal plane and to minimize the possibility of thermal injuries to the skin due to the use of energy, situations that are more frequent at the level of the umbilical scar at the moment of its disconnection. It is advisable to place a finger of your hand pressing on the navel, to delimit the umbilical scar, facilitating this surgical gesture. Thermal or ischemic damage can occur in any sector of the dissection (Fig. 16.2), especially in thin patients, so it is recommended to release the TCS attached to the aponeurosis with the lowest possible energy intensity [3].

16.2 Postoperative Complications

Postoperative complications were recorded in 15.5% of cases (Fig. 16.3).

There are several factors that we believe are important to take into consideration before performing surgery, to optimize results, minimize complications, and speed

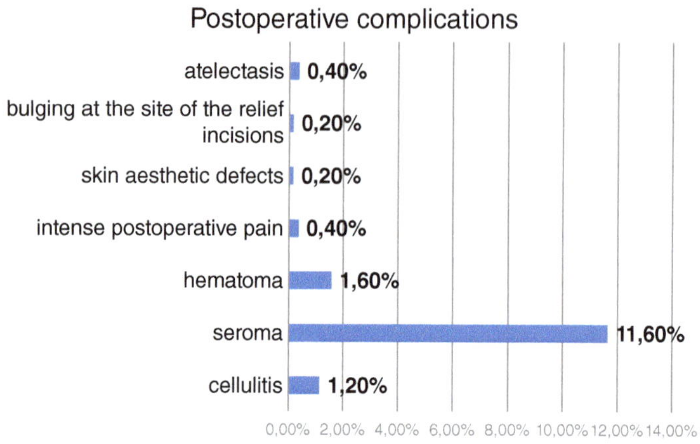

Fig. 16.3 Postoperative complications

up recovery times. They are correct diet; stop smoking, 1–2 months before and after surgery; hypopressive exercises, resolve, as far as possible, pre-existing pathologies; correct the use of drugs (NSAIDs, corticosteroids, contraceptives, etc.). The most common complication is seroma. The seroma is a topic of permanent discussion and controversy due to the divergent and often contradictory opinions regarding the etiological factors, the elements that contribute to its formation, and the therapeutic conduct.

Therefore, preventative management begins 2 months before surgery. We do this by preparing the abdominal wall with a physiokinetic treatment with hypopressive gymnastics, core strengthening, and manual lymphatic drainage. It is essential to prepare the skin with adequate hydration using moisturizing creams high in vitamin A and E. Furthermore, we indicate a complex of vitamins A, E, and C orally and continue for 30 days after surgery. This would produce better microvascular and lymphatic circulation of the abdominal wall, which would promote lymphatic drainage and reduce edema and postoperative seroma, resulting in benefits for better healing.

Vitamin A is involved in the formation and regeneration of cells and repairs damaged cells. This renewal process visibly improves the condition and appearance of the skin.

Vitamin E has antioxidant power. This delays premature aging and deterioration of skin cells and the appearance of wrinkles on the skin.

Vitamin C acts as an antioxidant, fighting free radicals. Furthermore, the body needs this vitamin to produce collagen, which is the protein responsible for the healing, elasticity, and resistance of the skin [3].

Despite all this preparation, postoperative seroma was evidenced in 10.6% of cases [3, 24]. Seromas were evaluated by clinical and ultrasound examination. Their management was conservative and physiokinetic in 96.8%, as they were small and oligosymptomatic or asymptomatic. Resolution occurred through open drainage through the suprapubic incision and placement of laminar latex drainage in 1% of cases (Fig. 16.4a), puncture aspiration in 0.8% (Fig. 16.4b), percutaneous drainage with placement of a pig-tail catheter in 0.6%, and spontaneous drainage through surgical accesses in 0.8% of cases.

There are also other factors associated with the appearance of the seroma, such as the temperature level of the energy used with electrocautery during the dissection of the subcutaneous tissue, the type of surgical approach, and the presence of a foreign body (mesh, sutures, adhesives, etc.). Seroma in endoscopic repairs has an incidence of 9.7% [24] to 12% [16, 25], and in dermolipectomies and liposuctions [26], it reaches 38% [26–30].

Fluid accumulation causes increased local pressure, which can lead to other complications such as spontaneous drainage of the seroma through the surgical wound, surgical wound dehiscence, and necrosis and may predispose to surgical site infection [26, 31–33] and the prosthesis or the possibility of developing chronic seromas with the formation of a fibrous capsule (Morell-Lavallen pseudocyst), which give rise to deformities of the abdominal wall [34], a condition that requires surgical treatment [31, 32, 35].

From a histopathological point of view, the factors that predispose to the appearance of the seroma are lymphatic ectasia, inflammatory exudate, and venulo-capillary vascular proliferation [26].

The serous fluid that forms under the dermoadipose flap after abdominoplasty appears to be an inflammatory exudate in the early postoperative period, which slowly transforms into an exudate with some lymph-like characteristics [36].

The use of energy used to dissect subcutaneous tissue is a controversial issue. In 1992, Kuzon et al. [37] from the University of Toronto carried out a comparative study on 38 patients undergoing abdominoplasty with low- and high-power electrosurgical devices. Overall and wound complication rates were not significantly different. The same situation was observed in our case series [3]. According to Jansen et al. [38], both open, laparoscopic, and endoscopic surgeries have shown positive results with a low rate of complications and recurrences. However, recommending that the first step in planning is pre-surgical physiotherapy, evidence is lacking on which regimen to use [1, 3, 38]. In turn, Fiori et al. [39] reported that minimally invasive surgery showed fewer complications and a shorter hospital stay than the open approach with a significant improvement in the quality of life after surgery and concluded that both open and laparoscopic surgeries are safe and effective for repairing DR associated or not with abdominal hernias, with low rates of recurrence and complications [3, 12, 16, 24, 39], demonstrating that open techniques, compared to laparoscopic approaches, were associated with a significantly higher rate of skin dehiscence (6.79% vs 2.86%) and hematoma formation (4.73% vs 1.09%) and at a significantly lower rate of postoperative seroma formation (2.47% vs 8.29%). No significant difference was observed in diastasis recurrence rates between open and laparoscopic repair (0.22 vs 0.63%) [3, 39, 40]. Another relevant and very controversial point is the use of a prosthesis in contact with the subcutaneous tissue to reinforce the anatomical restitution of the linea alba. Among the hypotheses proposed by Claus et al. as causes of seroma formation, the main highlights are extensive subcutaneous dissection and the location of the onlay mesh [3, 41]. In our

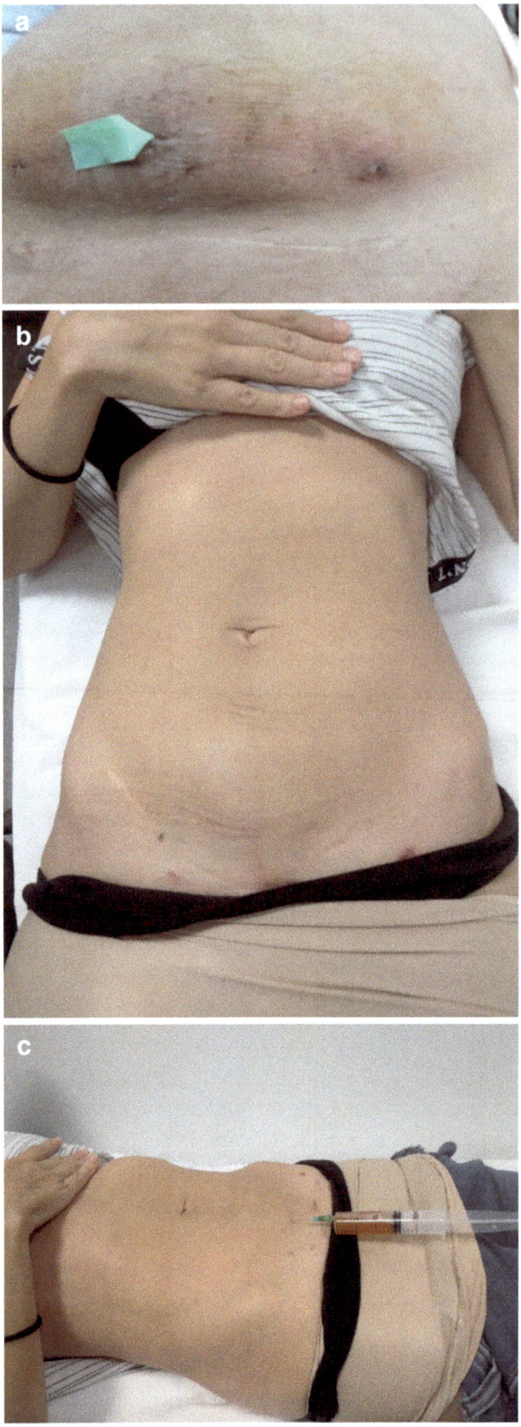

Fig. 16.4 (**a**) Open seroma drainage. (**b**) Localized seroma and (**c**) Puncture-aspiration drainage

series, a wide dissection of the preaponeurotic space was performed from the xiphoid appendage to the pubis and both anterior axillary lines. A large prosthesis was used, on average 22 × 15 cm, and the density of the mesh was light and of medium weight in 97.6%; comparing the types of prostheses and the width of the dissection, the percentage of seromas does not seem to increase [3]. Timmermans et al. in 2014 [42] found no statistical differences when comparing the percentage of postoperative seroma after DR repair with or without prosthesis, as well as mesh placement in the supra-aponeurotic and preperitoneal plane [3, 42].

The use of drains in the postoperative period of surgery with dermoadipose flaps or in abdominoplasties is a subject of analysis in multiple works and still without consensus. Vinicio et al. in 2002 [43] presented a study in which they evaluated the presence of abdominal fluid after performing dermolipectomies without the use of drainage, with passive drainage, and with active drainage, observing that the use of active suction drains is necessary to reduce the rate of seromas and proposing that the cause of seroma formation is multifactorial (large spaces, dissection, insufficient hemostasis, incorrect use of electrocautery, and inadequate abdominal compression) [3, 43].

In our series the use of drains was systematic, one or two drains depending on the surgeon's preference, which were removed after an average of 7 days and when the secretion was less than 30 cc/day for 2 consecutive days. Furthermore, no differences were evident in the length of time drains remained in place between normal weight patients and obese patients, coinciding with the work of Rincón-Rubio et al. [3, 44]. However, authors such as Borile et al. [45] believe that there is no difference in the use or otherwise of drains and recommend not using them, stating that their prolonged use favors the increase in local infections and thromboembolic incidents [3, 44, 45].

A very important issue is the use of a postoperative belt. Choosing the correct sheath, material, size, and position and correct compression are important factors; therefore it is essential to try it before surgery to determine its comfort, adapt it to each case, and evaluate it in different positions, since it is an element that will be used between 30 and 60 days. Correct use reduces the postoperative seroma, avoids skin imperfections or wrinkles, minimizes the shear between the subcutaneous cellular tissue and the aponeurosis-prosthesis, promotes adhesion, and provides greater postoperative safety and comfort [3, 10, 12, 24]. It has been observed in some patients that the use of a belt or sun exposure during the immediate postoperative period can cause transient vasomotor changes in the skin, expressed as erythema on the anterior abdominal wall [3, 46].

The second most common complication was hematomas (1.6% [3] and 2.4% [24] of cases). 62.5% were resolved with conservative management because they were small and without clinical significance. Three cases required surgical interventions: an ultrasound-guided percutaneous drainage, one with transumbilical drainage and toilet (Fig. 16.5a), and one case of giant hematoma was resolved with preaponeurotic re-endoscopy with evacuation and washing of the neocavity [3]. Ecchymosis is a discoloration of the skin produced by the infiltration of blood into the subcutaneous tissues or by the rupture of the subcutaneous capillaries and is an

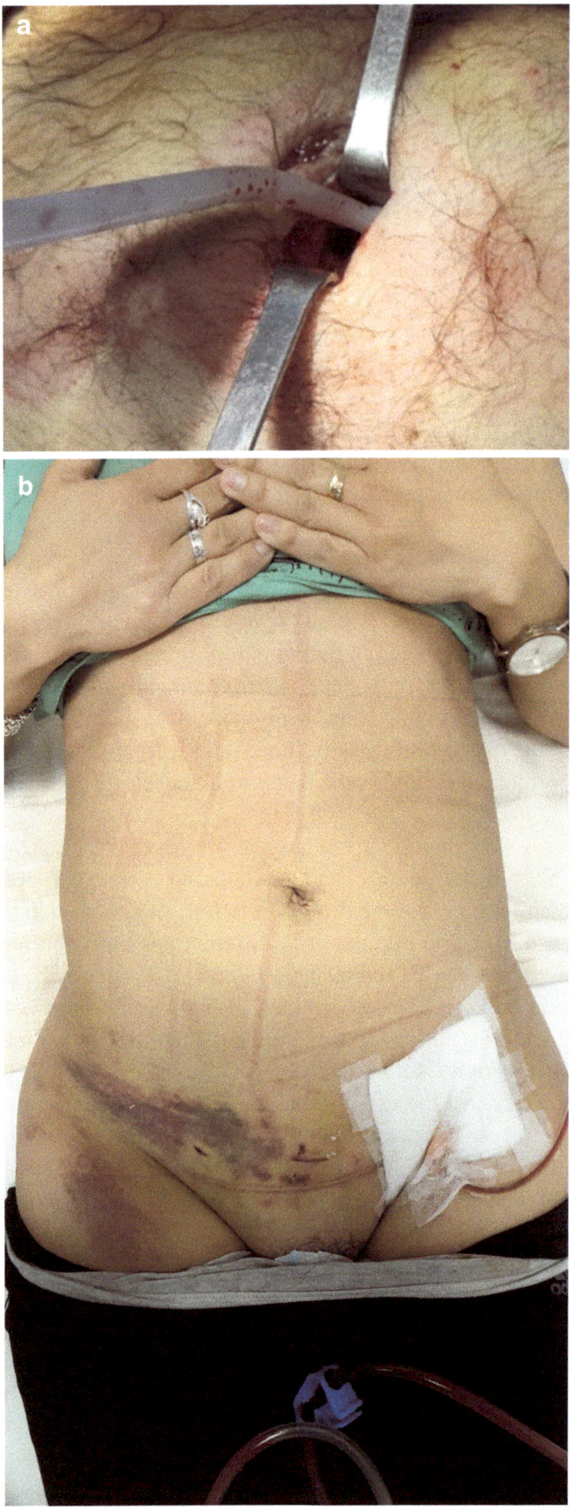

Fig. 16.5 (**a**) Transumbilical open hematoma drainage. (**b**) Ecchymosis in the left lower abdomen and root of the left thigh

entity not to be confused with hematomas (Fig. 16.5b). It generally resolves spontaneously through reabsorption and metabolism of the infiltrated blood without requiring surgical treatment.

Cutaneous hyposthesia of the anterior abdominal wall occurred in 100% of our patients in the immediate postoperative period [3], a situation also described by Van Uchelen et al. in 71% of cases [47]. Total recovery of skin sensitivity occurs from the periphery to the umbilical region, generally during the 6 months following surgery [3, 10–12, 23, 47].

We used local cold across the entire abdominal wall, from the operating room, a tactic that has given us good results and appears to reduce the postoperative seroma rate by minimizing the inflammatory response of electrocautery and surgical trauma, an observation by the authors that calls for future work for confirmation. A similar effect could be achieved by the low temperature of CO_2, which produces vasoconstriction during the procedure [3].

Pain management is a factor of great importance, both during surgery and after surgery, to promote a good level of postoperative comfort. The mean postoperative pain level at the time of discharge from the institution was 3/10, according to the visual analog scale (VAS). Discriminated pain was 2.5/10 ± 1.6 when the prosthesis was fixed with adhesive compared to 3.85/10 ± 1.76 when tacks were used [3].

In the immediate and medium postoperative period of REPA, we perform a dermatofunctional physiokinetic treatment with the aim of controlling postoperative edema and pain, avoiding the appearance of seromas and fibrosis as secondary complications [3, 48], containing the abdomen to avoid breaking the suture or muscle fibers during the healing process and educating the patient regarding postoperative care management. We use resources such as manual lymphatic drainage (MLD), compression system placement, neuromuscular taping (NMT) (Fig. 16.6a, b), and home cryotherapy.

The physiotherapy treatment protocol was implemented in the first instance with sessions lasting approximately 45 min. Manual lymphatic drainage maneuvers were applied, and then the neuromuscular taping tape was positioned with a lymphatic application technique, with 3 cm anchors, without stretching, in the shape of a fan,

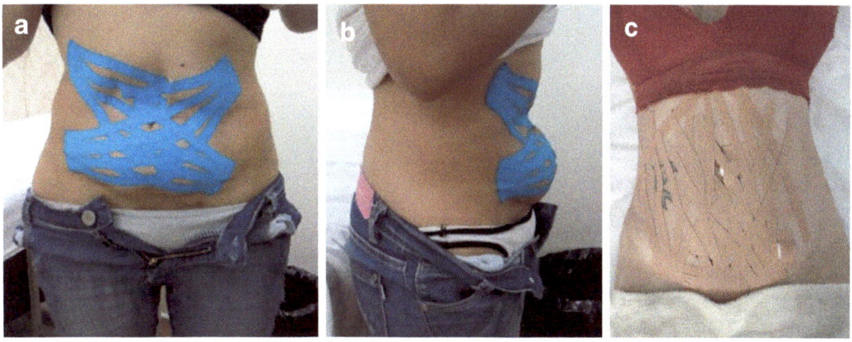

Fig. 16.6 (**a**, **b** and **c**) Neuromuscular Taping (TNM) for seroma management

cutting the tape into four strips, and crossing them in the center of the abdomen [3], and finally the positioning of the compression system was carried out, with or without selective compression, depending on the case [3, 12]. The treatment was daily, once a day, 5 days a week, for 10 sessions. Furthermore, starting from the first session, the patient was evaluated by filling out a form, where the medical history and the measurements of the abdominal circumference were taken, recording as a reference in three different points, to evaluate the edema after the first session, at least three times a week. The patient was asked to apply cryotherapy compresses three times a day for 20 min at home.

According to what patients report, we can state that the preoperative and postoperative physiokinetic treatment allows them to improve daily physical activity and physical exercises, have a possibly faster recovery of skin sensitivity with less sensation of swelling, and, in general, the general improvement of postoperative wellbeing [3, 23–25].

Postoperative infections were highlighted as omphalitis 2.2% and SSI (surgical site infection) (Fig. 16.7) and cellulitis 1.2% [3]. Similar situation was documented by Cuccomarino et al. with 2.4% [24].

The cases resolved with antibiotic therapy. A case of necrotizing fasciitis, requiring aggressive surgical debridement, antibiotic therapy, and negative pressure therapy, has been described. An important recommendation is the correct handling of the prosthesis, sutures, and mesh fixation elements, to reduce the risk of postoperative infection [3, 10–12, 23]. Other isolated complications were a case of skin defect with skin wrinkles in the subcostal region [3, 24], a patient with swelling on the left flank in the area of the muscle section, and an atelectasis.

Relapse occurred between 0.8% [3] and 2.4% [24]. The associated situations were respiratory infection with cough attacks and periumbilical hematoma, giant hematoma, surgical site infection, and two cases with use of 2–0 gauge suture in DR greater than 5 cm. Köhler et al. [49] recommend preoperative verification of DRA associated with midline hernias, as these patients benefit from midline repair with mesh, reducing the recurrence rate. Similarly, Van Uchelen states that midline plication alone, as a single surgical gesture, is not sufficient to repair umbilical and epigastric hernias associated with DRA, demonstrating in his work a 40% recurrence of DRA by studying patients with ultrasound and 5-year follow-up [47, 50].

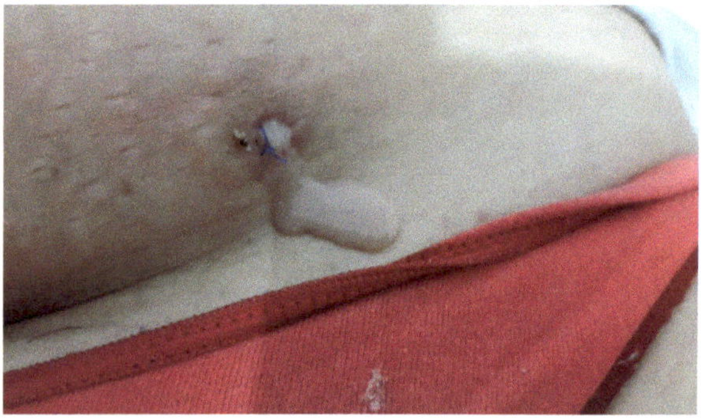

Fig. 16.7 Infection of the surgical site, trocar access in the left iliac fossa

References

1. Olsson A, Kiwanuka O, Wilhelmsson S, Sandblom G, Stackelberg O. Surgical repair of diastasis recti abdominis provides long-term improvement of abdominal core function and quality of life: a 3-year follow-up. BJS Open. 2021;5(5):zrab085. https://doi.org/10.1093/bjsopen/zrab085.
2. Brauman D. Diástasis de rectos: anatomía clínica. Plast Reconstr Surg. 2008;122:1564–9.
3. Juárez Muas D, Palmisano EM, Pou Santonja G, González Higuera LG, Martínez Maya JD, Domínguez G, Ayala Acosta JC, Blanco M, Cuccomarino S, Cabral Castelli ML. Morbilidad a corto y largo plazo de la reparación endoscópica preaponeurótica en la diástasis de los rectos asociada o no a hernia de la línea media: estudio pros- pectivo, multicéntrico e internacional. Rev Hispanoam Hernia. 2023;11(3):111–7.
4. Hills NF, Graham RB, McLean L. Comparación de la función de los músculos del tronco entre mujeres con y sin diástasis de los rectos abdominales al año posparto. Phys Ther. 2018;98:891–901.
5. Benjamin DR, Frawley HC, Shields N, van de Water ATM, Taylor NF. Relación entre la diástasis del músculo recto abdominal (DRAM) y las disfunciones musculoesqueléticas, el dolor y la calidad de vida: una revisión sistemática. Fisioterapia. 2019;105:24–34.
6. Keshwani N, Mathur S, McLean L. Relación entre la distancia interrectal y la gravedad de los síntomas en mujeres con diástasis de los rectos abdominales en el período posparto temprano. Phys Ther. 2018;98:182–90.
7. Parker MM, Dugan S. Diástasis del recto abdominal y dolor y disfunción lumbopélvica: ¿están relacionados? J Salud de la Mujer Fisioterapia. 2009;33:15–22.
8. Doubkova L, Andel R, Palascakova-Springrova I, Kolar P, Kriz J, Kobesova A. Diástasis de los músculos rectos del abdomen en pacientes con dolor lumbar. J Rehabilitación musculoesquelética de espalda. 2018;31:107–12.
9. Liaw LJ, Hsu MJ, Liao CF, Liu MF, Hsu AT. Las relaciones entre la distancia entre los rectos medida por imágenes de ultrasonido y la función de los músculos abdominales en mujeres posparto: un estudio de seguimiento de 6 meses. J Orthop Sports Phys Ther. 2011;41:435–43.
10. Juárez Muas D, Cuccomarino S. Reparación Endoscópica Preaponeurótica (REPA). Munual Práctico de Cirugía endoscópica de Pared Abdominal. Ezequiel Palmisano y Col. 1° ed. Ed. Autores de Argentina. Bs. As. 2020. 14:159–70.
11. Juárez Muas D, Verasay G, García WM. Reparación endoscópica prefascial de la diástasis de los rectos: descripción de una nueva técnica. Rev Hispanoam Hernia. 2017;5(2):47–51.
12. Juárez MD. Hernioplastia umbilical laparoscópica asociada a diástasis de los rectos. In: Schlottmann F, Sadava EE, editors. Cirugía Laparoscópica: Técnica Quirúrgica en Cirugía General. Editorial Medica Panamericana. Argentina. 2023. p. 51–69.
13. Emanuelsson P, Gunnarsson U, Strigård K, Stark B. Complicaciones tempranas, dolor y calidad de vida después de la cirugía reconstructiva para la diástasis del músculo recto abdominal: un seguimiento de 3 meses. J Plast Reconstr Aesthet Surg. 2014;67:1082–8.
14. Emanuelsson P, Gunnarsson U, Dahlstrand U, Strigård K, Stark B. La corrección quirúrgica de la diástasis del recto abdominal (ARD) reduce el dolor y mejora la fuerza de los músculos de la pared abdominal: un ensayo prospectivo y aleatorizado que compara la reparación con malla retromuscular con la autoreparación de doble fila. -suturas de retención. Cirugía. 2016;160:1367–75.
15. Olsson A, Kiwanuka O, Wilhelmsson S, Sandblom G, Stackelberg O. Estudio de cohorte sobre el efecto de la reparación quirúrgica de la diástasis sintomática de los rectos abdominales sobre la función del tronco abdominal y la calidad de vida. Abierto BJS. 2019;3:750–8.
16. Juárez Muas D. Preaponeurotic endoscopic repair (REPA) of diastasis recti associated or not to midline hernias. Surg Endosc. 2019;33(6):1777–82. https://doi.org/10.1007/s00464-018-6450-3.
17. Cándido G, Lo T, Janssen PA. Factores de riesgo para la diástasis de los rectos abdominales. J Asociación Cuadro Fisiother Salud de la Mujer. 2005;97:49–54.

References

1. Olsson A, Kiwanuka O, Wilhelmsson S, Sandblom G, Stackelberg O. Surgical repair of diastasis recti abdominis provides long-term improvement of abdominal core function and quality of life: a 3-year follow-up. BJS Open. 2021;5(5):zrab085. https://doi.org/10.1093/bjsopen/zrab085.
2. Brauman D. Diástasis de rectos: anatomía clínica. Plast Reconstr Surg. 2008;122:1564–9.
3. Juárez Muas D, Palmisano EM, Pou Santonja G, González Higuera LG, Martínez Maya JD, Domínguez G, Ayala Acosta JC, Blanco M, Cuccomarino S, Cabral Castelli ML. Morbilidad a corto y largo plazo de la reparación endoscópica preaponeurótica en la diástasis de los rectos asociada o no a hernia de la línea media: estudio pros- pectivo, multicéntrico e internacional. Rev Hispanoam Hernia. 2023;11(3):111–7.
4. Hills NF, Graham RB, McLean L. Comparación de la función de los músculos del tronco entre mujeres con y sin diástasis de los rectos abdominales al año posparto. Phys Ther. 2018;98:891–901.
5. Benjamin DR, Frawley HC, Shields N, van de Water ATM, Taylor NF. Relación entre la diástasis del músculo recto abdominal (DRAM) y las disfunciones musculoesqueléticas, el dolor y la calidad de vida: una revisión sistemática. Fisioterapia. 2019;105:24–34.
6. Keshwani N, Mathur S, McLean L. Relación entre la distancia interrectal y la gravedad de los síntomas en mujeres con diástasis de los rectos abdominales en el período posparto temprano. Phys Ther. 2018;98:182–90.
7. Parker MM, Dugan S. Diástasis del recto abdominal y dolor y disfunción lumbopélvica: ¿están relacionados? J Salud de la Mujer Fisioterapia. 2009;33:15–22.
8. Doubkova L, Andel R, Palascakova-Springrova I, Kolar P, Kriz J, Kobesova A. Diástasis de los músculos rectos del abdomen en pacientes con dolor lumbar. J Rehabilitación musculoesquelética de espalda. 2018;31:107–12.
9. Liaw LJ, Hsu MJ, Liao CF, Liu MF, Hsu AT. Las relaciones entre la distancia entre los rectos medida por imágenes de ultrasonido y la función de los músculos abdominales en mujeres posparto: un estudio de seguimiento de 6 meses. J Orthop Sports Phys Ther. 2011;41:435–43.
10. Juárez Muas D, Cuccomarino S. Reparación Endoscópica Preaponeurótica (REPA). Munual Práctico de Cirugía endoscópica de Pared Abdominal. Ezequiel Palmisano y Col. 1° ed. Ed. Autores de Argentina. Bs. As. 2020. 14:159–70.
11. Juárez Muas D, Verasay G, García WM. Reparación endoscópica prefascial de la diástasis de los rectos: descripción de una nueva técnica. Rev Hispanoam Hernia. 2017;5(2):47–51.
12. Juárez MD. Hernioplastia umbilical laparoscópica asociada a diástasis de los rectos. In: Schlottmann F, Sadava EE, editors. Cirugía Laparoscópica: Técnica Quirúrgica en Cirugía General. Editorial Medica Panamericana. Argentina. 2023. p. 51–69.
13. Emanuelsson P, Gunnarsson U, Strigård K, Stark B. Complicaciones tempranas, dolor y calidad de vida después de la cirugía reconstructiva para la diástasis del músculo recto abdominal: un seguimiento de 3 meses. J Plast Reconstr Aesthet Surg. 2014;67:1082–8.
14. Emanuelsson P, Gunnarsson U, Dahlstrand U, Strigård K, Stark B. La corrección quirúrgica de la diástasis del recto abdominal (ARD) reduce el dolor y mejora la fuerza de los músculos de la pared abdominal: un ensayo prospectivo y aleatorizado que compara la reparación con malla retromuscular con la autoreparación de doble fila. -suturas de retención. Cirugía. 2016;160:1367–75.
15. Olsson A, Kiwanuka O, Wilhelmsson S, Sandblom G, Stackelberg O. Estudio de cohorte sobre el efecto de la reparación quirúrgica de la diástasis sintomática de los rectos abdominales sobre la función del tronco abdominal y la calidad de vida. Abierto BJS. 2019;3:750–8.
16. Juárez Muas D. Preaponeurotic endoscopic repair (REPA) of diastasis recti associated or not to midline hernias. Surg Endosc. 2019;33(6):1777–82. https://doi.org/10.1007/s00464-018-6450-3.
17. Cándido G, Lo T, Janssen PA. Factores de riesgo para la diástasis de los rectos abdominales. J Asociación Cuadro Fisiother Salud de la Mujer. 2005;97:49–54.

18. Lee D, Hodges PW. Comportamiento de la línea aAlba durante una tarea de curl-up en diástasis del recto abdominal: un estudio observacional. J Orthop Sports Phys Ther. 2016;46:580–9.
19. Thabet AA, Alshehri MA. Eficacia del programa de ejercicios de estabilidad central profunda en mujeres posparto con diástasis de rectos abdominales: un ensayo controlado aleatorio. J Musculoesqueleto Neuronal Interact. 2019;19:62–8.
20. Carlstedt A, Bringman S, Egberth M, Emanuelsson P, Olsson A, Petersson U, et al. Manejo de la diástasis de los músculos rectos del abdomen: recomendaciones para las directrices nacionales suecas. Scand J Surg. 2021;110(3):452–9. https://doi.org/10.1177/1457496920961000.
21. Reinpold W, Köckerling F, Bittner R, Conze J, Fortelny R, Koch A, et al. Clasificación de la diástasis del recto: propuesta de la Sociedad Alemana de Hernia (DHG) y la Sociedad Internacional de Endohernia (IEHS). Cirugía Frontal. 2019;6:1–6.
22. Ranney B. Causas, reconocimiento y reparación de la diástasis de rectos y la hernia umbilical. SDJ Med. 1990;43:5–8.
23. Muas DM, Palmisano EM, Santoja GP, Paz OR. Adjuvant botulinum toxin for endoscopic management (preaponeurotic endoscopic repair) of severe diastasis recti. Int J Abdom Wall Hernia Surg. 2021;4:45–50.
24. Cuccomarino S, Bonomo LD, Aprà F, Toscano A, Jannaci A. Preaponeurotic endoscopic repair (REPA) of diastasis recti: a single surgeon's experience. Surg Endosc. 2022;36(2):1302–9. https://doi.org/10.1007/s00464-021-08405-1. Epub 2021 Mar 4. PMID: 33661382.
25. Juárez Muas DM, Palmisano E, Pou Santoja G, Cuccomarino S, González Higuera G, Mayo P, Martínez Maya JD, Domínguez G, Ayala Acosta JC, Chichizola A. Reparación endoscópica preaponeurótica (REPA) como tratamiento de la diástasis de los músculos rectos asociada o no a hernias de la línea media. Estudio multicéntrico. Rev Hispanoam Hernia. 2019;7(2):59–65.
26. Moretti E, Gómez GF, Monti J, Vázquez G. Investigación de seromas postliposucción y dermolipectomía abdominal. Cir plást iberolatinoam. 2006;32(3):151–60. http://scielo.isciii.es/scielo.php?script=sci_arttext&pid=S0376-78922006000300001&lng=es
27. Smith MM, Lin MP, Hovsepian RV, Wood D, Nguyen T, Evans GR, Wirth GA. Postoperative seroma formation after abdominoplasty with placement of continuous infusion local anesthetic pain pump. Can J Plastic Surg = Journal canadien de chirurgie plastique. 2009;17(4):127–9. https://doi.org/10.1177/229255030901700411.
28. Smith MM, Hovsepian RV, Markarian MK, et al. Continuous-infusion local anesthetic pain pump use and seroma formation with abdominal procedures: is there a correlation? Plast Reconstr Surg. 2008;122:1425–30.
29. American Society of Plastic and Reconstructive Surgeons 2000/2005/2006 National Plastic Surgery Statistics: Cosmetic and Reconstructive Procedure Trends. www.plasticsurgery.org.
30. Teimourian B. Management of seroma in abdominoplasty. Aesthet Surg J. 2005;25:510–1.
31. Nassif TM, Silveira FGL, Assunção LF, Garcia ERBR, Sanches VM. Analysis of risk factors for the formation of seroma in classical abdominoplasty. Rev Bras Cir Plást. 2018;33(2):156–60.
32. Keramidas EG, Rodopoulou S, Khan U. Pseudo-cyst formation after abdominoplasty combined with liposuction: a case report and review of the literature. Eur J Plast Surg. 2006;28:400–2. https://doi.org/10.1007/s00238-005-0796-1.
33. Ersek RA, Schade K. Subcutaneous pseudobursa secondary to suction and surgery. Plast Reconstr Surg. 1989;85(3):442–5.
34. Zecha PJ, Missotten FE. Pseudocyst formation after abdominoplasty—extravasations of Morel-Lavalleé. Br J Plast Surg. 1999;52(6):500–2. https://doi.org/10.1054/bjps.1999.3154.
35. Fernández García A, Fernández Pascual C, Santoyo Gil-López F, Alonso RS. Morel-Lavallee pseudocyst after abdominoplasty without liposuction. Cirplást iberolatinoam. 2009;35(2):163–8.
36. Andrades P, Prado A. Composición del seroma postabdominoplastia. Aesth Plast Surg. 2007;31:514–8. https://doi.org/10.1007/s00266-007-0078-3.
37. Kuzon W, Crawford R, Binhammer P, Fielding C, Knowlton R, Levine R. Effect of electrosurgical technique on wound healing and early complication rate following abdominal dermolipectomy. Ann Plast Surg. 1996;37(3):245–50.

38. Jessen ML, Öberg S, Rosenberg J. Treatment options for abdominal rectus diastasis. Front Surg. 2019;6:65. https://doi.org/10.3389/fsurg.2019.00065.
39. Fiori F, Ferrara F, Gobatti D, Gentile D, Stella M. Surgical treatment of diastasis recti: the importance of an overall view of the problem. Hernia. 2021;25(4):871–82. https://doi.org/10.1007/s10029-020-02252-0. Epub 2020 Jun 20. PMID: 32564225.
40. ElHawary H, Barone N, Zammit D, Janis JE. Closing the gap: evidence-based surgical treatment of rectus diastasis associated with abdominal wall hernias. Hernia. 2021;25(4):827–53. https://doi.org/10.1007/s10029-021-02460-2. Epub 2021 Jul 28. PMID: 34319467.
41. Claus C, Malcher F, Cavazzola LT. Comment to: TESLAR for treatment of umbilical/para-umbilical hernia and rectus abdominus diastasis is associated with unacceptable persistent seroma formation. Should subcutaneous endoscopic mesh placement be abandoned? Hernia. 2020;24(6):1411–2.
42. Timmermans L, de Goede B, van Dijk SM, Kleinrensink GJ, Jeekel J, Lange JF. Meta-analysis of sublay versus onlay mash repair in incisional hernia surgery. Am J Surg. 2014;207(6):980–8.
43. Vinicius M, Mendonça L, da Motta MP. Incidência de Hematoma e Seroma em Abdominoplastia com e sem uso de Drenos. Rev Soe Bras Cir Plást São Paulo. 2002;17(1):69–74.
44. Rincón-Rubio L, Cemborain-Valarino M, Gutiérrez-Barrozo K, Gil-Masroua B, Bookaman-Salazar A. Manejo del drenaje aspirativo en dermolipectomía abdominal en pacientes postbariátricos. Cirugía Plástica Ibero-Latinoamericana. 2018;44(1):37–45. https://doi.org/10.4321/s0376-78922018000100007.
45. Borile G, Pavelecini M, Dreher R. The use of suction drains in abdominal dermolipectomy: a randomized clinical trial. Plast Reconst Surg. 2008;121(4):228e–9e.
46. Hanssen A, Palmisano EM, Hanssen DA, Hanssen RA, Daes JE. Vasomotor changes in abdominal skin after endoscopic subcutaneous/Preaponeurotic repair of diastasis recti (REPA). Int J Surg Case Rep. 2020;75:182–4. https://doi.org/10.1016/j.ijscr.2020.08.056.
47. van Uchelen JH, Kon M, Werker PM. The long-term durability of plication of the anterior rectus sheath assessed by ultrasonography. Plast Reconstr Surg. 2001;107(6):1578–84. https://doi.org/10.1097/00006534-200105000-00046.
48. Chi A, Lange A, Guimares MVTN, Santos CB. Prevention and treatment of ecchymosis, edema, and fibrosis in the pre-, trans-, and postoperative periods of plastic surgery. Rev Bras Cir Plast. 2018;33(3):343–54.
49. Köhler G, Luketina RR, Emmanuel K. Sutured repair of primary small umbilical and epigastric hernias: concomitant rectus diastasis is a significant risk factor for recurrence. World J Surg. 2015;39:121–6. https://doi.org/10.1007/s00268-014-2765-y.
50. Hickey F, Finch JG, Khanna A. Una revisión sistemática sobre los resultados de la corrección de la diástasis de los rectos. Hernia. 2011;15(6):607–14. https://doi.org/10.1007/s10029-011-0839-4.

MIX
Papier aus verantwortungsvollen Quellen
Paper from responsible sources
FSC® C105338
www.fsc.org

If you have any concerns about our products,
you can contact us on
ProductSafety@springernature.com

In case Publisher is established outside the EU,
the EU authorized representative is:
Springer Nature Customer Service Center GmbH
Europaplatz 3, 69115 Heidelberg, Germany

Printed by Libri Plureos GmbH
in Hamburg, Germany